C000185272

Athletic Development

Athletic Development: A Psychological Perspective is an examination of the psychological factors that help or hinder the development of participants in sport. This includes influences such as families, coach-athlete interactions, and transitional episodes on an individual's pathway in sport.

This edited collection of topical chapters shines a unique psychological perspective on the athlete's development through sport. It explores a range of contemporary themes that influence athlete's development including:

- An introduction to athletic development which orientates a holistic, psychological perspective of the athletic development process.
- Social influences on athletic development, which explores the impact of varied social influences (e.g., coach, family, peers, school) on sports participation and performance from a psychological perspective.
- Athlete wellbeing, which explores various aspects influencing mental health and welfare as an athlete progresses through their sports career.

The book combines key theory with illustrative case studies, to analyse the complexities of athletic development. It takes a critical perspective highlighting some of the debates and controversies in these areas and uses spotlight boxes in each chapter to focus on questions or topics of particular interest. *Athletic Development: A Psychological Perspective* is a key reader for all students in the fields of sport and exercise psychology, sport coaching, and related sport science subjects.

Caroline Heaney is a Senior Lecturer in Sport and Fitness at The Open University. She is a British Association of Sport and Exercise Sciences (BASES) Accredited Sport and Exercise Scientist and a Health and Care Professions Council (HCPC) registered Sport and Exercise Psychologist, and has provided sport psychology support to athletes from club to elite level.

Nichola Kentzer is a Lecturer in Sport and Fitness at The Open University. She is an experienced academic who specialises in sport psychology and education. She is a BASES Accredited Sport and Exercise Scientist and an HCPC registered Sport and Exercise Psychologist, and has provided sport psychology support to a broad range of athletes.

Ben Oakley is a Professor in Sports Performance Education at The Open University and has previously lectured at Portsmouth and Southampton Solent Universities. Formerly, he worked as a national coach in windsurfing, which included attending the Olympic Games twice. He sits on the advisory board for the *Applied Coaching Research Journal* and has been an external examiner at five other universities.

Athletic Development
A Psychological Perspective

Edited by Caroline Heaney,
Nichola Kentzer, and Ben Oakley

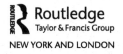 Routledge
Taylor & Francis Group

NEW YORK AND LONDON

 The Open
University

First published 2022
by Routledge
52 Vanderbilt Avenue, New York, NY 10017

and by Routledge
2 Park Square, Milton Park, Abingdon, Oxon, OX14 4RN

Routledge is an imprint of the Taylor & Francis Group, an informa business

© 2022 The Open University

The right of Caroline Heaney, Nichola Kentzer, and Ben Oakley to be identified as the authors of the editorial material, and of the authors for their individual chapters, has been asserted in accordance with sections 77 and 78 of the Copyright, Designs and Patents Act 1988.

All rights reserved. No part of this book may be reprinted or reproduced or utilised in any form or by any electronic, mechanical, or other means, now known or hereafter invented, including photocopying and recording, or in any information storage or retrieval system, without permission in writing from the publishers.

Trademark notice: Product or corporate names may be trademarks or registered trademarks, and are used only for identification and explanation without intent to infringe.

Library of Congress Cataloging-in-Publication Data
A catalog record for this book has been requested

ISBN: 978-0-367-72103-9 (hbk)
ISBN: 978-0-367-72102-2 (pbk)
ISBN: 978-1-003-15345-0 (ebk)

Typeset in Baskerville and Futura
by Apex CoVantage, LLC

Contents

Figures

Tables

Boxes and Case Studies

About the Contributors

Daniel J. Brown is a Chartered Psychologist of the British Psychological Society and a Senior Lecturer in Sport and Exercise Psychology at the University of Portsmouth, UK. Daniel's current research centres on the psychology of human excellence and wellbeing. Specifically, his work focuses on understanding and facilitating thriving in humans, athlete transitions and developmental experiences, and the development and assessment of interventions used in sport and performance psychology.

Iain Greenlees is Professor of Applied Sport Psychology at The University of Chichester. He is also an Associate Lecturer with The Open University. He has published widely in sport psychology and has a specific interest in the psychological determinants of sporting performance. His research interests include motivation in sport, group dynamics, personality in sport, and the effectiveness of sport psychology interventions. Iain is a Health and Care Professions Council (HCPC) registered Sport and Exercise Psychologist with over 20 years' experience.

Caroline Heaney is Senior Lecturer in Sport and Fitness at The Open University. She is an HCPC registered Sport and Exercise Psychologist with over 20 years of applied experience. She has an interest in the psychology of sport injury, mental health in sport, and career transitions in sport. Her research focuses on the psychological aspects of sport injury and she has published a range of journal articles and book chapters related to this topic.

Joanna Horne is a Staff Tutor in Psychology at The Open University. She is an experienced academic with a teaching specialism in research methods and statistics. Jo also teaches sport and exercise psychology and has a research interest in engagement in physical activity, and the barriers and facilitators to physical activity faced by particular subsets of the population.

Karen Howells is Senior Lecturer in Sport and Exercise Psychology at Cardiff Metropolitan University and an Associate Lecturer at The Open University. She is a British Psychological Society (BPS) Chartered Sport Psychologist and a HCPC Practitioner Psychologist who has worked in a diverse range of sports and at multiple levels. Her research interests include responses to adversity, adversarial growth, the post-Olympic blues, mental health in elite athletes, and applied sport psychology.

Sophia Jowett is Professor of Psychology at Loughborough University. Her research work revolves around interpersonal relationships, leadership, and communication in sport and coaching. This research has been funded by research councils, government, and charity agencies. Her research has been widely published in a range of scientific journals, book chapters, monographs, and conferences. This research has informed coach development across the world. She is associate fellow of the BPS.

Nichola Kentzer is a Lecturer in Sport and Fitness at The Open University, who specialises in sport psychology and education. She has an interest in the wellbeing and the professional development of students, teachers, coaches, and sport psychologists. She is a British Association of Sport and Exercise Sciences (BASES) Accredited Sport and Exercise Scientist and an HCPC Practitioner Psychologist, currently providing sport psychology support to equestrian athletes.

Candice Lingam-Willgoss is Senior Lecturer in Sport and Fitness at The Open University. She has spent 20 years working as an academic in higher education specialising in sport and exercise psychology. She has an interest in exercise adherence, negative exercise behaviours, career transitions, and winter sports.

Robert Morris is currently a Lecturer in Sport Psychology at the University of Stirling. Robert is a BASES Accredited, BPS Chartered, and HCPC registered Sport and Exercise Psychologist. Robert is also an applied practitioner in sport psychology, providing support to a range of team, national, international, and Olympic athletes. In addition, Robert conducts research on a number of areas related to sport psychology, including talent development and transitions, dual careers, and mental health in sport.

Ben Oakley is Professor of Sports Performance Education at The Open University. His expertise is in leading online learning projects with a sports performance and welfare focus and he has worked on BBC, FIFA, Sport England, and UK Coaching initiatives. His research has investigated elite sport policy, the developmental influences of champion athletes, and online learning effectiveness.

Jessica Pinchbeck is Senior Lecturer in Sport and Fitness at The Open University. She is an experienced academic who specialises in sport sociology. She has an interest in the psychosocial factors that influence sports participation. Specific research interests include qualitative research into the role of the family in youth sports participation and factors that influence female sports participation.

Daniel J. A. Rhind is a Reader in Psychology at Loughborough University. He specialises in safeguarding human rights in, around, and through sport. He is interested in issues related to athlete welfare, wellbeing, and how organisational cultures can serve to facilitate or prevent abuse.

Katelynn Slade is a Doctoral Researcher in Sport Psychology at Loughborough University. Her research is focused on challenging interactions in high performance sport and how they are perceived and managed independently and together by coaches and athletes. She has an interest in wellbeing, empowerment, and relationships in sport.

Lauren R. Tufton is a Lecturer in Sport Psychology, Physical Education, and Coaching at Buckinghamshire New University, and she is an Applied Sport and Exercise Psychologist in training with the BPS. Her research areas of interest include creativity in sport, and the application of coach-athlete relationship theory to equestrian sport partnerships.

Editors' Acknowledgements

The editors would like to thank the following people for their help in reviewing and preparing the chapters: Steph Doehler, Lindsay Duffy, Iain Greenlees, Candice Lingam-Willgoss, Ben Langdown, Jim Lusted, Kieran McCartney, Bharti Mistry, Helen Owton, Simon Penn, Jessica Pinchbeck, Simon Rea, Alex Twitchen, Gavin Williams, and Nigel Wright.

Introduction

Ben Oakley, Caroline Heaney, and Nichola Kentzer

The catalyst for this book was a fruitless search for a text that would support our Open University teaching of psychological aspects of an athlete's development and their sporting careers. We concluded that since contemporary and applied insights were so important, we ought to curate our own book with the help of other researchers in the field. So much has changed in the past decade that Dan Roan, the BBC sports editor, called it 'the decade that shook' sport (Roan, 2020). Our experience of searching for such a text suggests that a sport psychology focused collection that includes mental health, athlete welfare, and other aspects of an athlete's journey is timely. Indeed, this has arguably become more significant with the ongoing effects of the global pandemic.

This book examines some of the main psychological influences on developing athletes and the research of effective and ineffective environments for training and growth. In this introduction we identify three choices we have made about the language used in the book and section titles before explaining some of the main themes in each section.

First is the deliberate choice to use 'athletic development' as opposed to talent development. This book aims to explore athletes developing in sport at all levels and environments, not just the performance context that 'talent' implies. Collins et al. (2012) used the term 'participant development' to convey breadth beyond high performance but this term has not been widely used since then. However, Collins et al. (2012) observed that development in sport is far from being a seamless straight-line progression from childhood to retirement: it is complex and messy. The term 'athletic development' is preferred here because it represents the dynamic and non-linear process with multiple pathways that individuals may take (Abbott & Collins, 2004). In the 2020s there is wide recognition of the importance of psychological aspects and the impact on the environment, key episodes, and transitions to athlete's progress (Stambulova et al., 2020), and whilst much of this work is focused on talented performers, we want to talk of athletic development more broadly. Chapter 1 delves deeper into the use of the term in the wider literature and explains how the book's distinct athletic development perspective is informed by a range of psychological aspects. There are thirteen different chapters beyond the opening and closing ones which represent the diversity of psychological perspectives reflected in the book title.

Second, athletic development often uses the journey metaphor. For instance, we use the term 'athlete journey' in two of our section titles. You will also see that the journey metaphor is often used in everyday career-related narratives in terms of progression and destinations (e.g. Inkson, 2007). We draw attention to these metaphors to emphasise how commonly they are used in athletic development: it emphasises direction and progress. If we want to reinforce that athletic development is dynamic and non-linear, we might say it is a journey along a winding road encountering bumps along the way, often with an uncertain destination. It is not perhaps until the obvious use of this type of language is highlighted that we see how ubiquitous it is in this field.

The third main choice is that a holistic approach to athletic development has been adopted and is part of the Section 1 title. The introduction to that section explains what is meant academically by 'holistic'. Here we very briefly describe it being about the whole person and from multiple perspectives. Needless to say, this book's psychological focus should be interpreted as part of broader biopsychosocial perspective. Notice in Section 2 we use a social psychology focus which closely connects with relationships and interpersonal influences.

Further discussion of the book's three main sections and their accompanying themes follows. In Section 1 you will find Chapters 1 to 5 which attempt to make sense of athletic development as a field of study. To achieve this, readers also need to understand the main research terminology used in studies; this is also an overall aim of the section. You will see how the research field has evolved over time to the multiple perspectives and studies represented in the book. The other theme covered, in Chapters 2, 3, and 4 is about how the study of athlete career transition has evolved. It is in these transition-related chapters that you see how athletic identity, social support, and psychological interventions are explored. These ideas, and the developments of them, reoccur in later chapters where they are applied to different athletic development perspectives.

Section 2, as the title suggests, has a social focus and explores the social environment in which an athlete develops, acknowledging the importance of having a more complete view of athlete paths in sport. The section examines the influence of this social setting that surrounds the athlete as they move along their athletic development journey. Collectively, Chapters 6 to 10 discuss the potential impact of the socially created environment and the key individuals who accompany or guide the athlete. In particular, there is an examination of the influence of an athlete's family and school environment, their relationship with their coach(es), and how the coach-created environment can affect their sporting experience.

Section 3 is focused on the theme of mental health during the athletic development journey. Applying the holistic approach taken by the book, this section acknowledges that the mental health of the athlete can be affected both positively and negatively by a multitude of factors inside and outside of the sporting environment. Increasingly the importance of mental health in athletes is being recognised at all levels of sporting participation. Chapters 11 to 14 seek to examine the prevalence of mental health difficulties in sport. The section also explores how sporting environments can be structured and developed to ensure that athletes are exposed to conditions where they can thrive and that protect their mental health and welfare.

In a time when change and uncertainty is particularly prevalent, understanding some of the psychologically informed insights of how athletes are helped or hindered in their athletic development is topical. This book will give you a range of conceptual tools and practical scenarios to make sense of your own and others' growth experiences in sport. Yet, there is still much more to understand about how individual athletes, social settings, and organisational influences can contribute to effective training and development.

REFERENCES

Abbott, A., & Collins, D. (2004). Eliminating the dichotomy between theory and practice in talent identification and development: Considering the role of psychology. *Journal of Sports Sciences*, *22*(5), 395–408.

Collins, D., Bailey, R., Ford, P. A., MacNamara, A., Toms, M., & Pearce, G. (2012). Three Worlds: New directions in participant development in sport and physical activity. *Sport, Education and Society, 17*(2), 225–243.

Inkson, K. (2007). *Understanding careers: The metaphors of working lives.* Sage Publications.

Roan, D. (2020, January 2). The 2010s—The decade that shook sport. *BBC Sport Website.* www.bbc.co.uk/sport/50955918

Stambulova, N. B., Ryba, T. V., & Henriksen, K. (2020). Career development and transitions of athletes: The international society of sport psychology position stand revisited. *International Journal of Sport and Exercise Psychology*, 1–27.

SECTION I

Athletic Development

A Holistic View of the Journey

Ben Oakley

The focus of this first section is to explore topics that span athletic careers that take a holistic view of athletic development. However, while 'holistic' means different things to different groups of academics and practitioners, an item they would all probably agree on is that a holistic, broad view of the athlete journey that avoids too narrow a perspective is beneficial. Over the years more sophisticated approaches to the study of athletic development have emerged. For example, Stambulova et al. (2020) identify that the study of athlete transitions was at first, from 1960–80, narrowly framed on the final athlete retirement transition: more holistic studies came to the fore from the new millennium onwards.

Whilst athlete development is not solely about transitions, it is in this field that three useful clarifications of the term holistic have emerged. The term holistic has been defined as follows:

- Viewing athletes as a whole person, i.e., a person does sport together with other life commitments (e.g., studies, work, family; Wylleman et al., 2013);
- An athlete's development as holistic, i.e., multidimensional elements complemented by psychological, psychosocial, academic-vocational, and financial layers interacting with each other (Wylleman, 2019);
- An athlete's environment as holistic, i.e., made up of interacting micro- and macro-levels as well as athletic and non-athletic domains (Henriksen et al., 2010).

So, in effect this section's focus is on topics which are multidimensional and apply to athletes' whole careers, considering the whole person as well as their whole environment. The section consists of five chapters; there is so much to cover under the title of holistic athletic development that it cannot all be discussed in this section, but the chapters effectively help set up and frame the rest of the book. The five chapters therefore provide an overall context of the research that is outlined in subsequent sections.

The first two chapters are distinctly multidimensional and broad in examining the growth and development of the psychological aspects of athletic development. In Chapter 1: *What Is*

Athletic Development? Ben Oakley evaluates what is meant by the term athletic development in this book drawing on use of the term in other sport contexts. The chapter describes how this book's athletic development perspective is informed by a range of ideas from psychology. The relationships between the psychological ideas are tentatively explored to describe a nuanced picture of one way of exploring the topic. To help frame the scope and extent of this book's coverage of psychological aspects of athletic development (e.g., motivational climate), a framework of athletic development is explained. We have adapted the work of Gagné who developed a Differentiated Model of Giftedness and Talent (DMGT) over three iterations (e.g., Gagné, 2015). The purpose of adapting and presenting this framework is to show the links between environmental, mental, welfare, and developmental ideas and processes. As part of this the role of chance in athletic development is also recognised.

This leads to Chapter 2: *How Did We Get Here? Exploring the Evolution of Athletic Development Perspectives*, in which Ben Oakley traces how the field of athletic development has evolved over time. The purpose of the chapter is to provide context for the different psychological perspectives often used and shows how subsequent chapters in this book link to each other and can be traced back to earlier foci. Exemplar study and review papers are used as reference points for this evolutionary account of eight perspectives, and the content of International Society of Sport Psychology (ISSP) 'Position Stands' add further evidence regarding the *timing* of when different perspectives became more prominent. The eight psychological perspectives discussed are: i) talent, ii) expertise, iii) developmental practice and play, iv) developmental environments, v) psychosocial skills and resources, vi) developmental transitions, vii) mental health, and viii) relationships with athletes (i.e. coaches/parents). Interpreting the field of athletic development's journey from early initial studies to these eight diverse perspectives helps readers make more sense of the field, especially for newcomers.

One of these eight psychological perspectives, that of developmental transitions, is addressed in the subsequent chapter since it closely fits to the holistic and journey focus of this section. As athletes progress through their sporting career they experience several career transitions, both expected and unexpected, which can impact on their mental wellbeing and athletic development. In Chapter 3: *Transitions on the Athlete Journey: A Holistic Perspective*, Robert Morris explores the various transitions faced by athletes and the potential psychological challenges of these. He discusses some of the main theoretical models that have been used in this field and explains the author's own research with colleagues (Drew et al., 2019) on the youth-to-senior transition. He uses this work to illustrate how ideas might be applied to other transitions; specifically, the suggestion that there are a series of transition variables that are underpinning features which influence the outcomes. The latter part of the chapter focuses on some of the key considerations for sport psychologists in supporting athletes in overcoming any challenges they face using a worked example.

In addressing transitions, it is also a timely opportunity to address the final stage all athletes face: that of retirement. Therefore, in Chapter 4: *Retirement From Sport: The Final Transition*, Candice Lingam-Willgoss examines how the prospect of retirement can be extremely daunting for an athlete especially since determining when to retire can be a difficult decision and one that sometimes the athlete has no control over. To help make sense of this topic four main theoretical perspectives on the retirement transition and the diverse causes of athlete retirement are explained. By framing retirement as a period of adaptation, a range of coping resources and strategies are explored that can help athletes navigate this final athlete transition.

These four chapters draw heavily on research studies and whilst some readers may be familiar with how athletic development is investigated, many newcomers will not. Therefore, in Chapter 5: *Researching Athletic Development,* Joanna Horne introduces research since the challenge of researching athlete careers, that often span 30 years or more, needs to be understood. This chapter outlines some of the methodological approaches adopted in research exploring aspects of athletic development. It addresses both qualitative and quantitative approaches and explores research design, research instruments, and data analysis, including a useful introduction to the terminology used in statistical analysis. Throughout the chapter reference is made to published research to illustrate examples of approaches, designs, and instruments used to collect data. Some of the research challenges in athletic development will become clearer to newcomers from the case studies which are drawn from the range of studies indicated in the evolution of the topic area in Chapter 2.

The chapters in this section of the book set the scene for the following sections and provide a valuable underpinning for understanding the psychological perspectives of athletic development, how it evolved and how it is researched. They represent one way of looking at this evolving field in recognising that physiological and social perspectives also have a role to play.

REFERENCES

Drew, K., Morris, R., Tod, D., & Eubank, M. (2019). A meta-study of qualitative research on the junior-to-senior transition in sport. *Psychology of Sport and Exercise, 45*. https://doi.org/10.1016/j.psychsport.2019.101556

Gagné, F. (2015). From genes to talent: The DMGT/CMTD perspective. De los genes al talento: la perspectiva DMGT/CMTD. *Revista de Educación, 368*, 12–37.

Henriksen, K., Stambulova, N., & Roessler, K. K. (2010). Holistic approach to athletic talent development environments: A successful sailing milieu. *Psychology of Sport and Exercise, 11*(3), 212–222.

Stambulova, N., Ryba, T., & Henriksen, K. (2020). Career development and transitions of athletes: The international society of sport psychology position stand revisited. *International Journal of Sport and Exercise Psychology*. https://doi.org/10.1080/1612197X.2020.1737836

Wylleman, P. (2019). A developmental and holistic perspective on transitioning out of elite sport. In M. H. Anshel (Ed.), *APA handbook of sport and exercise psychology: Volume 1. Sport psychology* (pp. 201–216). American Psychological Association.

Wylleman, P., Reints, A., & De Knop, P. (2013). A developmental and holistic perspective on athletic career development. In P. Sotiriadou & V. De Bosscher (Eds.), *Managing high performance sport* (pp. 191–214). Routledge.

CHAPTER 1

What Is Athletic Development?

Ben Oakley

It appears to be a relatively simple two-word combination but deciding exactly what athletic development means is not as simple as it might appear. There is no universally accepted definition of the term. The purpose of this chapter is to discuss some of the judgements that are required to arrive at an appropriate understanding of athletic development. The chapter explains how this book's distinct athletic development perspective is informed by a range of ideas from psychology. The relationship between these ideas is explored to describe a complex, nuanced picture of one way of exploring the topic. Along the way the role of chance in athletic development is also acknowledged. As a starting point for this discussion we examine what previous attempts have been made to define athletic development and what can be gleaned from this work.

EXPLORING DIFFERENT PERSPECTIVES

Often when people use 'athletic' it denotes ideas around physical, sporting, or performance dimensions whilst 'development' invokes notions of growth, improvement, and learning. To explore this further Figure 1.1 is used to show how four different concepts that relate to athletic development are expressed, namely: physical literacy, long-term athletic development, talent development, and youth athletic development.

In the top left quadrant of Figure 1.1, the International Physical Literacy Association (IPLA) focuses on how 'physical activities for life' grew from physical educators' interest in the roles of movement and athleticism amongst young people. They suggest movement and athleticism are important parts of an individual's experience and development journey and lay the foundation for an active life (e.g., Whitehead, 2010).

There is commonality in the description of outcomes of 'confidence' and 'physical competence' between the physical literacy perspective and the long-term athletic development position statement from the National Strength and Conditioning Association (NSCA) in the bottom left quadrant of Figure 1.1 (Lloyd et al., 2016). The NSCA, as you would expect from a strength and conditioning perspective, emphasises physical training functions of athletic development including enhancing physical performance and injury reduction. It is worth noting that an original long-term athlete development (LTAD) model (Balyi & Hamilton, 2004) was adopted by some organisations in an effort to more closely align training prescription with the tempo of maturation. However, parts of this LTAD model have been heavily critiqued academically for lack of evidence (e.g., Bailey et al., 2010).

The two perspectives on the left side of Figure 1.1 (Physical Literacy and Long-Term Athletic Development) both suggest the importance of movement foundations and developing life-long

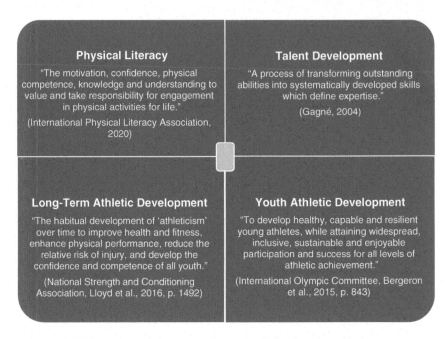

Physical Literacy

"The motivation, confidence, physical competence, knowledge and understanding to value and take responsibility for engagement in physical activities for life."

(International Physical Literacy Association, 2020)

Talent Development

"A process of transforming outstanding abilities into systematically developed skills which define expertise."

(Gagné, 2004)

Long-Term Athletic Development

"The habitual development of 'athleticism' over time to improve health and fitness, enhance physical performance, reduce the relative risk of injury, and develop the confidence and competence of all youth."

(National Strength and Conditioning Association, Lloyd et al., 2016, p. 1492)

Youth Athletic Development

"To develop healthy, capable and resilient young athletes, while attaining widespread, inclusive, sustainable and enjoyable participation and success for all levels of athletic achievement."

(International Olympic Committee, Bergeron et al., 2015, p. 843)

FIGURE 1.1 Four different perspectives that relate to athletic development

healthy habits and that these lead to improvement in the lives of individuals. However, you might detect a contrasting holistic tone (IPLA) compared to one more focused on performance (NSCA). For example, the IPLA talks of the need to 'value and take responsibility for engagement' which suggests a focus on the overall experience of, and relationship with, movement compared to the NSCA's focus on distinct outcomes.

The perspectives on the right-hand side of Figure 1.1 perhaps more explicitly focus on development, starting with talent development in the top right quadrant. Generally, no one organisation represents the field of talent development; there are many possible definitions and stakeholders. One prominent author often referenced in sport cited here is Gagné (2004) who describes talent development as a systematic *process* from his background in education. Viewed this way, talent development is very unlikely without a deliberate development and learning process to transform potential into expertise. This arguably applies to most performance domains such as music, dance, and drama, as well as sport. Likewise, those from physical literacy or a strength and conditioning perspective also discuss the importance of deliberate learning processes.

Thinking about this book's definition of athletic development one question to resolve is: how much should athletic development solely be about achieving expertise or other broader ranges of aspiration? The International Olympic Committee's (IOC) consensus statement on youth sport perhaps helps respond to this question (Bergeron et al., 2015; see bottom right of Figure 1.1). The second half of the statement has a focus on youth athletic development's goal. It claims youth athletic development aims to achieve "sustainable and enjoyable participation and success for all levels" (Bergeron et al., 2015, p. 843); this is very different from the focus on expertise in talent development. A perspective that encompasses all levels of achievement is a practical framing to use as we consider how to articulate this book's definition of athletic development.

THIS BOOK'S PERSPECTIVE ON ATHLETIC DEVELOPMENT

As we move towards how this book will use the term athletic development it is useful to examine each part discretely (i.e. 'athletic' and 'development').

Athletic

In this book we have a clear focus on competitive sport. Thinking about the athletic aspect of competitive sport a useful reference point is the NSCA's definition of athleticism: "the ability to repeatedly perform a range of movements with precision and confidence *in a variety of environments* [our emphasis], which require competent levels of motor skills, strength, power, speed, agility, balance, coordination, and endurance" (Lloyd et al., 2016, p. 1491). When the NSCA position statement describes long-term athletic development as the habitual development of athleticism over time and relates it to confidence and competence it is about movements people acquire through diverse environments and a balanced sporting life. We deliberately refer to a balanced sporting life since this implies one in which athletes experience diversity in a range of sporting movements and contexts.

Our intention, as editors, is that 'athletic' also includes the sustainable and enjoyable participation in competitive sport and success for all levels (cf. Bergeron et al., 2015). However, what standards might athletic 'success' be referenced against? A self-referenced standard of success might be achieving a first (e.g., swimming 500 metres or running 5 kilometres). Alternatively, externally referenced success might be against a recognised threshold time or team selection (e.g., competing at a certain level, team, or league). We suggest that achieving externally referenced standards is often a feature used to define athletic development outcomes. We evaluate some of these ideas with the help of case study scenarios in the next section.

Development

Development implies a focus on learning and developmental processes and *relationships* that help athletes transform any potential they have into healthy, resilient, and sustainable participation (Bergeron et al., 2015). Development also involves enhancing physical, social, and psychological skills (Bailey et al., 2010). This book's psychological focus often explores social relations and the learning environments created by others. Gagné (2015) describes this as the psychological influence of significant persons in the athlete's immediate environment such as family, coaches, and mentors. The learning, development, skills, and relationships are likely to have most impact over a period of time, but any evidence of the minimum duration required for relationships to influence development is inconclusive.

Elements that help summarise this book's perspective of athletic development are listed here. These partly arise from the preceding discussion. We propose that athletic development involves at least these important elements:

1. sustained coaching relationships over a period of time;
2. outcomes of confidence and competence in sports performance;
3. sustainable sport participation and success at a range of levels;

A proposed fourth element is evaluated in the following section. This fourth element suggests that a person's self-identification as an athlete should be considered. This is often called athletic identity and it might be one of multiple identities to which they relate. This suggests athletic development involves:

4. the participant being likely to self-identify as 'an athlete' (an athletic identity).

Applying these four elements to case study scenarios will help evaluate how development processes contribute.

Applying This Book's Use of Athletic Development

This section outlines two cases of athletic development trajectories in order to see how they might fit against the four elements (1–4) listed previously. The cases of Jofra and Azumah (see Figure 1.2) provide focus for further discussion and clarification and they deliberately address adult participation in sport. Adult cases highlight that athletic development is not neat linear progression from childhood and people follow varied routes.

Jofra and Azumah's cases outline how they have developed towards their current sports involvement. We discuss the extent that their athletic development fits against each element in turn.

1. Sustained coaching interactions are a feature of the athletic development process and Azumah has, it is assumed, been coached in gymnastics, football and basketball along with her current coaching relationships at the football club. A sustained coaching relationship is more open to debate in Jofra's case since the support is remote and of limited duration.

2. There is a contrast in the extent to which Jofra and Azumah can be said to exhibit sporting confidence and competence outcomes. Azumah's experience of childhood gymnastics, football, and basketball from the age of 7 does suggest an athletic development journey in which competence and confidence in varied movements and competitive sport has been established. Jofra's journey in competitive running is not so sustained and his case does not fit this element so well.

3. The level that each aspire to are very different in that Jofra has run his first 5km and now is targeting two marathons: he has set his own success standards. In contrast Azumah's aspiration is to achieve semi-professional team selection: this is an external success standard involving the team coach's judgement. Azumah's case study perhaps helps illustrate that, often, achieving external referenced success is considered as a feature of athletic development. Such a standard is not currently evident in Jofra's case.

4. The fourth athletic identity–related element suggests a person's self-identification as an athlete should be considered. For example, Azumah appears to identify herself as an athlete (footballer) but Jofra appears to describe his participation as a passionate pursuit. A more detailed conversation with both would be required to confirm this.

As you can see it is not always easy to precisely define athletic development: there are some grey areas. The case studies illustrate two people who have come to their current sport later in life. Azumah brings some elements from her previous experience in gymnastics—some movement competence.

JOFRA

AZUMAH

Jofra's interest in sport at school was negligible but now, at the age of 45, he is committed to distance running. At age 41 he completed a 'Couch to 5K' plan via a mobile app which contains training plans that gradually progress toward a 5-kilometre run over nine weeks. He completed three 5km races in his first year and gradually increased his distances and now, in his fourth year, he is undertaking two marathons, including one in Boston, USA. All of this has been achieved through online coaching and advice along with running groups and friendships he has developed. He now describes himself as: "An NHS worker and parent who is passionate about running". His personal best at 5K is 22 minutes. His goal of completing his first marathon has been met in year 3; he is starting to think about breaking a time of 4 hours this year.

Four Athletic Development Elements to Consider:

1. Sustained coaching relationships over a period of time;

2. Outcomes of confidence and competence in sports performance;

3. Sustainable sport participation and success at a range of levels;

4. The participant being likely to self-identify as 'an athlete' (an athletic identify).

Azumah, at the age of 25, describes herself as: "A late blooming and improving top footballer". She was on a regional gymnastics squad from ages 7 to 11 but then stopped since she lost interest and was keen on a range of other sports. For instance, in football and basketball she achieved some success on her school team and local representative squads. She continued playing football at a modest level but at 23 years of age was noticed and invited to train alongside a semi-professional club, whom she now plays for regularly. She has engaged with coaching and strength and conditioning guidance at the club over the last few years.

FIGURE 1.2 Two fictional athletic development trajectories (Jofra and Azumah) set beside four athletic development elements.

The case studies highlight how complex athletic development is and we must not assume it refers to a path that starts in childhood and therefore may be confused with talent development.

One way of summarising our use of athletic development in this book is this: it is a process; the process of turning mental and physical potential into varied athletic outcomes, often in competitive sport. Athletic development is about an individual's experience of that process and some of the main psychological factors involved. For us, Azumah's case is more within the scope of this book's athletic development perspective than Jofra's.

The purpose of this first half of the chapter has been to recognise how applying the athletic development term is not straightforward and emphasise a development process. In the following section a possible framework for extending this understanding and making links between the book's chapters is suggested which reinforces parts of the preceding discussion. This represents the book's interpretation of the field of study; it is not the only approach.

A FRAMEWORK OF ATHLETIC DEVELOPMENT

One of the secondary aims of this chapter is to explain how the book's athletic development perspective is informed by a range of ideas from psychology that address development processes. These are illustrated in a schematic representation in Figure 1.3. The framework is not meant to represent all the possible variables of athletic development, but it does tie together the main psychological ideas explored in this book. There are a range of authors who have conceptualised talent or athletic development (e.g., Starkes & Ericsson, 2003; Simonton, 2017; Schinke et al., 2018; Stambulova et al., 2020). For Figure 1.3 we have adapted the work of Gagné, an educationalist who developed a Differentiated Model of Giftedness and Talent (DMGT) over three iterations (Gagné, 2000, 2004, 2015). With its consideration of natural abilities, environmental and mental catalysts, wellbeing, the developmental journey, and chance, this framework can be described as multidimensional and as reflecting the complexity of the athletic development process.

Here we explain each field (box) of our framework from left to right and how it relates to this book. The role of chance is illustrated further once the framework contents have been explained.

Natural Abilities

Start by looking at the left-hand side of the figure where natural abilities encompass physical and mental potential, often called talent, which can be considered as the 'raw material' that each athlete possesses (Gagné, 2015).

Environmental Catalysts

Moving to the right you encounter four boxes with components labelled 'Environmental Catalysts', 'Mental Catalysts', 'Wellbeing', and 'The Development Journey'. Two of these, 'environmental' and 'mental' catalysts affect the athletic development process, either positively or negatively (Gagné, 2015).

Under Environmental Catalysts, 'social influences' refers to the larger scale psychosocial environment encompassing the educational and group motivational climate of which an athlete is a part (two chapters discuss these: Chapters 8 and 10). The 'individual relationships' section includes, as previously mentioned, the psychological influence of significant persons in the athlete's immediate environment. Gagné (2015) states that it includes parents and siblings, coaches, peers, mentors, and even figures adopted as role models by athletes. Five chapters connect with these: Chapters 6, 7, 8, 9, and 10.

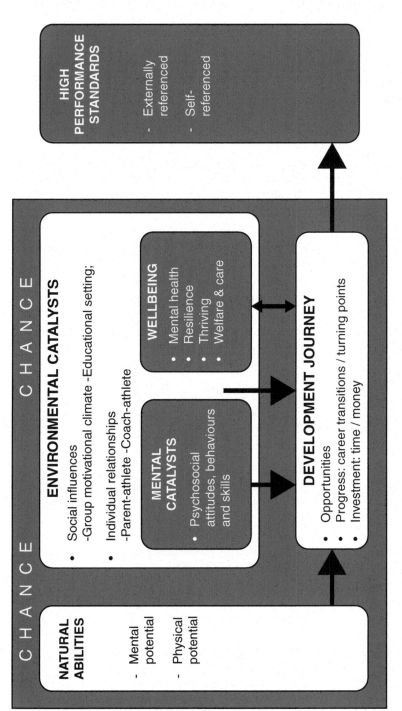

FIGURE 1.3 This book's framework of athletic development

Source: Adapted from Gagné, 2015, p. 19

Mental Catalysts

The mental catalysts in the framework refer to an individual's psychosocial attitudes, behaviours, and skills that support their development. Psychological skills have been associated with sporting development and success stemming from many decades of research (an early example being Orlick & Partington, 1988) and, more recently, the relationship between skills and the ability to respond to transitions and career challenges has been recognised (e.g., Collins & MacNamara, 2018). Likewise, psychological constructs such as an athletes' conscientiousness or persistence (e.g., Duckworth, 2016) are known to contribute to sustaining effort and practice regimes that support positive outcomes. As Gagné (2015) observes long-term aspirational goals "require intense dedication, as well as daily acts of will power to maintain practice through obstacles, boredom, and occasional failure" (p. 22). No one chapter in this book encompasses the full range of attitudes, behaviours, and skills but many closely connect with these mental catalysts. For example, Chapters 2 and 12.

Wellbeing

Wellbeing is an important consideration when examining athletic development. The reason being that wellbeing and illbeing dynamically interact with the catalysts to help or hinder development (Gagné, 2015). Wellbeing has a range of positive or negative aspects that can contribute to, or harm, an athlete's development, but four (mental health, resilience, thriving, and welfare/care) have been selected in this book since there are significant and growing bodies of research for each. Notice the deliberate bidirectional arrow pointing both ways from/to the development journey inferring that wellbeing influences development in a two-way relationship. Four chapters connect with this: Chapters 11, 12, 13, and 14.

The Development Journey

At the bottom of the figure, the 'development journey' refers to the series of structured activities leading to specific high-performance standards, often over a significant period of time (e.g., the inclusion in a squad and training programme that Azumah is a part of). The complexity of the process could warrant a whole separate book but for simplicity it is broken down into three components here.

- 'Opportunities' refers to the competitive and training resources/activities that are available to an individual, which will vary from athlete to athlete. This is not directly addressed in a separate chapter, but it is implied throughout the book.
- 'Progress' refers to how athletes negotiate critical moments, such as career transitions and turning points in their development, often using psychological skills in doing so. An individual's response to and resilience in these critical moments is crucial to their development (e.g., Collins & MacNamara, 2018). Transitions are addressed holistically, as something that happens throughout athletic careers, in Chapters 4 and 5.
- 'Investment' refers to the amount of time that an athlete invests in training when they consciously specialise in a sport. Financial resources may be needed for equipment, facility access, travel, and competition costs. This again varies according to an athlete's circumstances. This is not directly addressed in a separate chapter but it is an implied understanding throughout the book.

Framework Summary

As we close and summarise the framework, we should bring attention to 'Chance' appearing at the top of the figure. As opportunities often depend on circumstances, luck and chance have an influence. We explore this in a little more detail with a spotlight in a moment.

The framework therefore provides a theoretically informed overview of athletic development that may eventually result in high performance standards, and the confidence and competence likely to arise during development. This possible final outcome is shown on the far right of Figure 1.3. Viewing the athletic development journey in this way with its catalysts and contributing elements, including recognition of the role of chance, provides a useful springboard for further study. The following illustrates the role of chance further.

Spotlight On: Chance in Athletic Development

There are at least two crucial 'rolls of the dice' that determine an individual's opportunities: his or her parents and background. Not only does chance determine genetic legacy, and therefore influences physical and mental abilities, it is also evident in the environment athletes develop within. The term "the social gradient" (Public Health England, 2017) is used to describe health and other opportunities that are determined by background and uneven socio-economic circumstances. These are illustrated in the sloped playing field analogy in Figure 1.4. However, this is not just true of health outcomes; it also extends to educational achievement and sports participation with

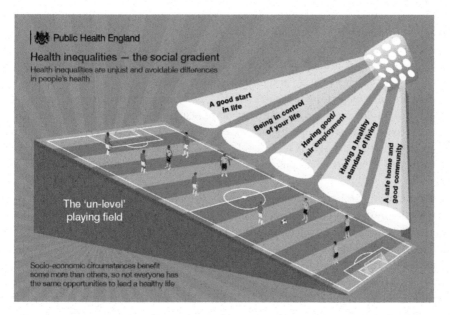

FIGURE 1.4 Illustrating the health inequalities as a result of the social gradient

Source: Public Health England, 2017

those from disadvantaged backgrounds less likely to play sport beyond school (Sport England, 2020).

When you were born may be another important element of chance that contributes to athletic achievement. The relative age effect (RAE) refers to the fact that relatively older athletes within an age year are often over-represented among age-group or elite sport squads (e.g., Cobley et al., 2009). For example, in the UK, where the school year starts in September, being born in July/August can often be a disadvantage in school sports because pupils will be the youngest and often smaller than their year group compared to relatively older more developed peers. The chance factor of when you are born can have an impact in early athletic development especially in sports in which size and strength are important.

However, recent research (e.g., McCarthy et al., 2016) has suggested that younger, later maturing athletes who manage to remain in an athletic development programme eventually become advantaged in comparison to their relatively older peers. It is claimed that they develop resilience to compensate for their relatively lagged physical development. This perhaps illustrates that a longitudinal perspective is required for researching athletic development and often psychology can contribute useful insights even to a physical phenomenon such as relative differences in maturation.

CLOSING THOUGHTS

Athletic development is defined differently by various professional groups ranging from sport and conditioning coaches (NSCA) and physical educators (IPLA) through to stakeholders and researchers focusing on performance success (IOC). This chapter's exploration of athletic development draws on the discussion of four elements to help illustrate distinctive features, namely: i) sustained coaching relationships, ii) outcomes of confidence and competence, iii) sustainable sport participation at a range of levels, and iv) athletic identity. These elements help determine what types of athlete developmental journeys are likely to be encompassed by this book's perspective.

To help frame the scope and extent of this book's coverage of psychological aspects of athletic development, a framework of athletic development has been presented and explained to show the links between environmental, mental, welfare, and developmental ideas and processes. As part of this the role of chance in athletic development was recognised.

Finally, athletic development is not a simple puzzle to be solved with A, plus B, plus C, plus D equalling athletic competence. It is a multidimensional phenomenon full of remaining uncertainties and individually different athlete paths. However much sense and order we try to apply we should recognise how it includes the vagaries of the human condition in relationships, genetics, environmental influences, and yes, at times, good fortune. This is what makes it so interesting to study and why this book aims to make a small contribution to furthering understanding, especially amongst those new to the topic.

REFERENCES

Bailey, R., Collins, D., Ford, P., MacNamara, Á., Toms, M., & Pearce, G. (2010). Participant development in sport: An academic review. *Sports Coach UK*, *4*, 1–134.

Balyi, I., & Hamilton, A. (2004). *Long-term athlete development: Trainability in childhood and adolescence. Windows of opportunity. Optimal trainability*. National Coaching Institute & Advanced Training and Performance.

Bergeron, M. F., Mountjoy, M., Armstrong, N., Chia, M., Côté, J., Emery, C. A., . . . & Malina, R. M. (2015). International Olympic Committee consensus statement on youth athletic development. *British Journal of Sports Medicine*, *49*(13), 843–851.

Cobley, S., Baker, J., Wattie, N., & McKenna, J. (2009). Annual age-grouping and athlete development. *Sports Medicine*, *39*(3), 235–256.

Collins, D. J., & MacNamara, A. (2018). *Talent development: A practitioner guide*. Routledge.

Duckworth, A. (2016). *Grit: The power of passion and perseverance* (Vol. 234). Scribne.

Gagné, F. (2000). Understanding the complex choreography of talent development through DMGT-based analysis. In K. A. Heller et al. (Eds.), *International handbook of giftedness and talent* (2nd ed., pp. 67–79). Elsevier.

Gagné, F. (2004). Transforming gifts into talents: The DMGT as a developmental theory. *High Ability Studies*, *15*(2), 119–147.

Gagné, F. (2015). From genes to talent: The DMGT/CMTD perspective. De los genes al talento: la perspectiva DMGT/CMTD. *Revista de Educación*, *368*, 12–37.

International Physical Literacy Association (IPLA). (2020). *International Physical Literacy Association homepage*. www.physical-literacy.org.uk/

Lloyd, R. S., Cronin, J. B., Faigenbaum, A. D., Haff, G. G., Howard, R., Kraemer, W. J., . . . & Oliver, J. L. (2016). National Strength and Conditioning Association position statement on long-term athletic development. *Journal of Strength and Conditioning Research*, *30*(6), 1491–1509.

McCarthy, N., Collins, D., & Court, D. (2016). Start hard, finish better: Further evidence for the reversal of the RAE advantage. *Journal of Sports Sciences*, *34*(15), 1461–1465.

Orlick, T., & Partington, J. (1988). Mental links to excellence. *The Sport Psychologist*, *2*(2), 105–130.

Public Health England. (2017, September 8). Closing the health gap and reducing inequalities. *Public Health Matters*. https://publichealthmatters.blog.gov.uk/2017/09/08/closing-the-health-gap-and-reducing-inequalities/

Schinke, R. J., Stambulova, N. B., Si, G., & Moore, Z. (2018). International society of sport psychology position stand: Athletes' mental health, performance, and development. *International Journal of Sport and Exercise Psychology*, *16*(6), 622–639.

Simonton, D. (2017). Does talent exist? Yes! In J. Baker, S. Cobley, J. Schorer, & N. Wattie (Eds.), *Routledge handbook of talent identification and development in sport* (pp. 11–18). Taylor & Francis.

Sport England. (2020). *Active Lives Survey 2018/19 report*. www.sportengland.org/know-your-audience/data/active-lives

Stambulova, N. B., Ryba, T. V., & Henriksen, K. (2020). Career development and transitions of athletes: The international society of sport psychology position stand revisited. *International Journal of Sport and Exercise Psychology*, 1–27.

Starkes, J. L., & Ericsson, K. A. (2003). *Expert performance in sports: Advances in research on sport expertise*. Human Kinetics.

Whitehead, M. (2010). *Physical literacy: Throughout the lifecourse* (1st ed.). Routledge.

CHAPTER 2

How Did We Get Here? Exploring the Evolution of Athletic Development Perspectives

Ben Oakley

Research fields don't just suddenly appear, they evolve over decades. The same is true of athletic development which started being widely studied in the 1990s. Knowing about the history and evolution of, and influences upon, a relatively new field is valuable in making more sense of it. The purpose of this chapter is to provide a broader context of the different psychological perspectives often used in studying athletic development. The chapter explores how psychological aspects of athletic development, as partly represented by the chapters in this book, link to each other and can be traced back to earlier foci.

The task of establishing 'how did we get here?' in this chapter is partly illustrated by the content of review/study papers or International Society of Sport Psychology (ISSP) 'position stands'. It is recognised that such position statements do not always represent the state of knowledge of a particular domain since they are often reflective of the interests of those who sit on society committees rather than the diverse views of a research community. Position statements and other papers are used here as an indication of *when* a research perspective has gained momentum. This chapter represents an interpretation of the topic of athletic development's journey from early initial studies to the diverse research described in this book. Mapping the evolution over time of some of the theoretical positions used in athletic development is primarily to help readers understand the field and provide a guide through it, particularly for newcomers.

GETTING STARTED

A useful starting point is the overview provided in Table 2.1 which shows eight different athletic development perspectives related to psychology drawn from Bruner et al.'s (2009) citation analysis of athletic development models, sport psychology position statements, and the sport psychology literature. The order in which they are presented in the table approximately relates to when the early research in each perspective gained prominence. For example, three established perspectives are indicated at the top of Table 2.1, whilst five active and still evolving perspectives are identified at the bottom of the table. These contemporary perspectives are more likely to include studies published in the last decade.

TABLE 2.1 Eight different athletic development perspectives with a psychological focus

Athletic Development Perspective	Main Psychological Focus	Example of Related Paper or Position Statement, Including Title
MORE ESTABLISHED RESEARCH PERSPECTIVES		
• **Talent and its identification**	Conceptualising the multidimensional (biological, psychological, social) basis of talent	Lidor et al. (2009) *To Test or Not to Test? The Use of Physical Skill Tests in Talent Detection and in Early Phases of Sport Development* [ISSP position stand]
• **Expertise: practice quality and quantity**	Cognitive psychology (e.g., information processing)	Helsen et al. (1998) "Team sports and the theory of deliberate practice" [paper]
• **Development: practice, play, and diversification**	Child and youth development	Côté et al. (2009). *To Sample or to Specialize? Seven Postulates About Youth Sport Activities That Lead to Continued Participation and Elite Performance* [ISSP position stand]
ACTIVE AND STILL EVOLVING RESEARCH PERSPECTIVES		
• **Developmental environments and culture**	Ecological psychology Youth developmental psychology	Mathorne et al. (2020) 'An "organizational triangle" to coordinate talent development: A case study in Danish swimming' [paper]
• **Psychosocial skills and resources**	Personal psychological strategies and behaviours	MacNamara et al. (2010) 'The role of psychological characteristics in facilitating the pathway to elite performance part 1: Identifying mental skills and behaviours' [paper]
• **Developmental transitions**	Holistic career and environment perspectives	Stambulova et al. (2020) *Career development and transitions of athletes: position stand revisited* [ISSP position stand]
• **Mental health**	Holistic career, identity and cultural sport psychology perspectives	Schinke et al. (2018). *Athletes' mental health, performance, and development* [ISSP position stand]
• **Relationships with athletes (e.g., coach and/or parent)**	Social psychology	Harwood and Knight (2015). 'Parenting in youth sport: A position paper on parenting expertise' [paper]

The aim of the table is twofold: firstly, to provide a pedagogic tool to alert readers of psychological perspectives that are perhaps new to them, and secondly, to demonstrate that there are a number of foci for researching athletic development. The table is not able to show the overlaps and links between each perspective: each perspective does not exist in isolation from the others.

The chapter is structured with a brief outline of the evolution of each perspective discussed in turn. This will explain that sometimes, even within each perspective, research has taken varied directions and there are relationships between perspectives as was demonstrated in Chapter 1 (see Figure 1.3).

TALENT AND ITS IDENTIFICATION

The field of athletic development has always been influenced by those studying elite athletes and excellence. For example, studies on Olympic athletes. One of the first to have an impact was de Garay and colleagues' (1974) research analysing the physical profiles of 1,265 athletes across 13 sports attending the 1968 Olympic Games in Mexico City. This investigation heightened awareness of distinct *anthropometrical* and *physical* profiles for successful Olympic athletes in different sporting events, i.e., ignoring psychology. This study contributed to the belief, now realised to be false (Lidor et al., 2009), that measuring children's physical characteristics enables the identification of athletes who have the potential to later succeed in specific sports or events after sufficient training. At the time the Cold War was at its height and many coaches and sport scientists started to believe that physical profiling of young children might yield advantages in finding talent and success in the global sporting arms race (Oakley & Green, 2001).

Since this type of 'talent and its identification' research has been conducted over many decades it is placed at the top of Table 2.1. Mero et al.'s (1990) investigation of strength, speed, and endurance capacities amongst pre-pubescent children, aged 10–13 years, is an example of continuing physiologically based research. Their study recommended that 'the parameters used in this investigation can be used for talent selection in sport' (p. 57). This demonstrates that this belief was still prevalent almost two decades after the original Mexico Olympic Games research.

Increasingly psychologists have critiqued a solely biological (i.e., physical) conceptualisation of talent in favour of a more multidimensional perspective that encompasses biological, psychological, and social aspects. An example of a biological focus is when physical tests are solely used to identify talent before adolescent growth has been completed. For instance, in 2004, Abbott and Collins proposed that psychology had a key role to play in understanding the development process of talented athletes and stressed the complex pathways and the multidimensional nature of sporting development and success. Then in 2009, the ISSP issued a position stand (Lidor et al., 2009) on the issue of testing. This stand observed that "no clear-cut evidence has been found to support the predictive value of physical skill tests in talent detection during development in sport" (p. 140). It also suggested, "additional factors such as psychological preparation and social support should also be included in order to obtain the most comprehensive picture of the ability [of athletes] . . . to attain a high level of proficiency" (Lidor et al., p. 144). This and other contributions provided a firm evidence base against physical testing before adolescence and supported the potential for psychology to contribute to understanding talent development.

EXPERTISE: PRACTICE QUALITY AND QUANTITY

In parallel to this growing acceptance that sport psychology could contribute to talent development, an influential body of work was already underway in mainstream psychology drawing on a cognitive perspective. Two groups of cognitive psychology researchers were influential in this period, but it took a while for their investigations to be more widely noticed by the sport and exercise science community. We outline each group's contribution here.

Chase and Simon (1973) investigated expertise in chess and focused on information processing by using an experimental approach to study cognitive mechanisms. They helped to initiate the detailed study of how expertise is developed which, for them, relied on understanding the role of practice quality and quantity. Ericsson and colleagues (1993) extended this earlier work on expertise in chess into another domain: with a focus on music. They studied violin players' expertise and asked violin players of four different skill levels (top potential international soloists, plus three other levels of skilled violin players) to estimate the amount of time they had engaged in a variety of practice activities throughout their music careers. By the age of 23, all participants in the study had engaged in violin lessons and practice for a decade or more. They found that 10,000 hours of practice is required to reach the highest standard of performance. But they also described the type of quality practice required as a very specific: they named this 'deliberate practice'. This is characterised as highly structured, requiring effort, focused to overcome weaknesses, and being carefully monitored, by others, to provide feedback.

It did not take long for sport psychology researchers to ask the question: 'How does this deliberate practice apply to sporting expertise?'. One of the first studies of sport training, practice and expertise was Helsen et al. (1998). This and subsequent studies (e.g., Young & Salmela, 2002) often focused on eliciting information from athletes through retrospective questionnaires. The main suggestion from these studies was that a relationship exists between the number of hours spent in relevant quality practice activities and the level of performance.

What followed a decade later was an interesting example of just one research finding (i.e., Ericsson et al.'s [1993] quantity of practice) being magnified by other authors. Three separate popular book authors arguably oversimplified how expertise could be achieved. Even now, well over a decade after these books were published, many coaches, parents, and athletes have heard that 10 years and 10,000 hours of practice are claimed to be required in order to become an elite athlete. Many still believe it to be true. The 10-year/10,000-hour rule, as it has come to be known, was propagated in popular 'talent' books such as *Outliers* by Gladwell (2008), *The Talent Code* by Coyle (2009), and *Bounce* by Syed (2010). Subsequent research and copious examples suggest that expertise can be achieved in shorter timescales and goes beyond practice hours as the key component. For example, Bullock et al. (2009) demonstrated how a rapid, intensive programme could produce a Winter Olympian in just 14 months. The multidimensional nature of talent development was also reinforced by Lidor et al.'s (2009) ISSP position stand.

DEVELOPMENT: PRACTICE, PLAY, AND DIVERSIFICATION

In contrast to measuring the quantity and quality of practice, the interest amongst some sport psychologists was on a more social perspective. Unlike Chase and Simon's (1973) quantitative study of chess players' expertise, Bloom's (1982) report of qualitative interviews with talented individuals in mathematics, art, and sport retrospectively described their entire development path, taking into consideration the influence of family, peers, teachers, and coaches. One of the first sport psychologists to draw on Bloom's work was Côté (1999) in his study on the influence of the family on talent development and the quality of their practice, including play-like, informal activities. Over the years Côté and colleagues have continued with further research emphasising children's development, autonomy, enjoyment, and diverse activities. These ideas are represented in the widely cited Developmental Model of Sport Participation (DMSP; Côté, 1999; Côté et al., 2003).

This model of effective athletic development places emphasis on social interaction and unstructured play, often without adults or coaches. Côté (1999) terms this 'deliberate play' and recognises the benefits of children flexibly organising their own games and practices—for example on a basketball court, in the backyard or garden, or at the skate park—which can often be more fun and diverse than formal practices. The impact of this research perspective has been a greater discussion about if, and when, it is appropriate for young athletes to specialise in one sport year-round. The influence of the DMSP now means that amongst academics and some coaches the advantages of sampling a range of sports rather than specialising on one in childhood are recognised (e.g., Bergeron et al., 2015). A decade after Côté's original 1999 paper, he was the lead author of a 2009 ISSP position stand in which seven postulates (propositions) about sampling or specialisation in youth sport were discussed (Côté et al., 2009; see Table 2.1, column 3). Interestingly, Côté published this position stand working with Lidor and Hackfort as authors; the very same authors of the physical talent testing ISSP position stand referred to earlier (i.e., Lidor et al., 2009).

Overall, to summarise this section, the developmental psychology–informed ideas from this development, practice, play, and diversification perspective go back more than three decades and are firmly established. These ideas often resonate through to the current research and practices in athletic development. In particular, relationships with parents and coaches and the influence of favourable environmental conditions around an athlete for them to flourish and develop (see Chapter 1, Figure 1.3). One possible critique of research on a single element, such as parents, coaches, or peers, is that it does not capture the integration of elements in the whole environment. It is therefore highly appropriate that it is to an environment perspective that we move to next, with Côté continuing to contribute.

ENVIRONMENT: FAVOURABLE CONDITIONS FOR ATHLETIC DEVELOPMENT

This perspective assumes that the environment that is designed and created in sport programmes can do a great deal to help or hinder the overall intent of a programme. The study of the environment that surrounds an athlete has a holistic focus on the overall atmosphere, relationships, culture, and organisational factors. Within sport psychology two contrasting perspectives have emerged: positive youth development and talent development environments.

Positive Youth Development

One perspective is based on positive youth development (PYD), which often includes community or recreational sport settings. PYD is a conception of development in which young people are viewed as having personal resources and strengths that can be developed (Lerner et al., 2005). Research has sought to identify features of youth programme environments both within and beyond sport that can be harnessed to foster positive change in personal resources such as confidence, belonging, and character (Lerner et al., 2005). Literature highlights the link between environment, development of personal resources and how need fulfilment relates to young people's wellbeing. For example, one of the most cited studies is from the US's National

---

Box 2.1 Eight Main Environmental Features That Facilitate Positive Youth Development

1. Physical and psychological safety.

2. Appropriate structure (i.e., clear expectations regarding rules and boundaries).

3. Supportive relationships.

4. Opportunities to belong.

5. Positive social norms (i.e., positive values such as fair play, cooperation, responsibility, empathy, and self-control).

6. Support of efficacy (the need for those supporting young people to develop autonomy, helping empower them and increasing their intrinsic motivation).

7. Opportunities for skill building.

8. Integration of family, school, and community efforts (i.e., to lessen dissonance).

Source: Adapted from NRCIM, 2002, pp. 90–91

Research Council and Institute of Medicine (NRCIM, 2002) which identified eight main features that should be present in the context of general community programmes to facilitate PYD (see Box 2.1).

Côté et al. (2014) extended this work and proposed the Personal Assets Framework (PAF) in sport. This suggests that sport experiences may, over time, impact on participant's personal assets (resources). These assets are their confidence (positive self-worth in sport), competence (a positive view of one's action in sport), connection (positive bonds with others), and character (respect for rules, integrity, and empathy). It is suggested that changes in these personal assets influence the individual's continued sport participation, performance, and development.

The PYD perspective is valuable since so much of the athletic development literature and research is dominated by talent development. However, a meta-analysis of qualitative research in PYD concluded that the literature is fragmented, and theory used sparingly (Holt et al., 2017). It appears this particular conception of athletic development may require clarification when compared to other perspectives, but PYD does offer some useful insights to coaches working with young people.

Talent Development Environments

A body of work has grown around the evaluation of talent development environments (TDEs) and understanding the influences upon effective design, goals, and coherence of a development programme. To begin to illustrate this, the work of Martindale et al.'s (2007) interview-based study will be used. They identified five generic characteristics of effective TDEs:

1. Long-term aims and methods—e.g., encouraging practices that help athletes stay in the sport, improve, and avoid too much emphasis on age-group (e.g., U15) success.

2. Wide-ranging coherent messages and support—e.g., consistent communication and support from coaches, parents, and an organisation's reward and selection systems.

3. Emphasis on appropriate development, not early success—e.g., de-emphasise winning as success and provide integrated teaching that builds responsibility, autonomy, and awareness.

4. Individualised and ongoing development—e.g., provide regular goal-setting and review sessions and identify, prepare for, and support key transitions.

5. Integrated, holistic, and systematic development—e.g., supporting athletes are aligned in their expectations and athlete lifestyle balance is promoted consistently.

Subsequently these researchers have developed, and refined, a questionnaire tool, the Talent Development Environment Questionnaire (Hall et al., 2019), to measure these characteristics. Also see Chapter 8 on creating an optimal motivational climate for effective coaching.

Another body of work has developed mainly by studying Scandinavian talent environments using a holistic ecological approach (e.g., Henriksen et al., 2010). The holistic ecological approach views athletic development as emerging out of daily interactions between an athlete and their environment and how these interactions mirror the culture of a development setting. It draws on a branch of psychology known as ecological psychology. This uses the human-environment system as unit of analysis and it has an emphasis on perceptual learning and development (Lobo et al., 2018). Henriksen et al. (2010) developed a framework, a 'working model', as a reference point in analysing different environments (see Figure 2.1).

Henriksen's research uses rich case studies of effective and ineffective talent development environments to show what components, processes, and cultural and organisational interactions stimulate athlete progress. The framework (Figure 2.1) is used to help articulate deep descriptions of what is observed by researchers. For instance, successful kayak, athletics, football, and swimming clubs, in addition to a national sailing squad and a less successful golf environment have all been analysed, including their distinctive features (2010–20; e.g., Mathorne et al., 2020).

Many of the ideas emerging from these detailed case studies are similar to Martindale et al.'s (2007) generic characteristics but it is worth drawing attention to three additional characteristics. One is evidence of *proximal role models* being significant for developing athletes; another is the importance of support for the development of *psychosocial skills* (see following section); and a third is training that allows for *diversification* of sporting and other activities (Mathorne et al., 2020). Notice that diversification is a theme originally identified by Côté (1999).

This psychosocial perspective offers rich insights into programme design decisions which help and hinder development. Next, we change our focus from the broad environment to studying the individual athlete.

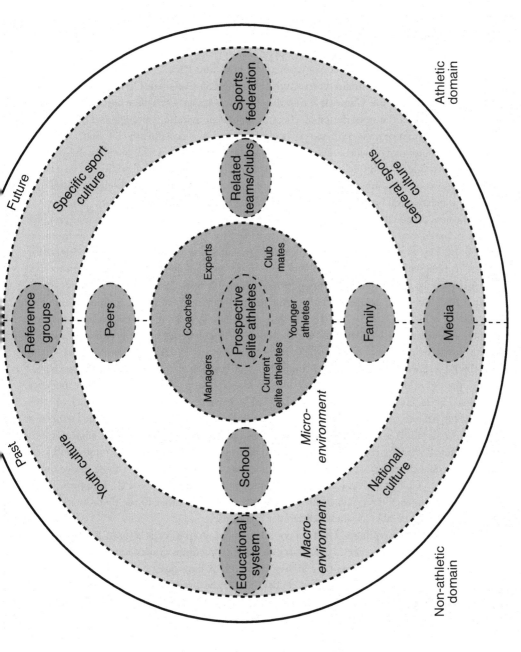

FIGURE 2.1 The athletic talent development environment working model

Source: Henriksen et al., 2010, p. 213

PSYCHOSOCIAL SKILLS AND RESOURCES

The psychological attitudes, skills, and resources (i.e., personal strategies and behaviours) of the individual athlete can have a significant bearing on athletic development (MacNamara et al., 2010). This section mainly focuses on psychological skills that support athletic development and we briefly touch, in less detail, on resilience.

Once again it was a study investigating Olympic athletes that heavily influenced the development of this aspect of sport psychology practice. Orlick and Partington's (1988) publication of their interview and questionnaire-based study involving 235 Canadian Olympians who participated in the 1984 Olympic Games in Sarajevo or Los Angeles has been often cited. The key result from this study was the importance of effective mental preparation strategies with attentional focus and performance imagery being particularly related to successful athletes. Sport psychologists' research into psychological skills continued with Gould et al.'s (1993) interview-based study on the United States 1988 Olympic Wrestling Team. Their work provided additional insights on how athletes cope with stress using a variety of coping strategies including thought control, task focus, and behavioural based strategies (e.g., following a pre-performance routine).

In the next decade the momentum for studying psychological aspects of performance grew. For example, Smith et al. (1995) developed a measurement tool: the Athletic Coping Skills Inventory (ASCI-28). This assesses seven psychological skills that athletes use to manage their sports performance (coping with adversity, coachability, concentration, confidence and achievement motivation, goal setting and mental preparation, peaking under pressure, and freedom from worry).

In a British context, detailed interview studies of Olympic athletes have also been conducted (e.g., Hardy et al., 2017) and a blend of psychological skills has been identified similar to the work mentioned earlier. The blend of skills and attitudes has been labelled by one group of researchers as the Psychological Characteristics of Developing Excellence (PCDE; MacNamara et al., 2010). This blend is shown on the left side of Table 2.2. The contents of the table are explained here.

On the right side of Table 2.2 are the important contributing factors, with positive, negative, and dual effects (Hill et al., 2019). The PCDE can be considered as a set of tools which are then deployed to achieve or counter the factors on the right side of the table. Amongst the factors four are positive, so athletes are encouraged to maximise and use these. The negative clinical indicators in Table 2.2 (in the right-hand column) may need skills to be deployed to counter and avoid them. Two dual effect factors (perfectionistic tendencies and fear of failure) can be drawn on but in moderation. Collins and MacNamara (2017) suggest the aim of their PCDE approach is to build combinations of these skills, which admittedly overlap, in order to use them in addressing challenges, and to be able use these skills under pressure.

The notion of responding to challenge or adversity is also part of a body of literature about resilience in sport (see Chapter 12). In sport psychology sometimes similar concepts or ideas exist but since they stem from different research groups and/or have different philosophical foundations they use a different term. Indeed resilience, and the preceding discussion about mental skills, resources, or characteristics, is perhaps an example of overlapping concepts. In the sport performance and welfare context Fletcher and Sarkar (2012) described resilience as: "the role of mental processes and behaviour in promoting personal assets and protecting an individual from the potential negative effect of stressors" (p. 675). Therefore, any discussion about the 'psychosocial skills and resources' perspective of athletic development might also encompass resilience-related research.

TABLE 2.2 The Psychological Characteristics of Developing Excellence (PCDE) and contributing factors

Skills and Attitudes (PCDE)	Contributing Factors		
	Positive Effect (i.e., 'maximise')	Dual Effect (i.e., 'in moderation')	Negative Effect (i.e., 'counter & avoid')
• Commitment • Focus and distraction control • Realistic performance evaluation • Self-awareness • Coping with pressure • Planning and self-organisation • Goal-setting • Quality practice • Effective imagery • Actively seeking social support	• Imagery & active preparation • Self-directed control & management • Seeking & using social support • Active coping	• Perfectionistic tendencies • Fear of failure	• Clinical indicators (e.g., eating disorders, anxiety, depression)

Source: Adapted from Collins & MacNamara, 2017; Hill et al., 2019

As we have seen the athletic development perspective in this section emphasises how equipped athletes are to overcome challenges and adversity in their paths. This type of focus is arguably one of the key perspectives in athletic development. We turn next to the developmental transitions perspective, since adapting to physical, mental, and social challenges lies at the heart of a transitional perspective of athletic development.

DEVELOPMENTAL TRANSITIONS

Athletic development through the athlete's lifespan involves transitions from initiation into sport all the way through the ups and downs of the journey to discontinuing the sport. These transitions are a focus of many studies. Much of the early sport psychology transition research examined retirement from elite sport (e.g., Werthner & Orlick, 1986). However, over time the field has progressed towards a 'holistic' perspective on the athlete's career rather than one solitary event in time (e.g., career termination). The ISSP position stand in 2020 provides a useful explanation of how this perspective has evolved over time in three stages (Stambulova et al., 2020; see Table 2.1). These 'initiation', 'growth', and 'establishment' stages are outlined here with slight adjustments to terms the original authors used for clarity in the context of this chapter.

The three stages this perspective has evolved through are:

- Initiation (1960s–80s)—The initial focus was on athletic retirement. This was conceptualised as a 'social death' linking retirement to a form of grieving and loss, influenced by thanatology and social gerontology models (Rosenberg, 1984). However, a shift to a transition as a form of adaptation resulted in a more positive view of athletic retirement.
- Growth (1990s)—This decade saw the perspective shift to a whole career perspective. Recognition of within-career transitions was conceptualised as 'a miniature lifespan course' and viewed as turning phases in which athletes cope with specific demands in order to continue in their sport. New frameworks emerged to help explain this revised perspective (e.g., Stambulova, 1994).
- Establishment (2000 to present)—A whole person and a whole environment view becomes more widely used. New conceptualisations included transitions being classified as normative (expected) and nonnormative (unexpected). Perhaps the most influential framework has been the holistic athletic career model (Wylleman, 2019; Wylleman & Lavallee, 2004).

As career transitions are discussed in detail in the following chapters (see Chapters 3 and 4) we will limit the discussion to the previous evolutionary outline. However, it is worth making some closing comments on the overlaps between developmental transitions and other perspectives covered in Table 2.1.

In 2009, Bruner et al. observed that there was minimal integration between the talent related and transition literature. For instance, whilst the study of transitions addresses psychological skills in overcoming challenges, the crossover of these ideas and concepts is often not made explicit. In contrast, a significant part of the transition literature closely connects to the impact of a favourable environment and culture in supporting transitions. For example, you may remember that environment and culture was illustrated in Figure 2.1 (Henriksen et al.'s, 2010; the athletic talent development environment working model).

Also, it is becoming clear that effective talent environments have features which ensure that they nourish athletes' development and mental health (Henriksen et al., 2019). Therefore, this suggests Chapter 11 on mental health has considerable relevance to transitions. It is to mental health perspectives that we turn to next.

MENTAL HEALTH

The athlete mental health perspective has become prominent due to greater awareness of the impact of mental health during athletic careers in recent years. In the 2017–19 period, a total of six position stands or statements were published in English signifying the intense activity and interest in this perspective. These statements ranged from national organisations (e.g., British Association of Sport and Exercise Sciences [BASES]) to international organisations (e.g., the International Olympic Committee [IOC] and ISSP). In this section, we aim to provide a brief introductory overview to this rapidly developing field.

Mental health is widely discussed in the media and is often viewed negatively, through an illness-based lens. This public discussion and negative perspective of mental health has contributed to its stigma and those involved in sport not fully understanding what mental health is exactly (Gorczynski et al., 2019). The ISSP position stand (Schinke et al., 2018) uses a definition of mental health from the United States Department of Health and Human Services: "a state of successful performance or mental function, resulting in productive activities, fulfilling relationships with other people, and the ability to adapt to change and to cope with adversity" (1999, p. 4). Mental health, similar to physical health, is often discussed in different position statements as a personal resource or asset that allows people to function, manage stress, and contribute or collaborate with others effectively. Chapters in this book that discuss the potential of athletic experiences to be positive and developmental are, for example, those on coach-athlete relationships (Chapter 6), motivational climate (Chapter 8), resilience (Chapter 12), thriving (Chapter 13), and welfare (Chapter 14).

The ISSP position stand identifies several risk factors associated with athletic development that can impact mental health. Researchers have addressed various forms of athletes' experiences, such as overtraining, injury, concussion, and depression (Schinke et al., 2018). These issues are considered from a broader biopsychosocial lens in athletic mental health research and can be seen as outcomes of, for example, competition overload, inefficient training, under-recovery, and poor balance in athletes' lives. A common denominator for these lies in stressors experienced by athletes and their stress appraisals (Schinke et al., 2018).

Schinke et al. (2018) explains that a link between stress experienced by athletes and identity-related concepts is often explored through the mental health perspective. The authors continue by describing how sport psychologists may consider identity if working with athletes who are culturally diverse and/or part of a minority, compared to their peers. Sometimes this diversity contributes to complex structures of athletes' identities including their race, ethnicity, nationality, gender, sexual orientation, education, and their relationship with sport. Researchers have identified that centralising some of these identities and marginalising others in athletes' environments prevents these people from expressing their uniqueness and can lead to identity crisis. Such athletes often have additional sources of stress dealing with such crises which can drain their mental health resources (Schinke et al., 2018).

We will not consider interventions or strategies in this brief overview as these are addressed in Chapter 11. However, a firm understanding of mental health is fundamental to athletic development since it interacts with the environmental and mental catalysts described in Chapter 1. Mental health literacy, promoting knowledge about mental health problems which aid recognition, management, or prevention, is cited in the ISSP position stand as one of the key strategies for addressing mental health. We have suggested mental health and welfare perspectives closely interact with the nature of relationships in the sport setting and this is what we address next.

RELATIONSHIPS WITH ATHLETES

A relationship perspective on athletic development provides an appropriate final perspective to outline since it resonates with the start of this chapter. Bloom (1982) and Côté (1999) both emphasised the importance of, and emotional support provided by, relationships with both coaches and parents of developing athletes. However, there are very few studies of the interactions between coaches, young athletes, and parents. Most of the athlete relationships research focuses on either coach-athlete or parent-athlete relationships. Here we briefly explore examples of influential studies of each.

Coach-Athlete Relationships

One of the early studies of coach-athlete relations was Mageau and Vallerand's (2003) use of a Self-Determination Theory (SDT) perspective in which coaches' autonomy-supportive behaviours and the psychological processes through which these have a positive influence on athletes' motivation were identified. Jowett and colleagues have generated momentum in the study of coach-athlete relationships. Their work is based on the combined social interdependence between the coach and the athlete using a 3+1Cs coach-athlete relationship model (e.g. Jowett & Meek, 2000; Jowett & Cockerill, 2003; Jowett, 2007). This widely cited model emphasises how effective coaching is complementary to athletes' needs, being committed to athletes, being close to them, and being co-orientated (perceptions of mutual trust). Jowett is a co-author of Chapter 6 on coach-athlete relationships.

Coach-athlete relationships have also been viewed from a sociological perspective in which, amongst other things, impression management, 'face', and showing care have been addressed (e.g., Jones, 2006; Jones, 2009). This type of literature does not study the coach-athlete dyad in isolation; it also considers the broader social and situational influences and histories of those interacting. This social lens shows how coaches are often in positions of power and authority and held in high esteem. Social accounts of coaching have often shown that whilst these power imbalances often mean that coaches are well placed to care for athletes, sometimes the power can be used oppressively in a way that harms relationships and wellbeing (Kuhlin et al., 2019).

Parent-Athlete Relationships

This balance in how relations may help or hinder athletes is also evident in parent-child relations in sport. Knight (2019) provides a brief overview of the history of sport parenting research which includes some work that has, like coach-athlete relationships, drawn on SDT to good effect. She describes the direction of the most recent investigations as focusing on one of three areas: the influence of parental involvement in youth sport, factors affecting parental involvement in youth sport, or strategies to promote high-quality parental involvement. Evidence suggests that a successful relationship between all three parties—athlete, parent, and coach—is particularly helpful for athletic development especially when effective interactions are able to reduce stress for children in the sport environment (Harwood & Knight, 2009). Chapter 9 explores the influence of the family, including parents, in more detail. As is evident, the athlete relationship perspectives illustrate how social and psychological views can all contribute to deeper understandings of athletic development.

As we bring the chapter to a close the brief spotlight box that follows conveys that athletic development perspectives from Table 2.1 do not exist on their own. Sport psychologists do not just focus on one perspective, they often draw on multiple perspectives simultaneously to gain a rounded view of possible causes and influences of athletes facing developmental challenges.

Spotlight On: Multiple Perspectives in Action

For this spotlight we examine an example of how a sport psychologist might draw on multiple perspectives, and consider the whole athlete, when working with Jo, an elite fencer, who has disclosed recent poor mental health. This followed Jo learning that funding cuts were going to be made in the national squad, and there was a chance she would be dropped from the programme.

The sport psychologist here might consider the *developmental transition perspective* that would allow them to understand how ineffective coping might lead to a crisis-transition outcome with subclinical symptoms (sadness, anxiety, decrease in self-esteem, etc.). Furthermore, if unresolved, Jo's symptoms might become clinical symptoms requiring long-term treatment (Schinke et al., 2018). Therefore, preventing crisis is important by helping him/her to increase awareness of transition demands.

The *psychosocial skills and resources perspective* would allow the sport psychologist to focus on identifying Jo's transitions and develop his/her necessary attitudes, behaviours, resources, and coping strategies. One avenue might be including consideration of their social support before and during transition plus deliberate reflection and learning from the experience after the episode to prepare for future challenges.

The *talent development environment perspective* would allow Jo and the sport psychologist to consider the environment in which Jo is training and performing. One possible focus might be to investigate the motivational climate in Jo's training group (see Chapter 8) as a possible factor for satisfying his/her basic psychological needs and maintaining their mental health (Schinke et al., 2018).

In summary, sport psychologists do not think unidimensionally about athletic development; with a case like Jo, they usually take a multidimensional view.

CLOSING THOUGHTS

The narrative of how athletic development research has arrived at where we are now is a rich, fascinating arc, often touching on studies of Olympic athletes, talent, their expertise, and the social and environmental influences on them. Who would have thought that initial interest in chess and violin players' quantity and quality of practice would end up transitioning into studies that acknowledge cognitive, developmental, motivational, and ecological psychology theories? There is a reasonable balance in athletic development between an analysis and measurement of the individual, their interactions, their environment, and their sporting career lifespan, including transitions. However, there are still a number of unanswered questions about how these different types of psychological inquiry interact with each other. In your reading of subsequent chapters, it helps to know broadly where the insights and type of investigations you are reading about have come from and fit into the bigger picture.

REFERENCES

Abbott, A., & Collins, D. (2004). Eliminating the dichotomy between theory and practice in talent identification and development: Considering the role of psychology. *Journal of Sports Sciences, 22*(5), 395–408.

Bergeron, M. F., Mountjoy, M., Armstrong, N., Chia, M., Côté, J., Emery, C. A., . . . & Malina, R. M. (2015). International Olympic Committee consensus statement on youth athletic development. *British Journal of Sports Medicine, 49*(13), 843–851.

Bloom, B. S. (1982). The role of gifts and markers in the development of talent. *Exceptional Children, 48*(6), 510–522.

Bruner, M. W., Erickson, K., McFadden, K., & Côté, J. (2009). Tracing the origins of athlete development models in sport: A citation path analysis. *International Review of Sport and Exercise Psychology, 2*(1), 23–37.

Bullock, N., Gulbin, J. P., Martin, D. T., Ross, A., Holland, T., & Marino, F. (2009). Talent identification and deliberate programming in skeleton: Ice novice to Winter Olympian in 14 months. *Journal of Sports Sciences, 27*(4), 397–404.

Chase, W. G., & Simon, H. A. (1973). Perception in chess. *Cognitive Psychology, 4*(1), 55–81.

Collins, D. J., & MacNamara, A. (2017). Making champs and super-champs—Current views, contradictions, and future directions. *Frontiers in Psychology, 8*, 823.

Côté, J. (1999). The influence of the family in the development of talent in sport. *The Sport Psychologist, 13*(4), 395–417.

Côté, J., Baker, J., & Abernethy, A. B. (2003). From play to practice: A developmental framework for the acquisition of expertise in team sports. In J. L. Starkes & K. A. Ericsson (Eds.), *Expert performance in sports: Advances in research on sport expertise* (pp. 89–113). Human Kinetics.

Côté, J., Lidor, R., & Hackfort, D. (2009). ISSP position stand: To sample or to specialize? Seven postulates about youth sport activities that lead to continued participation and elite performance. *International Journal of Sport and Exercise Psychology, 7*(1), 7–17.

Côté, J., Turnidge, J., & Evans, M. B. (2014). The dynamic process of development through sport. *Kinesiologia Slovenica, 20*, 14–26.

Coyle, D. (2009). *The talent code: Unlocking the secret of skill in maths, art, music, sport, and just about everything else.* Random House.

de Garay, A., Levine, L., & Carter, J. E. (1974). *Genetic and anthropological studies of Olympic athletes.* Academic Press.

Ericsson, K. A., Krampe, R. T., & Tesch-Römer, C. (1993). The role of deliberate practice in the acquisition of expert performance. *Psychological Review, 100*(3), 363–406.

Fletcher, D., & Sarkar, M. (2012). A grounded theory of psychological resilience in Olympic champions. *Psychology of Sport and Exercise, 13*, 669–678. https://doi.org/10.1016/j.psychsport.2012.04.007

Gladwell, M. (2008). *Outliers: The story of success.* Little, Brown and Co.

Gorczynski, P., Gibson, K., Thelwell, R., Papathomas, A., Harwood, C., & Kinnafick, F. (2019). The BASES expert statement on mental health literacy in elite sport. *The Sport and Exercise Scientist, 59*, 6–7.

Gould, D., Eklund, R. C., & Jackson, S. A. (1993). Coping strategies used by US Olympic wrestlers. *Research Quarterly for Exercise and Sport, 64*(1), 83–93.

Hall, A. J., Jones, L., & Martindale, R. J. (2019). The Talent Development Environment Questionnaire as a tool to drive excellence in elite sport environments. *International Sport Coaching Journal, 6*(2), 187–198.

Hardy, L., Barlow, M., Evans, L., Rees, T., Woodman, T., & Warr, C. (2017). Great British medallists: Psychosocial biographies of super-elite and elite athletes from Olympic sports. In *Progress in brain research* (Vol. 232, pp. 1–119). Elsevier.

Harwood, C. G., & Knight, C. J. (2009). Stress in youth sport: A developmental investigation of tennis parents, *Psychology of Sport and Exercise, 10*(4), 447–456.

Harwood, C. G., & Knight, C. J. (2015). Parenting in youth sport: A position paper on parenting expertise. *Psychology of Sport and Exercise, 16*, 24–35.

Helsen, W. F., Starkes, J. L., & Hodges, N. J. (1998). Team sports and the theory of deliberate practice. *Journal of Sport and Exercise Psychology, 20*(1), 12–34.

Henriksen, K., Schinke, R., Moesch, K., McCann, S., Parham, W. D., Larsen, C. H., & Terry, P. (2019). Consensus statement on improving the mental health of high performance athletes. *International Journal of Sport and Exercise Psychology, 18*(5), 553–560. https://doi.org/10.1080/1612197X.2019.1570473

Henriksen, K., Stambulova, N., & Roessler, K. K. (2010). Holistic approach to athletic talent development environments: A successful sailing milieu. *Psychology of Sport and Exercise, 11*(3), 212–222.

Hill, A., MacNamara, Á., & Collins, D. (2019). Development and initial validation of the Psychological Characteristics of Developing Excellence Questionnaire version 2 (PCDEQ2). *European Journal of Sport Science, 19*(4), 517–528.

Holt, N. L., Neely, K. C., Slater, L. G., Camiré, M., Côté, J., Fraser-Thomas, J., MacDonald, D., Strachan, L., & Tamminen, K. A. (2017). A grounded theory of positive youth development through sport based on results from a qualitative meta-study. *International Review of Sport and Exercise Psychology, 10*(1), 1–49.

Jones, R. L. (2006). Dilemmas, maintaining "face," and paranoia: An average coaching life. *Qualitative Inquiry, 12*(5), 1012–1021.

Jones, R. L. (2009). Coaching as caring (the smiling gallery): Accessing hidden knowledge. *Physical Education and Sport Pedagogy, 14*(4), 377–390.

Jowett, S. (2007). Interdependence analysis and the 3+1Cs in the coach-athlete relationship. In S. Jowett & D. Lavallee (Eds.), *Social psychology in sport* (pp. 15–27). Human Kinetics.

Jowett, S., & Cockerill, I. M. (2003). Olympic medallists' perspective of the athlete–coach relationship. *Psychology of Sport and Exercise, 4*(4), 313–331.

Jowett, S., & Meek, G. A. (2000). The coach-athlete relationship in married couples: An exploratory content analysis. *The Sport Psychologist, 14*(2), 157–175.

Knight, C. J. (2019). Revealing findings in youth sport parenting research. *Kinesiology Review, 8*(3), 252–259.

Kuhlin, F., Barker-Ruchti, N., & Stewart, C. (2019). Long-term impact of the coach-athlete relationship on development, health, and wellbeing: Stories from a figure skater. *Sports Coaching Review*, 1–23.

Lerner, R. M., Brown, J. D., & Kier, C. (2005). *Adolescence: Development, diversity, context, and application* (Canadian ed.). Pearson.

Lidor, R., Côté, J., & Hackfort, D. (2009). ISSP position stand: To test or not to test? The use of physical skill tests in talent detection and in early phases of sport development. *International Journal of Sport and Exercise Psychology, 7*(2), 131–146.

Lobo, L., Heras-Escribano, M., & Travieso, D. (2018). The history and philosophy of ecological psychology. *Frontiers in Psychology*, *9*, 2228. https://doi.org/10.3389/fpsyg.2018.02228

MacNamara, Á., Button, A., & Collins, D. (2010). The role of psychological characteristics in facilitating the pathway to elite performance part 1: Identifying mental skills and behaviors. *The Sport Psychologist*, *24*(1), 52–73.

Mageau, G. A., & Vallerand, R. J. (2003). The coach–athlete relationship: A motivational model. *Journal of Sports Science*, *21*(11), 883–904.

Martindale, R. J., Collins, D., & Abraham, A. (2007). Effective talent development: The elite coach perspective in UK sport. *Journal of Applied Sport Psychology*, *19*(2), 187–206.

Mathorne, O. W., Henriksen, K., & Stambulova, N. (2020). An "organizational triangle" to coordinate talent development: A case study in Danish swimming. *Case Studies in Sport and Exercise Psychology*, *4*(1), 11–20.

Mero, A., Kauhanen, H., Peltola, E., Vuorimaa, T., & Komi, P. (1990). Physiological performance capacity in different prepubescent athletic groups. *Journal of Sports Medicine and Physical Fitness*, *30*(1), 57–66.

National Research Council and Institute of Medicine. (2002). *Community programs to promote youth development*. National Academy Press.

Oakley, B., & Green, M. (2001). The production of Olympic champions: International perspectives on elite sport development systems. *European Journal for Sports Management*, 83–105.

Orlick, T., & Partington, J. (1988). Mental links to excellence. *The Sport Psychologist*, *2*(2), 105–130.

Rosenberg, E. (1984). Athletic retirement as social death: Concepts and perspectives. In N. Theberge & P. Donnelly (Eds.), *Sport and the sociological imagination* (pp. 245–258). Texas Christian University Press.

Schinke, R. J., Stambulova, N. B., Si, G., & Moore, Z. (2018). International society of sport psychology position stand: Athletes' mental health, performance, and development. *International Journal of Sport and Exercise Psychology*, *16*(6), 622–639.

Smith, R. E., Schutz, R. W., Smoll, F. L., & Ptacek, J. T. (1995). Development and validation of a multidimensional measure of sport-specific psychological skills: The Athletic Coping Skills Inventory-28. *Journal of Sport and Exercise Psychology*, *17*(4), 379–398.

Stambulova, N. B. (1994). Developmental sports career investigations in Russia: A post-perestroika analysis. *The Sport Psychologist*, *8*(3), 221–237.

Stambulova, N. B., Ryba, T., & Henriksen, K. (2020). Career development and transitions of athletes: The international society of sport psychology position stand revisited. *International Journal of Sport and Exercise Psychology*. https://doi.org/10.1080/1612197X.2020.1737836

Syed, M. (2010). *Bounce*. Collins.

United States Department of Health and Human Services. (1999). *Mental health: A report of the surgeon general*. US Department of Health and Human Services, National Institute of Health & National Institute of Mental Health.

Werthner, P., & Orlick, T. (1986). Retirement experiences of successful Olympic athletes. *International Journal of Sport Psychology*, *17*(5), 337–363.

Wylleman, P. (2019). A developmental and holistic perspective on transitioning out of elite sport. In M. H. Anshel, T. A. Petrie, & J. A. Steinfeldt (Eds.), *APA handbook of sport and exercise psychology, Volume 1. Sport psychology* (pp. 201–216). APA handbooks in psychology series. American Psychological Association.

Wylleman, P., & Lavallee, D. (2004). A developmental perspective on transitions faced by athletes. In M. R. Weiss (Ed.), *Developmental sport and exercise psychology: A lifespan perspective* (pp. 503–523). Fitness Information Technology.

Young, B. W., & Salmela, J. H. (2002). Perceptions of training and deliberate practice of middle distance runners. *International Journal of Sport Psychology*, *33*, 167–181.

CHAPTER 3

Transitions on the Athlete Journey

A Holistic Perspective

Robert Morris

> *Throughout my career I have been through so many transitions, when I looked at them they appeared terribly daunting. . . . But it is how you look at them and every one I've experienced I have come out with new skills. . . .*
>
> Alex Danson, former GB women's hockey captain
> (Lingam-Willgoss & Heaney, 2020)

As athletes progress through their sporting career they experience several career transitions, both expected and unexpected, which can impact on their mental wellbeing and athletic development. Such transitions may include, for example, the junior-to-senior transition, transitions to another club or training group, and retirement from sport. This chapter will explore varied transitions faced by athletes and the potential psychological challenges of these. It will discuss theoretical models and empirical research on within-career transitions, with a case study used to contextualise the potential challenges athletes may face and the potential ways to manage the process.

THE CASE OF DAN

To conceptualise the complexity of within-career transitions and illustrate the various factors which may influence the process, here we outline the case of Dan: a rugby player who is going through the transition to senior sport, one of the many transitions athletes may face during their careers (see Case Study 3.1). Dan is also having to manage other facets of his life, meaning that his focus is not purely on his sport transition, creating further challenges.

CASE STUDY 3.1

Dan (Rugby)

Dan is an 18-year-old rugby player who has just signed his first professional contract with a team that competes in the Premiership. The team which he plays for is very supportive of young players moving up from the youth team to first team. Dan has played for several rugby teams in the past and has, in recent times, dedicated approximately 30 hours every week to training to support his development, knowing that if he performs well, the team he is now with will give him an opportunity to stake a claim for a regular first team place.

He has recently moved away from home for the first time, in preparation for training full-time with his team. He has a fear of being away from his parents and siblings who have supported him throughout his youth career. He is also moving away from his friends, many of whom he has grown up with and spent time with doing various hobbies including, for instance, watching rugby, going cycling, and playing in the park. Dan has also had a number of injuries recently and, although he believes he has a very good chance of being a successful player and having a lengthy career, he wants to explore the possibility of carrying on his education at university and exploring potential career options he could have post-retirement.

Dan's case is common—athletes often experience several concurrent and competing transitions, which combine to create a difficult process. Research has started to conceptualise the types of transitions that Dan is experiencing. This literature has identified that there are several transitions in the context of athletes' careers which may influence their development. These transitions have unique characteristics which may need to be considered when implementing support to assist athletes as they go through these processes.

MODELS OF TRANSITION

Transitions can be classified as normative transitions, which are those which are predictable and anticipated (e.g., the junior-to-senior transition; Sharf, 1997) and non-normative transitions, which are those which are unexpected (e.g., a career-ending injury; Wylleman & Lavallee, 2004). As non-normative transitions are difficult to predict, they are not easily depicted in any transition frameworks or models (Wylleman & Lavallee, 2004). There have, however, been several normative career transition models. For example, initial models (e.g., Bloom, 1985; Côté, 1999) have suggested that there are a series of stages that athletes will go through in their athletic careers including initiation, development, mastery, and retirement phases.

The Holistic Athlete Career Model

Wylleman and Lavallee (2004) and Wylleman et al. (2013) expanded upon previous work outlining normative transitions at the athletic level by also considering non-athletic domains. They suggest that athletes may experience different stages of development in five domains: athletic, psychological, psychosocial, academic/vocational, and financial (Wylleman et al., 2013). Their model is shown in Figure 3.1. It highlights the stages of transition with bold vertical rectangles representing the anticipated transitions which may occur throughout athletes' careers. The age ranges represented are guidelines that may not apply to all sports (e.g., gymnasts may enter the mastery stage and retire from sport earlier).

Athletic Level

The athletic level outlined by Wylleman and Lavallee (2004) and Wylleman et al. (2013) suggest that there are four normative transitions athletes go through. The first, the transition into competitive sports (the initiation stage), occurs at the age of approximately 5 or 6. This is where the athlete will be introduced to formal versions of the sport and potentially start to compete in a more organised training and competition environment. Typically athletes transition to the development stage at the age of 12 or 13; this is the phase where athletes engage in an intensive level of training and competition with a specific focus on development for performance gains (e.g., to develop skills to win competitions). At approximately 18 or 19 years old, athletes undergo the junior-to-senior transition. This is where athletes progress into the mastery stage of performance. In this stage, athletes compete at the elite level of sport and dedicate most of their athletic time

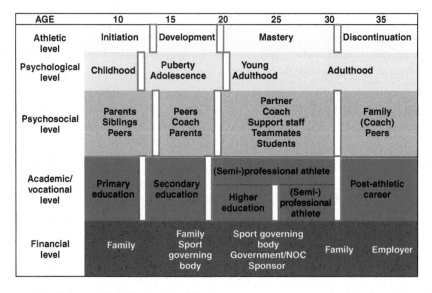

FIGURE 3.1 The Holistic Athlete Career Model representing transitions and stages faced by athletes at athletic, psychological, psychosocial, academic/vocational, and financial levels

Source: Wylleman et al., 2013

to training and competition; it is also during this stage that athletes may experience several other transitions, including changes of coach, relocation, injury, change of weight category, deselection, and change of sport discipline/playing position. The final transition which occurs is the transition from the mastery stage to the discontinuation stage. The discontinuation stage is where athletes terminate training and competing in their sport (discussed in Chapter 4).

Psychological Level

Wylleman and Lavallee (2004) and Wylleman et al. (2013) outline three stages of psychological development athletes will go through with concurrent transitions between them (childhood, adolescence, young adulthood/adulthood). Wylleman and colleagues identify that following a period of time at the childhood level, which is characterised by the degree of their interest in competitive sport and their understanding of their role, responsibility, and relationships within their sport, athletes will transition into a stage of adolescence at approximately 12 years of age. During adolescence, athletes are confronted with several developmental tasks which have to be managed effectively to ensure maturity, including managing and developing new and more mature relationships with peers, developing a masculine or feminine role in society, and attaining emotional independence from parents and others (Wylleman & Lavallee, 2004; Wylleman et al., 2013). Athletes also start to develop an athletic identity at this time. Following this development of self-identity, at the age of approximately 20, athletes will then transition into young adulthood/adulthood. During this transition and within the young adulthood/adulthood stage, athletes will continue to engage in tasks associated with managing and developing more mature relationships and development of self-identity (i.e., establish identities which are determined by the key facets in their lives).

Psychosocial Level

The psychosocial level of Wylleman et al.'s (2013) model outlines the social networks which are important for athletic development relevant to their athletic career stage. By understanding the changes in psychosocial network which occur throughout athletic development, athletes and support practitioners can identify and utilise support more effectively. This level of the model was based on earlier athletic family and marital relationships frameworks (e.g., Hellstedt, 1995; Coppel, 1995) and suggests that, concurrent with the initiation stage of the athletic level, until the age of 13, parents, siblings, and peers are the most influential people in (athletic) development. Following the transition into the development and adolescence stages of the athletic and psychological levels, respectively, peers, coaches, and parents are considered key to athlete development. Between 22 and 29 years old, concurrent with the mastery and young adulthood/adulthood stages of athletic and psychological levels, respectively, relationships with partners and coaches are considered influential. Finally, from the age of 29 (approximately) onwards, relationships with family members and coaches are of primary influence.

In addition to the importance of the changes themselves which occur during the transitions from one stage to the next, another key element of the changing social network is the changing function and role which such support provides. For example, research shows that the quality and content of athletes' relationships with coaches can change during the various athletic stages. Specifically, for instance, Bloom (1985) revealed that during the initiation stage, coaches reward young children for the effort they put in, rather than for the result itself. This positive reinforcement may encourage the children to remain in sport. During the development stage, Bloom (1985) identified that coaches adapt their support and become more focused on emphasising and developing the technical proficiency, discipline, and hard work of the young athletes. In the mastery stage, coaches place greater demands on their athletes in terms of outcomes and results (Bloom, 1985).

Academic/Vocational Level

At the academic/vocational level, the model outlines the transitions into (a) primary school between the ages of 4 and 7, (b) secondary school at the age of 12 or 13, (c) a combined higher education and (semi-)professional sport stage or a (semi-)professional athlete status at age 18 or 19, and (d) post-athletic career at the age of 30. Wylleman and Lavallee (2004) and Wylleman et al. (2013) emphasised that the transition into (semi-)professional sport may occur at an earlier stage for some athletes. Additionally, they emphasise that athletes who have semi-professional status may also have to have additional vocational employment to fund their sport, creating additional pressure to balance competing demands on time.

Financial Level

The final level of the model outlines the sources of financial support throughout and after their careers. Specifically, it outlines the importance of financial support from family in the early stages of athletes' careers, the shift in support from family to sport governing body, national Olympic Committees, private organisations, and/or sponsors at the end of the developmental stage and during (elite) sport careers, back to family support towards the latter end of their sporting career and into early retirement, and finally to employer support post-career. Again, these changes in support occur concurrently to transitions at the athletic, psychological, psychosocial, and academic-vocational levels.

Understanding Dan's Case Using the Holistic Athlete Career Model

The Holistic Athlete Career Model (Wylleman et al., 2013) is useful in helping evaluate the case of Dan. When we consider Dan's situation, we see that he is experiencing transitions at a variety of layers across the model. Specifically, Dan is experiencing the

a) junior-to-senior transition at the athletic level;
b) the transition from adolescence to adulthood at the psychological level;
c) changes in who he receives support from and differences in the type of support provided at the psychosocial level;
d) the possibility of moving to university at the academic/vocational level; and
e) changes in who he receives income from and the amount he receives at the financial level.

The model represents a step towards a holistic approach to athletic development and helps practitioners to provide support in cases like Dan's because it suggests that a broader understanding of athletes' lives is important. Although it is valuable to consider each layer of the model on its own merits (e.g., the challenges within each of five domains), Wylleman et al. (2013) posited that there may be interaction among the different levels in the model. This means that it is possible that more than one transition may occur concurrently across these domains, as is the case with Dan, which could have an adverse effect on overall development.

The term transition has been extensively used to describe many of the changes which occur during an athletic career. However, some argue that the term transition may be inappropriate when considering these constructs. The spotlight box that follows explores this claim.

Spotlight On: Transition or Critical Moments?

Nesti et al. (2012) argue that the term transition could easily be interpreted as signifying something "that is relatively smooth, steady and relatively easy to negotiate" (p. 25). Nesti et al. (2012) suggest that a more appropriate phrase may be "critical moments" (p. 25) as it has connotations of being dramatic in nature, which many of the transitions in the current chapter may be considered as. Critical moments have been described as anxiety-inducing occasions associated with important changes in athletes' identities.

They can be described in positive or negative terms and can be centered on personal, professional, or vocational matters, amongst other elements. Indeed, critical moments can range from being non-events to large, one-off events, and can be planned or unintentional. They may have a negative or positive effect on a person's sense of self (self-awareness and self-knowledge; Nesti et al., 2012). Ultimately a critical moment will, according to Nesti et al. (2012), involve the subjective lived experience of the individual and invoke an emotional response and be dependent on timing (i.e., the individual's personal and contextual circumstances at the time).

EXPLAINING THE PROCESS OF WITHIN-CAREER TRANSITIONS

In addition to predicting when transitions will occur, frameworks have also been proposed as a means of explaining the process which occurs when going through specific transitions. In a review of literature, Drew et al. (2019) identified that most transition research is underpinned by one main model describing and explaining transitions in sport: Stambulova's (2003) athletic career transition model. Other models which underpin transition research have included the model of human adaptation to transition (Schlossberg, 1981); the differentiated model of giftedness and talent 2.0 (Gagné, 2009); job demands-resources model (JD-R; Demerouti et al., 2001); the athletic talent development environment model (ATDE; Henriksen, 2010); the ecological model of human development (Bronfenbrenner, 1979); and the cognitive theory of stress and coping (Folkman & Lazarus, 1980).

One framework, which has been offered as a progression of these theories of transition, is the individual, external, cultural model of the junior-to-senior transition (see Drew et al., 2019). The authors posit that there are a series of transition preconditions and variables that are underpinning features which influence the outcomes that athletes may experience. These features can be found at the:

- individual (e.g., motivation to succeed),
- external (e.g., level of social support available),
- or cultural levels (e.g., values and beliefs emphasised in the environment).

These factors can be either facilitative or debilitative to development. See Figure 3.2, which outlines the framework and the key features therein.

Transition Preconditions

The preconditions outlined in this framework (on the left of Figure 3.1) may influence the subsequent athlete experiences. Athlete identification refers to initial awareness that the athlete may be about to undergo or is capable of undergoing the transition. For example, when considering transitions, such as transitioning to a new training group, a new team, or a new competition (e.g., moving from the European Tour to the Professional Golfers Association Tour), there is the need for initial identification that the athlete has the possibility to be successful. This identification may be self-selection via achieving a pre-requisite level or may be via coach selection. Without identification the subsequent transition experience may not occur or a different transition experience may occur.

Drew et al.'s (2019) proposed environmental pre-conditions also may or may not include support, including financial, social, and material provision. For instance, when considering relocation transitions in sports, such as canoeing, there is the need to have access to appropriate specialised

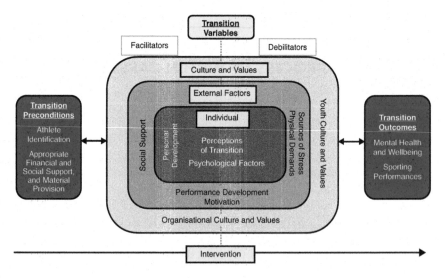

FIGURE 3.2 The individual, external, cultural model of the junior-to-senior transition

Source: Drew et al., 2019

training facilities and equipment (e.g., boats). Broadly, the pre-existing conditions available for a transition may influence, both positively and negatively, the potential success athletes may have when going through this process.

Transition Variables

With the existing preconditions present, athletes' transitions are then influenced by a series of variables shown in a series of central rectangles in Figure 3.1. These variables are at the individual (e.g., motivation to succeed), external (e.g., level of social support available), or cultural levels (e.g., values and beliefs emphasised in the environment) and can be either facilitative or debilitative to development. For example, in Dan's case, at the *individual level*, variables which would facilitate his development include the extent of focus he has on his personal development. The possible dual facilitative or debilitative aspect might include his perceptions of the transition in which, if he has positive yet realistic perspective of what he has to manage, he is more likely to experience a positive transition and outcome (see Drew et al., 2019) and vice versa if he has a negative perspective. If athletes have a perspective of a transition that they believe to be particularly easy or difficult, expectations may not match reality, making the process more challenging (Drew et al., 2019).

At the *external level*, it is suggested that social support is, generally, facilitative of transition; appropriate emotional, financial, and social support can ensure that athletes are able to seek out help where required. Contrastingly, sources of stress, such as demands and expectations from fellow athletes around how successful the team should be and increased physical demands (e.g., training demands), can have a debilitative effect if not managed. Also at the *external level* 'performance development motivation' refers to motivators depending upon athletes' expectations and initial transition experiences. For instance, when first making the transition in Dan's case, if he performs well, performance may become facilitative to transition due to increased confidence. The opposite effect may occur with early poor performance making transition more difficult.

The *culture and values level* refers to the varying influence of youth culture and values and/or organisational culture and values. Youth culture and values refers to the broader youth culture and values present; this may include aspects of development and socialisation (e.g., partying and drinking) which may be debilitative should athletes engage in this type of behaviour during transition. Organisational culture and values refer to the specific organisation within which the athlete trains and competes, and the key culture and values they emit, which may be either facilitative or debilitative. For instance, if there is a change of coach within a team, the specific organisational culture and values which are a prominent part of the environment may change. For the athletes in a team, this change may be facilitative (i.e., their values and beliefs match more closely to the new coach) and result in increased confidence and performance. For other athletes on the team, however, it may be debilitative.

Possible Interventions

Throughout the transition, interventions may have a positive effect on the process (Drew et al., 2019). Interventions which have been proposed as potentially having an influence on transition include: (1) development and utilisation of coping strategies, (2) mentoring/modelling, and (3) education programmes.

Coping strategies are the internal resources which athletes develop and utilise to manage the demands being placed upon them throughout transitions. This could include, for instance, their knowledge and experience of previous transitions based upon what helped them to manage previous transitions and what did not (see Morris et al., 2015). Other coping strategies which may be developed and utilised include emotional regulation, listening to music, problem solving, and problem-focused coping (Morris et al., 2015).

Mentoring/modelling refers to the 'buddying up' of athletes with senior peers or someone who has gone through the transition previously; this can help the athlete as they are able to see modelled the expected behaviours and key skills and knowledge required (Pummell & Lavallee, 2018). Education programmes focused on helping athletes, coaches, teammates, parents, sport science staff, and friends/peers to understand their role and how to cope with the demands of the process can help to increase athletes' readiness and knowledge of the transition (see Drew et al., 2019; Pummell & Lavallee, 2018). Education interventions have focused on mental skills, developing independence and responsibility, and potential performance and lifestyle adjustments (see Drew et al., 2019).

Transition Outcomes

Once the transition is negotiated, there are a number of possible outcomes which fall under *mental health and wellbeing* and *sporting performances* categories on the right side of Figure 3.2 (Drew et al., 2019). In relation to mental health and wellbeing, athletes may experience positive outcomes, including increased levels of health and wellbeing and daily functioning (e.g., happiness). Contrastingly, negative mental health and wellbeing consequences may occur; for some, transitions may result in feelings of being overwhelmed and maladaptive behaviours (e.g., depressed mood). Athletes may also experience feelings which are in between these extremes, where they are still able to function normally in everyday life.

In relation to performance, it is not uncommon for athletes to experience initial performance decreases as a result of transition; this is primarily when athletes are becoming used to their 'new' context or situation and are engaging in a change in demands that are being placed upon them (see Drew et al., 2019). For example, if athletes are changing weight category or their playing position within a team, they may not be familiar with some of the challenges they may experience which may result in them feeling uncertain about their capability to perform well. Thereafter, athletes may continue to experience negative performance outcomes as a result of transition or engage in more adaptive and positive behaviours, resulting in positive performance outcomes.

Understanding Dan's Case Using the Drew et al. (2019) Model

In addition to understanding Dan's case, using Wylleman and Lavallee (2004) and Wylleman et al.'s (2013) work, the individual, external, cultural model of the junior-to-senior transition (Drew et al., 2019) can also be useful in evaluating Dan's experience. The model posits that when going through a transition, there will be several factors which need to be considered (such as the individual, external, and cultural variables), and many types of interventions which may be appropriate. In Dan's case, consideration can be given to aspects of his transition highlighted by the model, like his (a) perceptions of the transition (individual), (b) his motivation to undergo the transition (individual), (c) sources of stress he may be experiencing (individual and external), (d) organisational values and beliefs (cultural), and (e) the interventions which may be most appropriate given these circumstances.

Dan perceives that he has a very good chance of becoming a senior player and is highly motivated to do so, having moved away from home and trained for approximately 30 hours per week to support his development. In addition, he also believes that the organisational values and beliefs (i.e., being supportive of youth development) will mean that he has a good opportunity to be successful in the senior team. There are, however, several sources of stress Dan is experiencing directly associated with his transition, including having a fear of being away from his friends and family as well as the impact of his recent injuries. These sources of stress can be managed using a range of interventions, including coping strategy development, mentoring, and/or education programmes, which can take place before or during transition.

The model used here to assess Dan's case provides a lens through which practitioners and athletes can start to conceptualise areas of strength and weakness in athletes' knowledge and skills which can be cultivated to support their development. In breaking the transition down in this manner, areas of development arguably become clear; specifically, in helping Dan to negotiate his transition, consideration needs to be given to how to help him manage the sources of stress he is experiencing so that they become facilitative rather than debilitative to development. This ability to manage sources of stress could be what ultimately results in a successful or unsuccessful transition.

RESEARCH EXPLORING KEY TRANSITION VARIABLES

Several empirical studies have focused on understanding athletes' transition experiences and the key variables associated with the process. Such work (e.g., Bruner et al., 2008) has highlighted that transitions can be positive and/or negative experiences for athletes, and, similar to what was proposed earlier in the models of transition, embody several competing variables which cross over athletic and non-athletic (e.g., psychosocial, educational) domains. The research has high-lighted several transitional challenges and demands, and the value of social support and internal resources in the process.

Throughout the empirical literature, it is regularly foregrounded that transitions can be a negative and/or challenging event; an event that may question who and what an athlete is and their ability to manage and cope effectively. For some, this can lead to the process being particu-larly demanding, leading them to have feelings of worry, isolation, and ultimately, wellbeing issues which may, in extreme cases, lead to maladaptive coping behaviours including drug and alcohol abuse (e.g., Morris et al., 2015, 2016). Contrastingly, a number of athletes report positive transi-tion experiences, highlighting the progression opportunities that the process offered them which they had not had before (see Pummell et al., 2008).

Challenges and barriers to transition identified in the literature have included higher technical and physical demands, the need to prove their value to new teammates where necessary, the need to build and establish new relationships with new coaches, managing educational demands, a lack of control over transition, and reduced confidence (e.g., Finn & McKenna, 2010). Additionally, athletes may be challenged by physical, philosophical, and/or cultural distance demands which can occur (e.g., Relvas, 2010). For instance, during deselection athletes may experience challenges with answering the question: Who am I? because their identity may no longer be clear to them. This may especially be prevalent in instances where they have spent many years training in pur-suit of sporting success, only to be deselected and told they are no longer of value to the team.

Empirical literature on transitions in sport have identified that there are several resources which athletes use to overcome challenges and barriers they may experience during transition.

These resources include excellent sporting skills (e.g., physical, technical, tactical, and psychosocial skills relevant to the sport; Morris & Deason, 2020); goal-directed attributes (e.g., a professional attitude; Drew et al., 2019); intelligence (e.g., emotional intelligence; Mills et al., 2012); and social competence (Drew et al., 2019).

Social support from family, friends, coaches, and teammates can also be a valuable mechanism for athletes. Specifically, support from these persons can ensure appropriate emotional, technical, and tangible provision is in place throughout any transition (Finn & McKenna, 2010). When support is provided to athletes which is emotional and facilitative to their development, it is more likely to support a positive transition as it may protect athletes from unrealistic expectations from key stakeholders (Jones et al., 2014). Where support is focused on performance outcomes, however, athletes are likely to experience enhanced difficulties during transition (Morris et al., 2015). During an injury transition, for instance, if support is focused on performance outcomes, there may be a lack of support for emotional and physical challenges of this process, with focus instead aimed at returning the athlete to performance level as soon as possible. This may mean that the injury recovery process happens too quickly, leaving the athlete vulnerable to further injuries and distress.

Understanding Dan's Case Using the Research

In addition to understanding Dan's case using transition-related models, the main research exploring key transition variables can also be useful in helping direct required support. One of the common variables identified in the research as being helpful is the social support, in particular from family, friends, coaches, and teammates who can provide appropriate emotional, technical, and tangible support. For Dan, as he has moved away from home, his opportunities to access support from friends and family has been reduced. Consideration, therefore, could be given to ensuring that Dan still receives appropriate support, which may not be forthcoming from the usual sources due to his relocation. This is especially important when transitions can lead to athletes questioning who they are and what they want to be, which can lead to further worry and isolation. Ultimately, if the appropriate support is not in place, or in this instance, there is no replacement for the regular support, Dan may suffer the consequences of worry and isolation (e.g., maladaptive behaviours).

When athletes get deselected, become injured, transition to a new club, or encounter many of the other transitions prevalent in an athletic career, support mechanisms can disappear or become unclear. In the spotlight box here, the question of who is responsible for transition is explored.

Spotlight On: Who's Responsibility Is It?

Consider the example of when athletes are deselected from a programme and may not receive support from the organisation that released them. This often leads to athletes feeling a sense of anger and disappointment towards the organisation, as Brown and Potrac (2009) discuss:

> [Athletes] perceived that there was little meaningful support made available to them once they had been notified of their deselection. Interestingly, the

participants displayed some anger when discussing this topic, as they felt that they had committed themselves to their clubs for a number of years only to be disposed of with little thought or care when they were considered as lacking the ability to progress to professional status. For example, David noted: 'The club didn't do anything really. All they are is talk and talk is cheap. They just want to get you out of the door and they don't want to see your face again. They just want to wash their hands of you. They don't lose any sleep over it. That makes me angry because I have given them everything for the past ten years and it's as though that counts for nothing.' (David) (p. 152).

This scenario can be viewed in two ways. Firstly, it is not uncommon for the academic literature to suggest that organisations should maintain a level of responsibility to support athletes when they deselect them (Brown et al., 2018). The suggestion is that they have used these athletes to better their organisation, but as soon as the athlete becomes disposable, they are let go without another thought and without providing the appropriate support in some cases. They have a moral responsibility to help deselected athletes maintain positive health and wellbeing. Contrastingly, it can be argued that when athletes are deselected, there are in a similar scenario as other members of the public in that when they get released from a job or their contract ends, they are left to manage things on their own with limited or no support. Which leads to the question: why does the responsibility lie with sports organisations to support athletes they deselect when other employers are not levied with the same responsibility?

ACADEMIC PRINCIPLE IN PRACTICE: DAN'S CASE SUMMARY

Throughout this chapter, we have drawn on Dan's case in addition to some key literature which may help reveal solutions for providing the best support for someone in his situation, or in a similar position. If we view his case in the context of the models and empirical literature highlighted, there are several factors which need to be considered when supporting him:

- Firstly, Dan is going through the transition to senior sport. This transition, in and of itself, can challenge athletes. There is the possibility of Dan experiencing increased expectations placed upon him to train and compete at a higher level; there is likely to be increased physical and mental demands placed upon him; he has to create new peer/friendship groups; plus he may have to cope with a reduction in confidence which may occur as a result being unable to negotiate such challenges (see Drew et al., 2019). In addition, Dan has experienced injuries recently, so a consideration of the additional challenges these might pose to his ability to train and compete fully may need to be considered.
- Secondly, Dan is experiencing the addition and adaptation to his broader social support environment, especially as a result of moving away from home. Having moved, Dan now needed to explore where and when he could call upon other social support mechanisms. These new

support mechanisms may include any partner, coaches, support staff, and teammates (see Wylleman & Lavallee, 2004; Wylleman et al., 2013); in Dan's circumstance, none of these relationships are established. Specifically, Dan lives alone, and is working with very new coaches, support staff, and teammates. His interpersonal skills and the approach he takes in developing these relationships will either help or hinder his development.

- Thirdly, Dan is also exploring the possibility of going to university. Specific considerations in this regard include, for instance, helping evaluate if this is the right decision at this stage, exploring what his options are in terms of study time and intensity (part or full time), in addition to course choice and future career aspirations. University may also present its own challenges in terms of youth culture and environment which may influence Dan's experience, specifically to what degree he nurtures relationships with university peers and has a social life (see Drew et al., 2019).

- Finally, each of the previous points also needs to be considered holistically. Although each individual element of Dan's life has its own challenges, as can be seen in both the literature (e.g., Wylleman & Lavallee, 2004; Wylleman et al., 2013) and in the current case, many of these elements can and do occur concurrently. Decisions made in one facet of Dan's life may influence others; for instance, if he chooses to go to university and have a social life there, he may be distracted from his sport and establishing himself in the squad. Dan may also be trying to develop a new social support group at the same time as both transitioning to senior sport and starting university. Although in some respects this may be facilitative to development (i.e., there are more people from which to gain support), it could have a hindering effect as there is less time to spend with each person to establish appropriate rapport.

In light of this summary, the three interventions outlined earlier—(1) development and utilisation of coping strategies, (2) mentoring/modelling, and (3) education programmes—may be appropriate in helping Dan with his transition. For him, enhancing coping strategies may include the development of key mental skills required to cope with the transition to senior sport and the demands this may present in terms of expected outcomes (e.g., resilience, motivation, anxiety control). Coping strategies also include his interpersonal skills to help him develop relationships with his new peers, coaches, and support staff. He will also require key problem-solving skills to help him determine if, when, and what his approach should be to entering higher education.

In relation to mentoring/modelling, a formal relationship with a senior peer may help Dan in several ways. Specifically, being mentored by a senior peer may mean that Dan has an avenue for developing important peer relationships with the rest of the squad and coaching and support staff and may also mean that Dan is able to get a sense from peers as to the expected behaviours in senior sport. If Dan is mentored by a senior who has previously been to university and/or moved away from home, he may also be able to explore his own current circumstances and compare and learn from his colleague's experiences. Doing so could mean Dan has greater self-awareness of some of the potential benefits and pitfalls of his situation.

Finally, an education programme which outlines to Dan the key challenges he may be about to experience, potential solutions to those challenges, and explores with him personalised solutions given his context may also be helpful. For example, by exploring and explaining to Dan the common features of the junior-to-senior transition and the challenges it may present, he may become more aware of what to expect, less nervous about the process, and, therefore, cope better when such instances do occur. Additionally, education on key strategies he may be able to utilise during transition, from which he can then choose and develop as necessary, can also help him to overcome transition difficulties.

Dan's case is not an uncommon one; athletes in transition often experience the process in a broader context which also needs to be considered. For others, the challenges and considerations may be different. Regardless, it is important these elements are examined so that the best individual solutions are available for all transitioning athletes.

CLOSING THOUGHTS

As athletes progress through their sporting career they experience several career transitions, both expected and unexpected, which can impact on their mental wellbeing and athletic development. This chapter has explored various transitions faced by athletes and the potential psychological challenges of these. It has covered theoretical models, transition into sport, and within-career transitions (e.g., changing teams) and considered strategies to ensure athletes have positive transitional experiences. In doing so, this chapter has highlighted some of the key considerations and challenges which may pose difficulties for athletes who are in transition, and some areas which need to be the key focus of intervention. Additionally, Dan's case uncovers the challenges which can be apparent when working with athletes during transition. In general, cases like Dan illustrate how difficult it can be to research this area since each athlete's experience is context- and biography-specific, meaning generalisability may not always be possible. Instead, transferring and extrapolating from case studies, as in this instance, may be more appropriate in determining how best to support athletes in transition.

REFERENCES

Bloom, B. S. (1985). *Developing talent in young people*. Ballantine Books.

Bronfenbrenner, U. (1979). *The ecology of human development: Experiments by nature and design*. Harvard University Press.

Brown, C. J., Webb, T. L., Robinson, M. A., & Cotgreave, R. (2018). Athletes' experiences of social support in their transition out of elite sport: An interpretive phenomological analysis. *Psychology of Sport and Exercise*, *36*, 71–80. http://doi.org/10.1016/j.psychsport.2018.01.003

Brown, G., & Potrac, P. (2009). You've not made the grade son: Deselection and identity disruption in elite level youth football. *Soccer and Society*, *10*, 143–159. https://doi.org/10.1080/14660970802601613

Bruner, M. W., Munroe-Chandler, K. J., & Spink, K. S. (2008). Entry into elite sport: A preliminary investigation into the transition experiences of rookie athletes. *Journal of Applied Sport Psychology*, *20*, 236–252. https://doi.org/10.1080/10413200701867745

Coppel, D. B. (1995). Relationship issues in sport: A marital therapy model. In S. M. Murphy (Ed.), *Sport psychology interventions* (pp. 193–204). Human Kinetics.

Côté, J. (1999). The influence of the family in the development of talent in sport. *The Sport Psychologist*, *13*, 395–417. https://doi.org/10.1123/tsp.13.4.395

Demerouti, E., Bakker, A. B., Nachreiner, F., & Schaufeli, W. B. (2001). The job demands–resources model of burnout. *Journal of Applied Psychology*, *86*(3), 499–512. https://doi.org/10.1037//0021-9010.86.3.499

Drew, K., Morris, R., Tod, D., & Eubank, M. (2019). A meta-study of qualitative research on the junior-to-senior transition in sport. *Psychology of Sport and Exercise, 45*. https://doi.org/10.1016/j.psychsport.2019.101556

Finn, J., & McKenna, J. (2010). Coping with academy-to-first-team transitions in elite English male team sports: The coaches' perspective. *International Journal of Sports Science and Coaching, 5*(2), 257–279. https://doi.org/10.1260%2F1747-9541.5.2.257

Folkman, S., & Lazarus, R. S. (1980). An analysis of coping in a middle-aged community sample. *Journal of Health and Social Behavior, 21*(3), 219–239. https://doi.org/10.2307/2136617

Gagné, M. (2009). A model of knowledge-sharing motivation. *Human Resource Management, 48*(4), 571–589. https://doi.org/10.1002/hrm.20299

Hellstedt, J. C. (1995). Invisible players: A family systems model. In S. M. Murphy (Ed.), *Sport psychology interventions* (pp. 117–146). Human Kinetics.

Henriksen, K. (2010). *The ecology of talent development in sport* [Unpublished doctoral dissertation]. University of Southern Denmark.

Jones, R., Mahoney, J., & Gucciardi, D. (2014). On the transition into Elite Rugby League. *Sport, Exercise, and Performance Psychology, 3*(1), 28–45. https://doi.org/10.1016/S0140-6736(13)61957-1

Lingam-Willgoss, C., & Heaney, C. (2020). The athlete's journey: Transitions through sport. *OpenLearn*. www.open.edu/openlearn/health-sports-psychology/the-athletes-journey-transitions-through-sport/content-section-overview?active-tab=description-tab

Mills, A., Butt, J., Maynard, I., & Harwood, C. G. (2012). Identifying factors perceived to influence the development of elite youth football academy players. *Journal of Sports Sciences, 30*(15), 1593–1604. https://doi.org/10.1080/02640414.2012.710753

Morris, R., & Deason, E. (2020). The transition from elite youth to elite adult professional soccer: A summary of current literature and practical applications. In J. Dixon, J. Barker, R. Thelwell & I. Mitchell (Eds.), *The psychology of soccer: More than just a game* (pp. 3–18). Routledge.

Morris, R., Tod, D., & Oliver, E. (2015). An analysis of organizational structure and transition outcomes in the youth-to-senior professional soccer transition. *Journal of Applied Sport Psychology, 27*(2), 216–234. https://doi.org/10.1080/10413200.2014.980015

Morris, R., Tod, D., & Oliver, E. (2016). An investigation into stakeholders' perceptions of the youth-to-senior transition in sport. *Journal of Applied Sport Psychology, 28*(4), 375–391. https://doi.org/10.1080/10413200.2016.1162222

Nesti, M. S., Littlewood, M. A., O'Halloran, L., Eubank, M., & Richardson, D. J. (2012). Critical moments in elite premiership football: Who do you think you are? *Physical Culture and Sport Studies and Research, 1*, 23–31. https://doi.org/10.2478/v10141-012-0027-y

Pummell, B., Harwood, C., & Lavallee, D. (2008). Jumping to the next level: Examining the within-career transition of the adolescent event rider. *Psychology of Sport and Exercise, 9*, 427–447. https://doi.org/10.1016/j.psychsport.2007.07.004

Pummell, E. K., & Lavallee, D. (2018). Preparing UK tennis academy players for the junior-to-senior transition: Development, implementation, and evaluation of an intervention program. *Psychology of Sport and Exercise, 40*, 156–164. https://doi.org/10.1016/j.psychsport.2018.07.007

Relvas, H. (2010). *A qualitative exploration of the transition from youth to professional football across Europe: A critique of structures, support mechanisms and practitioner roles* [Unpublished doctoral dissertation]. Liverpool John Moores University.

Schlossberg, N. K. (1981). A model for analyzing human adaptation to transition. *The Counseling Psychologist, 9*, 2–18. https://doi.org/10.1177%2F001100008100900202

Sharf, R. S. (1997). *Applying career development theory to counseling.* Brooks/Cole Publications.

Stambulova, N. B. (2003). Symptoms of a crisis-transition: A grounded theory study. In N. Hassmen (Ed.), *Svensk Idrottspykologisk Förening* (pp. 97–109). Örebro University Press.

Wylleman, P., & Lavallee, D. (2004). A developmental perspective on transitions faced by athletes. In M. Weiss (Ed.), *Developmental sport and exercise psychology: A lifespan perspective* (pp. 503–524). Fitness Information Technology.

Wylleman, P., Reints, A., & De Knop, P. (2013). A developmental and holistic perspective on athletic career development. In P. Sotiriadou & V. De Bosscher, (Eds.), *Managing high performance sport* (pp. 191–214). Routledge.

CHAPTER 4

Retirement From Sport
The Final Transition

Candice Lingam-Willgoss

You have already been introduced to the term 'transition' and explored the range of transitional experiences that athletes may encounter during their career. Now it is time to turn your attention to the final stage in the athlete's journey, retirement from sport. Elite athletes experience retirement much earlier than any other career (Knights et al., 2019), and as professionals working in sport settings it is important that we understand the wide range of emotions that can be experienced and may characterise this period of time in an athlete's life. For some the experience is positive and navigated successfully but for others it can present more of a challenge, eliciting emotions such as depression, loneliness, and low self-esteem (Wylleman, 2019). Just knowing when it is the right time to retire can be a difficult decision and in some cases a decision that the athlete feels they have little control over. For example, Olympic Gold Medallist Nicola Adams retired from boxing due to the fear of adversely affecting her eyesight if she received any more severe impact to the eye area.

In retirement, athletes have to adjust to several psychological, social, and vocational changes as they confront a life outside of the sporting environment. This has required research to take a more holistic perspective on retirement by viewing it in the context of a broader process rather than a stand-alone event (Wylleman, 2019). As you move through this chapter you will examine retirement from several theoretical perspectives, explore some of the most common reasons for retirement as well as look at what factors can facilitate a more positive transition out of sport. Before then, read Case Study 4.1 where you are introduced to Mila, a retired tennis player.

CASE STUDY 4.1

Mila (Former Tennis Player)

Mila was a professional tennis player with a successful career and was one of the top 100 players in the world. Her tennis career involved a highly demanding schedule of training, competition, and travel. At the age of 30, she had not yet achieved her goal of being one of the top 20 players in the world. She was also starting to feel constantly tired and less motivated to train and compete. Mila carried on with competition for another year, but her drive to continue training faltered and she dropped further down in the rankings. She had also been discussing with her husband the prospect of starting a family, which had not been possible with her training and competition schedule. At 31 years old, she decided it was time to retire from the sport to focus on starting a family and possibly a new career. However, she had not made any definitive plans for her retirement from the sport.

When Mila did retire, she thought it would be a relief from the pressure of her schedule, giving her time to do many other things. Instead, she felt like she had failed and had lost the identity she had for many years as a tennis professional. She also became distant from the many tennis friends with whom she had spent a considerable part of her life on the competitive tour circuit. She had no career to fill her time and had not been immediately successful with becoming pregnant. She was feeling bored, depressed, and anxious about where her life was going. Her husband and family were very supportive and encouraged her to see a psychologist. This helped her to focus on the positive aspects of her tennis career and to make plans for her new life. She started to regularly exercise doing activities she enjoyed and decided to help with youth coaching at a local tennis club. Mila also had a strong interest in physiotherapy, having experienced injury and rehabilitation during her tennis career. She decided to achieve her tennis coaching qualifications and study to become a physiotherapist which provided her a new focus.

What the case study illustrates is how retirement from sport isn't a straightforward process and often, as in Mila's case, no one single factor leads an athlete to decide to retire. A combination of factors including age, decreased performance, and loss of motivation in addition to just feeling like it was time to retire contributed to Mila's decision to step away from tennis. We will be relating to Mila and her experiences throughout the chapter, but first we look at some key theoretical perspectives that are often referred to when exploring retirement from sport.

THEORETICAL PERSPECTIVES ON RETIREMENT FROM SPORT

Many researchers have attempted to conceptualise the process of transition, specifically retirement from sport, resulting in the development of several models and theories which fall into four broad categories (Lavallee et al., 2015):

1. models of death and dying (thanatological);
2. models of ageing (social gerontological);
3. models of human adaptation to transition;
4. conceptual models of career transitions in sport.

Developing an insight into these different theoretical approaches will help you develop your academic understanding of this area and facilitate a deeper appreciation of the complexities of athlete transition.

Thanatology

Thanatological models suggest that retirement from sport bears similarities to death and dying, and is a form of loss or social death (Rosenberg, 1984). Social death refers to the concept of being treated as if you were dead, something particularly salient for athletes who often experience a loss of identity and feelings of isolation following retirement (Brewer, 1993). This is also linked to social awareness concepts that were originally developed through research with terminally ill patients but have some application when looking at retirement from sport. Glaser and Strauss (1965) identified four varied levels of awareness related to this that can be applied to the athletic experience:

1. closed awareness, where the athlete is unaware of imminent retirement;
2. suspected awareness, where the athlete suspects something due to subtle changes;
3. mutual pretence, where all those around an athlete know retirement is imminent, but no one acknowledges it;
4. open awareness, where all involved acknowledge retirement is near.

We can suggest based on existing evidence that those athletes who have an open awareness are more likely to have a more positive transition out of sport, potentially due to both planning and free choice, two concepts we look at later in the chapter.

Perhaps the best known thanatological theory is Kübler-Ross' (1969) stages of death/grief model which has frequently been used to explain how athletes process negative change events, such as injury or retirement. This theory suggests that while mourning the end of their career, the athletes will drift in and out of these emotional stages: denial, anger, bargaining, depression, acceptance, and reorganisation (Kübler-Ross, 1969). For example, in the case study on Mila, her low mood resonates with some of these stages. However, like some of the other models discussed, this theory is based on the assumption that retirement always demands serious adjustment that will have negative implications. While anecdotally there is some support for this theory there is still little academic support evident for this explanation, with researchers suggesting that while athletes may exhibit some of these emotions they are unlikely to be in such a rigid order (e.g., Udry et al., 1997).

Social Gerontology

Where theories of thanatology relate experiences to social death, social gerontological models focus on the study of the ageing process with a prime focus on the way that society and older people interact. In the context of retirement from sport five theories have been identified as most relevant. These are illustrated in Figure 4.1.

Broadly, models and theories within social gerontology address the way in which the athlete adapts to the social reorganisation faced at the retirement stage. Burgess' (1960) activity or substitution theory posits that roles that are lost are replaced or substituted by others that allow activity levels to remain and continue. In a similar way, continuity theory (Atchley, 1976) suggests that it is about shifting or re-directing focus to another interest. Specifically in the context of sport, it suggests that athletes who see their athletic role as more important than any other will find retirement more of a challenge than those who have a more balanced perspective and are able to shift their athletic focus to other interests (Lavallee, 2007). There is an element in each of these theories that

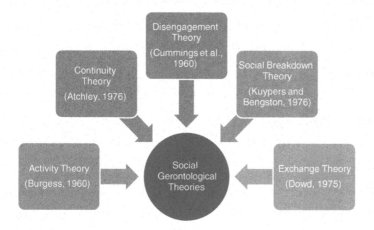

FIGURE 4.1 Social gerontological theories

relates to the way Mila eventually substitutes her role as an athlete with regular exercising and coaching. Disengagement theory offers a contrast: it is a more structured and functional theory suggesting that the process of withdrawal due to age is a mutually beneficial and positive experience for both individual and culture (Cummings et al., 1960 as cited in Lavallee, 2007).

While these theories may have some applications to sport they are still somewhat limited (Gordon & Lavallee, 2011). Later theories, such as the social breakdown theory (Kuypers & Bengtson, 1973), suggest that the loss of a role can carry with it a change in identity due to a shift in external labelling which, if not positive, can lead to the individual withdrawing from society. This has close links to the concept of athletic identity, including Mila's experience, being a strong predictor of whether retirement from sport is positive or negative (Martin et al., 2014). In contrast to this, Dowd's (1975) exchange theory views this process in a more positive light and has strong links to activity theory (Burgess, 1960), suggesting that through rearrangement and reordering successful transition is achieved. This theory when linked to sport emphasises the importance of preparation and retirement planning which can allow for reorganisation to be in place before the athlete leaves their sport. Notice how this relates to Mila's go-with-the-flow approach which resulted in a negative initial transition.

Transition Models

The somewhat negative lens with which gerontology and thanatology view transition is unsurprising, as both tend to view retirement in isolation rather than as the final stage in a more holistic process. Wholly more positive in nature are the types of transition models, which you covered in depth in Chapter 3, which see the final stage of the athlete's career—retirement—as a *process* not a single event. For example, Schlossberg's (1981) transition model of human adaption to transition identifies three interacting factors that influence the transition experience: 1) characteristics of the individual, 2) perception of transition, and 3) characteristics of the pre-transition and post-transition environments. This theory illustrates the phenomenological (i.e., personal lived experience) nature of retirement as it is as much about the individual variables that influence transition as it is about the transition itself.

Conceptual Models

Conceptual models of career transition in sport are generally viewed as far more helpful to our understanding of transition and retirement from sport (Lavallee et al., 2015). These models are more comprehensive and sport specific, such as Taylor and Ogilvie's (1994) model of adaptation to career transition. This model allows reflection on the entire retirement process including causes, factors influencing adaptation, coping resources, and quality of adjustment and interventions, as illustrated in Figure 4.2.

The strength of this model in contrast to those discussed earlier is largely due to its sport-specific focus and integration of earlier theory and contemporary research (Lavallee et al., 2015). Throughout this chapter we will explore some of the factors illustrated by Taylor and Ogilvie's model (1994) in more detail, starting with causes of career termination (retirement) which are listed at the top of Figure 4.2.

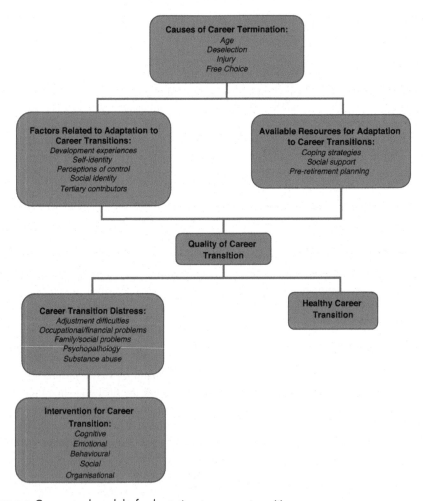

FIGURE 4.2 Conceptual model of adaptation to career transition

Source: Taylor & Ogilvie, 1994, cited in Lavallee et al., 2015

CAUSES OF RETIREMENT

In order to fully understand the psychological impact of retirement it is important to appreciate why athletes retire. This combined with an understanding of the context of their retirement experience underpins the longer-term impact on the athlete. As Figure 4.2 illustrates, there are four factors that are most commonly cited as causes of retirement: age, deselection, injury, and free choice.

Age

One of the most common causes of retirement can be linked to age due to the decline in performance that characterises the ageing process. This may also signify a time when other factors start to become a priority such as parenthood (as evident with Mila).

Deselection

A product of the potential decline in performance that comes with age can lead to an athlete no longer being able to achieve the training and performance demands of their sport, leading to deselection. This was touched on in Box 4.1; while Mila didn't face deselection in the technical sense, she did start to drop her ranking position reflecting her performance decline and inability to compete at her previous level.

Injury

Perhaps the most common transition experienced by an athlete during their career is that of injury. This transition typically carries with it a number of negative psychological responses (e.g., Ivarsson et al., 2017). Samuel and Tenenbaum (2011) reported that for high-level athletes, injury was the most frequently experienced non-normative transition and a very common cause of career termination and abrupt retirement (Park et al., 2013). The unplanned nature of injury means that when it results in retirement it can cause significant adjustment difficulties leaving athletes vulnerable to feelings of isolation, anxiety, and depression as well as many other negative responses (Walker & Heaney, 2013).

Free Choice

For some athletes the decision to retire from sport is a planned and very deliberate (free) choice with research suggesting that, from a psychological perspective, this results in a much smoother transition as athletes are more likely to have a clear retirement plan in place (Young et al., 2006). This links closely to a later section in the chapter dedicated to planning and preparation which are both key to ensuring a positive transition out of sport (Knights et al., 2019). Free choice can relate to several factors; for example, our case study athlete, Mila, realised she was not going to be able to achieve her goal of making the top 20 and was ready to focus on other aspects of her life. There are also several other factors linked to free choice that can influence why an athlete decides to retire some of which are illustrated in Figure 4.3.

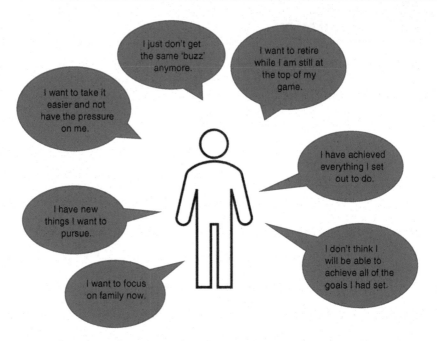

FIGURE 4.3 Other causes of retirement from sport

Source: Lingam-Willgoss & Heaney, 2020

Retirement Causes: Summary

Regardless of the reason for retirement for each athlete this transition will result in very different psychological, social, and physical implications. For example, where deselection may result in an athlete feeling forced to retire with a lack of control over their future and feelings of distress, free choice may mean retirement is more planned and controlled. These differences have led to retirement experiences being categorised more broadly as chosen or enforced with research frequently citing that the best time to retire is when the athlete feels ready (i.e., 'free choice'; Ryan, 2019). However, for many athletes the decision is taken away from them when the retirement comes completely unexpectedly (e.g., serious injury) resulting in a perceived lack of control and, as such, psychological distress is much more common for athletes in this situation (Park et al., 2013).

CONTRIBUTARY FACTORS TO ADAPTATION TO RETIREMENT

While the potential psychological impact of retirement can depend on whether it is chosen or enforced, the literature identifies several factors that can influence the way an athlete responds which we look at in this next section:

- athletic identity;
- perception of control;
- level of competition; and
- the type of sport.

Athletic Identity

Athletic identity has been defined "as the degree to which an individual identifies with the athlete role and is a much more conscious aspect of self-concept" (Brewer et al., 1993, p. 237). This represents a pivotal concept when exploring retirement as well as transitions more broadly. While a high level of athletic identity can be positive, it can also be a key factor in determining the degree of difficulty experienced when adjusting to retirement and is often cited as the strongest predictor of the quality of retirement at any competitive level. Having a strong athletic identity might limit an individual from possessing a multi-dimensional self-concept and, as such, they will see themselves almost exclusively as an athlete. An exclusive athletic identity can predispose athletes to being more vulnerable to adjustment difficulties such as heightened levels of stress and anxiety (Martin et al., 2014). This was partly reflected in Mila's post-retirement feelings. Giannone et al. (2017) explored similar situations with 72 varsity-level athletes and concluded that higher athletic identity was a potential risk factor for developing certain psychiatric symptoms such as depression and anxiety.

In contrast, athletes who develop a more multi-dimensional identity are better equipped in retirement as they have other 'roles' so leaving their sport is navigated in a more balanced way. Lally's (2007) research examined multi-dimensional identity with findings suggesting that athletes who had already redefined themselves prior to retirement have protected themselves from a major identity crisis. This redefining of self relates closely to several of the social gerontology theories discussed earlier in this chapter. Having something else to focus on and a wide range of interests makes successful transition more likely (Burgess, 1960; Dowd, 1975) as we eventually saw in Mila's case.

Perception of Control

The culture of competitive sport is one that encourages athletes to work with controllable variables and, where possible, be in control of nearly all aspects of their life—for example, their training schedule. Retirement from sport is no different and the degree of perceived control that an athlete has over their decision to leave sport can determine how they respond to their retirement (Park et al., 2013). Closely linked to the earlier notion of chosen retirement, research suggests that athletes who feel in control of their transition out of sport have much more successful adjustment to post-athletic life (Stambulova, 2016), while athletes who feel out of control can display a range of pathologies such as anxiety, depression, and substance abuse (Lavallee et al., 2015). For example, if you refer back to Mila: she made the decision to retire from tennis based on several factors and felt in control of her decision. Arguably, she initially perceived being out of control in terms of her new life.

The Type of Sport

While research looking at the differences in retirement experiences across multiple sports is still limited (Knights et al., 2016), findings do suggest that differences are evident; for example, team versus individual sports, the sport's level of popularity, and salaries (if any) can all impact how athletes navigate retirement. One of the reasons for this may be the way that athletes, even in retirement, can feel governed by the same social norms that they learnt in their sport. For example, research looking at this situation within the world of gymnastics has found that retired gymnasts hold on to winning and being perfect as values in their lives after sport (Cavallerio et al., 2017). Gymnastics is also a good example of an early specialisation sport which can see particularly unequal power in coach/athlete relationships, where albeit often inadvertently, coaches seek to diminish potential distractions by encouraging a sole focus on gymnastics. This can result in a lack of time and opportunity to develop alternative identities as an adolescent and may make transitioning out of sport more challenging. This is echoed by the work of Clowes et al. (2015) who concluded that gymnasts represent a vulnerable group in terms of their susceptibility to negative transitional experiences especially during retirement.

Experiences of the transition into retirement can also be very different in late specialisation sports. Lagimodiere and Strachan's (2015) research into male hockey and rugby players noted that despite both being team sports, the social support networks for both pre- and post-retirement were varied. This research went on to illustrate how those involved in more popular team sports (i.e., football compared to handball) may experience more adjustment struggles stemming from a combination of their higher level of athletic identity, a stronger connection to community, and loss of public esteem and support.

Level of Participation

A final factor that can have a bearing on the quality of the retirement experience relates to the level at which the athlete competes. Research suggests that athletes who compete at the elite level not only have a stronger commitment towards training and higher levels of athletic identity (Park et al., 2013) but also have more career events—for example, moving to a higher level, major accomplishments, injury, deselection, and changes in public perception—that can disrupt their athletic engagement and adjustment and require personal change (Samuel & Tenenbaum, 2011). This research also recognised how, due to other implications related to finance, position, and status, elite athletes also considered change events as much more significant which requires special consideration. It is also important to recognise that amateur athletes have their own unique challenges, in part due to juggling multiple roles and identities as sport is not their full-time job. This is something focused on by MacCosham et al. (2015) who looked at the experiences of amateur athletes in competitive sport and claimed that athletes at this level reported a sub-optimal leisure lifestyle, meaning that they were unsuccessful in balancing casual leisure with serious leisure. The challenge at lower levels is that the athlete is often juggling work, as well as their sport, and as such it consumes all of their free time, leading to the development of a very uni-dimensional structure to their lives and identity.

HELPING ATHLETES COPE: RESOURCES AND SUPPORT

The process of transitions in sport require athletes to 'cope' with changes, whether those events are positive or negative, planned or unplanned. Where planned transitions are less likely to result in negative or challenging situations some, such as injury, can see the athlete facing what Stambulova (2000) terms a 'crisis situation'. In these crisis situations, one can see that athletes adopt different coping strategies: avoidance (potentially withdrawing from activity), acceptance (adapting and compromising to stay in situation), or fighting (changing attitude and situation).

What become clear from the evidence is that, regardless of the strategy adopted, there are some key factors that play a fundamental role in the way the athlete will cope. Four of these strategies are included in Figure 4.4 which illustrates the underpinning factors integral to a positive transition from professional sport.

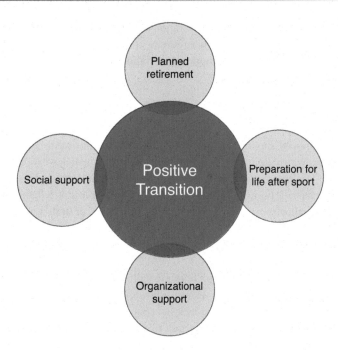

FIGURE 4.4 The positive transition model from professional sport

Source: Knights et al., 2019

We look at these factors in more detail in the next sections.

Planning and Preparation for Life After Sport

The importance of preparation and planning for a life after sport is frequently cited as fundamental to ensuring a positive transition out of sport. The significance of this type of forward planning complements the holistic approach now taken to retirement seeing it as an inevitable stage of a wider process that makes up the athlete's journey (Wylleman, 2019). In the context of elite sport it is now quite common for high-level athletes to engage with 'athlete lifestyle' or 'performance lifestyle' professional support programmes. These programmes provide structured and formal support that helps prepare athletes for career transitions by encouraging the development of a broader, more diverse perception of identity early on in their career which can result in a much more positive transition out of elite sport (e.g., Torregrosa et al., 2015; Cosh et al., 2015). Furthermore, any form of retirement planning is something that managers, coaches, agents, sponsors, and family should all be involved in, working with athletes to identify potential roles outside of sport that capitalise on their strengths and interests (Martin et al., 2014). Retirement planning can also facilitate a negative to positive shift in perception which has been found to be a key resource for a positive transition (Kuettel et al., 2017). For example, this approach can enable athletes to see positives such as increases in free time, decreased injury risk, and removal of competitive stress (Martin et al., 2014). Furthermore, research suggests that when key interventions are applied throughout the early retirement stages they can be of additional benefit to the athlete's wellbeing if the athlete has had suitable preparation and displays readiness (Park et al., 2013). In Mila's experience, she struggled early in her retirement due to a lack of a clear plan and focus, but once she had received some formal support from family and a psychologist her transition was much smoother.

Social and Organisational Support

The importance of social support within the athlete network has received extensive research attention due to the overwhelming positive impact it has been found to have on athletes, especially during retirement (Wylleman et al., 2013). An athlete who is well supported is much more likely to adapt and experience a positive retirement from sport regardless of whether that support is structured and within their sport (e.g., coach or sport psychologist) or unstructured and from their wider network outside sport (e.g., family and friends). However, studies into social support still suggest that there is a stigma attached to asking for 'help', due to cultural norms related to physical and mental toughness that underpin sporting excellence (Tibbert et al,. 2015). Even in retirement it seems that these qualities of being tough both mentally and physically remain a salient part of the individual's identity and feel at odds with the elite athlete identity they have developed. This perhaps explains why athletes will tend to seek out support from those within their sport rather than from those outside. However, it is important to note that by developing wider social circles outside of sport, a more varied identity can develop and transition can be navigated in a much more positive way resulting in a healthier adjustment to their new life (Brown et al., 2018). For example, those athletes who have already started to focus on new careers that will form the basis of their retirement are likely to have started to develop a new social network in these domains. For example, hockey Olympic Gold Medallists Helen Richardson-Walsh and Alex Danson both studied for degrees during their careers so they had something else on which to focus. Brown et al. (2018) also concluded that the people who provided the support could have an impact on the quality of the transition experience: if the athlete feels genuinely cared for and understood, the experience tended to be much more positive.

The personnel who provide support was studied by Lagimodiere and Strachan (2015). They identified some different outcomes in support between the immediate team personnel (e.g., coaches, team colleagues) and other more detached members of the sports organisation. The latter was deemed more positive. In high-performance sport organisations around the world there is also similar variety in experiences as dos Santos et al.'s (2016) investigation illustrates. Their study with 379 Brazilian Olympic athletes reported that 74.1% of those sampled felt that there was still a lack of information available about retirement and a further 59% had concerns about what would happen after retirement.

Other Strategies

You were introduced to a range of strategies that can help athletes navigate career transitions in Chapter 3 (development and utilisation of coping strategies, mentoring/modelling, and education programmes), and these can also benefit athletes during retirement. Other strategies that can facilitate a positive transition out of sport include counselling, cognitive restructuring (e.g., replacing negative thoughts with positive ones), stress management techniques, and projective techniques (e.g., where the individual projects their thoughts/feelings onto an imaginary person or situation; Wylleman et al., 2004). The challenge with some of these approaches is that they can require more formal support from an accredited sport psychologist and may take time to implement effectively. As was the case for Mila.

You may recognise that a key theme when examining retirement is athletes surrounding themselves with the right people, whether this is for emotional support (family members) or more professional advice (performance lifestyle consultants/sport psychologists). This reflects how, within elite sport, there are potentially extensive support networks around the athlete, and this network in some cases may also have to adapt and adjust to a change when an athlete retires (e.g., parents of young athletes). As we near the end of this chapter we switch focus to exploration of the perspectives of those who make up the support network around the athlete. In the spotlight box that follows, there is a summary of a research paper that has analysed the impact that retirement can have on parents and partners.

Spotlight On: Parents' and Partners' Experiences of Athlete Retirement

A qualitative study by Brown et al. (2019) investigated the experiences of seven athletes' parents and partners during the process of transition out of elite sport. The aim of the study was to understand how parents and partners managed their role during the transition process.

Purposive sampling was used to select parents and partners of former elite athletes. The participants were required to have experienced all, or a significant part of, the former athletes' careers in elite sport and their transition into retirement. Four long-term partners (one male and three females) and three parents (one male and two females) were included in the study. The former athletes had competed in individual summer Olympic sports at an international level for 5 to 15 years (mean = 12.50, SD = 3.88). At the time of the study, the former athletes had been retired for a relatively long period of time, between 3 and 12 years (mean = 6.42, SD = 3.90). Semi-structured interviews were used and the data from the interview transcripts were analysed according to the principles of interpretative phenomenological analysis.

Parents and partners reported that the start of the transition was a difficult and uncertain time. They experienced sadness, anger, and worry about the end of the athletes' career which was often under negative circumstances such as non-selection. Parents and partners felt they had lost their own identity which had been deeply linked to the athletes' career and their sporting success. They appeared to experience their own transition alongside the athlete, including a significant sense of loss. There was evidently a conflict between supporting the athletes' transition and simultaneously managing their own transition as a parent or partner.

Emotional support was the main support provided by parents and partners to athletes and was used to understand changes, discuss the way forward, and promote togetherness. The transition process and the provision of support often extended over a long period with a significant amount of uncertainty around the athlete finding a suitable career and financial security. Fortunately, as the transition progressed over time, parents and partners were able to use their reflection on the experience in a positive way to foster personal and athlete relationship growth.

Brown et al. (2019) acknowledge a key limitation of the study. The single interview undertaken with each participant may not have been sufficient to gain complex information about their transition experiences. Furthermore, the interviews relied on the historical recall of experiences which means that important details may not have been disclosed due to memory or emotional barriers.

In conclusion, the study found that an athlete's transition out of sport had a significant impact on parents and partners who experienced their own transition which mirrored the athletes' in many ways. This resulted in negative effects on their wellbeing, particularly in the early stages of transition, but also promoted some positive development in the longer term.

MOVING ON: LIFE AFTER SPORT

Even with the challenges that retirement from sport can present, with careful planning and preparation this can signal a new and exciting time for an athlete. Ryan (2019) discussed how this approach which has placed retirement as a process rather than an event (Torregrosa et al., 2004) can in fact result in high levels of thriving and minimal post-sport adjustment. There are countless examples of athletes having highly successful 'second' careers following their retirement, either within sport or in other domains. For example, Mila made a decision to use her level of experience and love of tennis to start coaching and study physiotherapy. This decision to stay within sport is not unusual and transitioning to a coaching or management career is a common next step—for example, Frank Lampard's successful transition from a player to a manager (Chroni et al., 2020). This move into coaching can allow athletes to maintain aspects of their athletic identity by remaining in a similar environment with a similar lifestyle and support networks. However, a career in coaching is far from the only option with research highlighting that athletes possess a plethora of transferable competencies developed during their years as athletes. For example, a deep knowledge of teamwork, performing under pressure, effective communication, a strong work ethic, goal-setting, and time management—all of which can be highly attractive to future employers (e.g., Wylleman, 2019).

CLOSING THOUGHTS

Upon completion of this chapter you will have developed a more detailed understanding of the complexities of retirement from sport. You have explored how retirement is potentially the most challenging transition an athlete will face and explored several factors that can impact this final stage of the athlete journey. Through this you should now have a better understanding not only of why some athletes may experience adjustment difficulties but also that there are several factors that can influence the quality of the retirement experience to make it a positive one. By viewing retirement as the final episode in a much broader sporting career process, and thus ensuring that athletes are receiving the right support and have planned and prepared for their retirement, a successful transition into the next stage of their lives can be achieved.

REFERENCES

Atchley, R. C. (1976). *The sociology of retirement*. Schenkman.

Brewer, B. W. (1993). Self-identity and specific vulnerability to depressed mood. *Journal of Personality*, *61*(3), 343–364.

Brewer, B. W., Van Raalte, J. L., & Linder, D. E. (1993). Athletic identity: Hercules' muscles or Achilles heel? *International Journal of Sport Psychology*, *24*(2), 237–254.

Brown, C. J., Webb, T. L., Robinson, M. A., & Cotgreave, R. (2018). Athletes' experiences of social support during their transition out of elite sport: An interpretive phenomenological analysis. *Psychology of Sport and Exercise*, *36*, 71–80.

Brown, C. J., Webb, T. L., Robinson, M. A., & Cotgreave, R. (2019). Athletes' retirement from elite sport: A qualitative study of parents and partners' experiences. *Psychology of Sport and Exercise*, *40*, 51–60.

Burgess, E. W. (1960). *Aging in western societies*. The University of Chicago Press.

Cavallerio, F., Wadey, R., & Wagstaff, C. R. (2017). Adjusting to retirement from sport: Narratives of former competitive rhythmic gymnasts. *Qualitative Research in Sport, Exercise and Health*, *9*(5), 533–545.

Chroni, S. A., Pettersen, S., & Dieffenbach, K. (2020). Going from athlete-to-coach in Norwegian winter sports: Understanding the transition journey. *Sport in Society*, *23*(4), 751–773.

Clowes, H., Lindsay, P., Fawcett, L., & Knowles, Z. R. (2015). Experiences of the pre and post retirement period of female elite artistic gymnasts: An exploratory study. *Sport and Exercise Psychology Review*, *11*(2).

Cosh, S., LeCouteur, A., Crabb, S., & Kettler, L. (2015). Career transitions and identity: A discursive psychological approach to exploring athlete identity in retirement and the transition back into elite sport. *Qualitative Research in Sport, Exercise and Health*, *5*(1), 21–42.

dos Santos, A. L. P., Nogueira, M., & Böhme, M. (2016). Elite athletes' perception of retirement support systems. *International Journal of Physical Education, Sports and Health*, *3*(1), 192–199.

Dowd, J. J. (1975). Aging as exchange: A preface to theory. *Journal of Gerontology*, *30*(5), 584–594.

Giannone, Z. A., Haney, C. J., Kealy, D., & Ogrodniczuk, J. S. (2017). Athletic identity and psychiatric symptoms following retirement from varsity sports. *International Journal of Social Psychiatry*, *63*(7), 598–601.

Glaser, B. G., & Strauss, A. L. (1965). Discovery of substantive theory: A basic strategy underlying qualitative research. *American Behavioral Scientist*, *8*(6), 5–12.

Gordon, S., & Lavallee, D. (2011). Career transitions. In T. Morris & P. Terry P (Eds.), *The new sport and exercise psychology companion* (pp. 567–582). Fitness Information Technology.

Ivarsson, A., Johnson, U., Andersen, M. B., Tranaeus, U., Stenling, A., & Lindwall, M. (2017). Psychosocial factors and sport injuries: Meta-analyses for prediction and prevention. *Sports Medicine*, *47*(2), 353–365.

Knights, S., Sherry, E., & Ruddock-Hudson, M. (2016). Investigating elite end-of-athletic-career transition: A systematic review. *Journal of Applied Sport Psychology*, *28*(3), 291–308.

Knights, S., Sherry, E., Ruddock-Hudson, M., & O'Halloran, P. (2019). The end of a professional sport career: Ensuring a positive transition. *Journal of Sport Management, 33*(6), 518–529.

Kübler-Ross, E. (1969). *On death and dying.* Scribner.

Kuettel, A., Boyle, E., & Schmid, J. (2017). Factors contributing to the quality of the transition out of elite sports in Swiss, Danish, and Polish athletes. *Psychology of Sport and Exercise, 29*, 27–39.

Kuypers, J. A., & Bengtson, V. L. (1973). Social breakdown and competence. *Human Development, 16*(3), 181–201.

Lagimodiere, C., & Strachan, L. (2015). Exploring the role of sport type and popularity in male sport retirement experiences. *Athletic Insight, 7*(1), 1.

Lally, P. (2007). Identity and athletic retirement: A prospective study. *Psychology of Sport and Exercise, 8*, 85–99.

Lavallee, D. (2007). Theoretical perspectives on career transitions in sport. In D. Lavallee & P. Wylleman (Eds.), *Career transitions in sport: International perspectives.* Fitness Information Technology.

Lavallee, D., Park, S., & Taylor, J. (2015). Career transition among athletes: Is there life after sports? In J. M. Williams & V. Krane (Ed.), *Applied sport psychology: Personal growth to peak performance* (7th ed., pp. 490–509). McGraw-Hill Education.

Lingam-Willgoss, C., & Heaney, C. (2020). The athlete's journey: Transitions through sport. *OpenLearn.* www.open.edu/openlearn/health-sports-psychology/the-athletes-journey-transitions-through-sport/content-section-overview?active-tab=description-tab

MacCosham, B., Patry, P., Beswick, C., & Gravelle, F. (2015). Leisure lifestyle and dropout: Exploring the experience of amateur athletes in competitive sport. *International Journal of Sport Management, Recreation and Tourism, 20*(2), 20–39.

Martin, L., Fogarty, G., & Albion, M. (2014). Changes in athletic identity and life satisfaction of elite athletes as a function of retirement status. *Journal of Applied Sport Psychology, 26*, 96–110.

Park, S., Lavallee, D., & Tod, D. (2013). Athletes' career transition out of sport: A systematic review. *International Review of Sport and Exercise Psychology, 6*(1), 22–53.

Rosenberg, E. (1984). Athletic retirement as social death: Concepts and perspectives. *Sport and the Sociological Imagination*, 245–258.

Ryan, L. (2019). *Flourishing after retirement: Understanding the sport career transition of New Zealand's elite athletes* [Doctoral dissertation]. The University of Waikato.

Samuel, R. D., & Tenenbaum, G. (2011). How do athletes perceive and respond to change-events: An exploratory measurement tool. *Psychology of Sport and Exercise, 12*(4), 392–406.

Schlossberg, N. K. (1981). A model for analyzing human adaptation to transition. *The Counselling Psychologist, 9*(2), 2–18.

Stambulova, N. B. (2000). Athlete's crises: A developmental perspective. *International Journal of Sport Psychology, 31*(4), 584–601.

Stambulova, N. B. (2016). Athletes' transitions in sport and life: Positioning new research trends within the existing system of athlete career knowledge. In R. J. Schinke, K. R. McGannon, & B. Smith (Eds.), *Routledge international handbook of sport psychology.* Routledge.

Taylor, J., & Ogilvie, B. C. (1994). A conceptual model of adaptation to retirement among athletes. *Journal of Applied Sport Psychology, 6*(1), 1–20.

Tibbert, S. J., Andersen, M. B., & Morris, T. (2015). What a difference a "mentally toughening" year makes: The acculturation of a rookie. *Psychology of Sport and Exercise, 17*, 68–78.

Torregrosa, M., Boixados, M., Valiente, L., & Cruz, J. (2004). Elite athletes' image of retirement: The way to relocation in sport. *Psychology of Sport and Exercise, 5*, 35–43.

Torregrosa, M., Ramis, Y., Pallarés, S., Azócar, F., & Selva, C. (2015). Olympic athletes back to retirement: A qualitative longitudinal study. *Psychology of Sport and Exercise, 21,* 50–56.

Udry, E., Gould, D., Bridges, D., & Beck, L. (1997). Down but not out: Athlete responses to season-ending injuries. *Journal of Sport and Exercise Psychology, 19*(3), 229–248.

Walker, N., & Heaney, C. (2013). Psychological responses to injury. In M. Arvinen-Barrow & N. Walker (Eds.), *The psychology of sport injury and rehabilitation* (pp. 23–39). Routledge.

Wylleman, P. (2019). A developmental and holistic perspective on transitioning out of elite sport. In M. H. Anshel (Ed.), *APA handbook of sport and exercise psychology: Volume 1. Sport psychology* (pp. 201–216). American Psychological Association.

Wylleman, P., Alfermann, D., & Lavallee, D. (2004). Career transitions in sport: European Perspectives. *Psychology of Sport and Exercise, 5,* 7–20.

Wylleman, P., Reints, A., & De Knop, P. (2013). Athletes' careers in Belgium: A holistic perspective to understand and alleviate challenges occurring throughout the athletic and post-athletic career. In N. B. Stambulova & T. V. Ryba (Eds.), *Athletes' careers across cultures* (pp. 51–62). Routledge.

Young, J. A., Pearce, A. J., Kane, R., & Pain, M. (2006). Leaving the professional tennis circuit: Exploratory study of experiences and reactions from elite female athletes. *British Journal of Sports Medicine, 40*(5), 477–483.

CHAPTER 5

Researching Athletic Development

Joanna Horne

> *[Y]ou should ensure that reading and evaluating research is done on a continual basis. . . . Try not to be put off by the complex statistical analyses employed, or by the seemingly impenetrable academic writing that is often used.*
>
> (Jones, 2015, p. 12)

Research is the systematic process of collecting and analysing information, in order to increase our knowledge and understanding of a topic. It involves generating a research question, identifying an appropriate research design, collecting and analysing the data, and reporting the results. Conducting research in athletic development maintains and enhances our understanding of this area, which informs our teaching and practice.

This chapter will primarily be useful to newcomers to research generally, or to specific research designs. It will introduce you to the main research *approaches* (the broad type of methodology), and some of the *designs* (the detailed procedure used to answer the research question) and *instruments* (the specific tools used to collect data) most commonly used in research into athletic development. The chapter will help you understand the findings of studies presented throughout this book and in your wider reading. It does not cover every research design, or teach you how to conduct research, but if you want to explore research in sport further, then Jones (2015) provides a comprehensive guide.

RESEARCH APPROACHES: QUANTITATIVE VERSUS QUALITATIVE

We start by outlining the two main methodological *approaches*—quantitative and qualitative research. The approach chosen will be informed by the researcher's philosophical assumptions, such as whether behaviour can be objectively measured, and the importance placed on the meanings of experiences and the nature of the research question.

What Is Quantitative Research?

Quantitative research comes from the assumption that behaviour can be observed and measured objectively (i.e., 'quantified'). It involves the scientific study of phenomena, using statistical techniques to analyse numerical data (e.g., test scores, Likert scales, physiological measures), with the aim of generalising the results to a population. For example, a researcher may use a state anxiety scale to collect numerical data regarding adolescent athletes' anxiety before and after moving to a higher level of competition.

We pause here to briefly explain three research terms. A *population* is all cases to which the research applies (e.g., adolescent athletes) and to which the findings may be generalised; a *sample* is a subset of the population, selected so that valid conclusions may be made about the nature of the population itself. A *hypothesis* contains a prediction, derived from theory, which can be tested through investigation; the experimental hypothesis (H_1) states an expected effect (e.g., 'Male athletes will score higher than female athletes on self-confidence'), whilst the null hypothesis (H_0) states no effect (e.g., 'There will be no differences in self-confidence between male and female athletes').

Quantitative research is based on deductive reasoning, whereby an explicit hypothesis is stated and then tested empirically (i.e., using objective measurements). If the findings are consistent with the hypothesis, then this supports the theory from which the hypothesis is derived. However, if the hypothesis is refuted, then this would be evidence against the theory. No single test of a hypothesis is enough to verify or falsify a theory, but several studies are used to build up a body of evidence regarding a theory's usefulness. Therefore, replication of research is vital within the scientific approach in order to show that the findings are reliable. This building up of evidence over time is apparent within varied athletic development perspectives (see Chapter 2).

What Is Qualitative Research?

Whereas quantitative research focuses on *quantifying* variables, qualitative research focuses on describing/categorising the *qualities* of data. Qualitative research comes from the assumption that it is the meanings of experience that are important and, as such, qualitative researchers are interested in gathering data that illuminates personal meaning and experiences. They most often try to gain naturalistic data in the form of observations, one-to-one interviews, focus groups, diaries, and data from open-ended questions. This means that the participants determine what information is generated, making the data very rich in meaning and ecologically valid (i.e., it relates well to the real world), but reliability (the extent to which data is consistent over time or when used by different testers) is difficult. For example, the researcher may conduct interviews or have focus group conversations to understand the nature of adolescent athletes' anxieties before and after moving to a higher level of competition.

Qualitative research is based on inductive reasoning, whereby the researcher will start with observations and data collection regarding a phenomenon, then look for patterns to generate a theory. Qualitative studies tend to generate large amounts of textual data and rely on researcher interpretation in the analysis of this data. They require the researcher to be reflexive—to be aware of the influence that they have had on the research process (e.g., how their background, values, and beliefs have impacted the interpretation of the data).

The key features, strengths, and weaknesses of the quantitative and qualitative approaches are shown in Table 5.1.

TABLE 5.1 Differences between quantitative and qualitative approaches

Feature	Quantitative	Qualitative
Concepts	Probability, causality	Experience, understanding, meaning
Reasoning	Generally deductive	Generally inductive
Sampling	Large, representative samples—random selection	Small samples/single cases—purposeful
Data	Numerical	Mainly text-based
Instruments	Questionnaires with closed questions, (Likert) scales, psychometric tests	Observations, interviews, focus groups, diaries, open-ended questionnaires
Setting	Controlled environment (e.g. laboratory)	Natural setting
Data analysis	Statistical—after end of data collection	Coding, identifying themes—may take place during data collection
Strengths	More objective, generalisable and reliable	Rich, meaningful data, high in ecological validity
Limitations	Low ecological validity	Difficult to generalise, complex, and time-consuming

Mixed Methods

Sometimes, a researcher may choose to draw on the strengths of both approaches by using a mixed-method approach (i.e., both quantitative and qualitative approaches). The earlier example of a researcher using a state anxiety scale to measure adolescent athletes' anxiety before and after moving to a higher level of competition will only show whether the level of anxiety changes, not the specific causes of the anxiety. So, the researcher may also conduct interviews, focus groups, or open-ended questionnaires to understand the nature of the athletes' anxieties. However, conducting a study with a mixed-methods approach can be costly and time-consuming.

RESEARCH DESIGNS

Once the researcher has generated their research question and/or hypothesis and has decided on their methodological approach (qualitative, quantitative, or mixed method), they then need to consider their research design (the detailed procedure used to answer the research question).

Cross-Sectional Designs

Cross-sectional designs are used to compare several non-manipulated groups (i.e., the participants fall naturally into these groups, rather than being assigned to them, e.g., age, gender, sport, nationality) at a single time point. In developmental psychology, they have been used to compare individuals of different age groups, which is quicker and easier than carrying out a longitudinal study of one sample repeatedly measured as they age. Clearly, this use can be applied to research in athletic development (see Box 5.1).

Box 5.1 Cross-Sectional Design Example—Pain, Athletic
Identity, and Depression in Retired Footballers

Using a cross-sectional design, Sanders and Stevinson (2017) aimed to identify factors that increase the risk of mental health difficulties after career termination in professional footballers. The sample included 307 retired male footballers.

Participants completed the Short Depression-Happiness Scale, the Pain Intensity Numerical Rating Scale, and the Athletic Identity Measurement Scale and reported their reasons for retirement. This allowed the researchers to compare participants with and without depressive symptoms.

Sanders and Stevinson (2017) found that those who met the criteria for clinically relevant depression (48 of the participants) were younger, more recently retired, and had higher athletic identity than those without depressive symptoms. They were also more likely to cite injury as the reason for retirement and report higher levels of injury-related pain.

Cross-sectional designs have the advantages of being reasonably quick and having low rates of attrition (i.e., participants dropping out of the study), but they are limited in that they do not identify developmental changes, only differences between groups, and cannot identify a causal relationship (i.e., that one variable affects another variable). To establish causality (the process by which one variable causes a change in another variable), an experimental design would be required.

Experimental Designs

An experimental design allows for the investigation of an Independent Variable (IV) on a Dependent Variable (DV), with minimal contamination from confounding variables, in order to determine cause and effect. The IV is the variable that is manipulated within an experiment, either through existing characteristics (e.g., elite vs. amateur) or experimenter manipulation (e.g., different training conditions)—the IV can then be identified as the cause of any effect on the variable that is being measured (the DV).

For example, a study may examine the effect of self-talk (IV) on athlete self-confidence (DV). If participants are assigned to different conditions of the IV (e.g., to an intervention group which is trained in the use of self-talk, or a control group which doesn't undergo the self-talk training), and other variables are controlled as well as they can be, then a difference in the DV (the athlete's self-confidence) is likely to be due to the IV (their use of self-talk). Often, measurements of the DV are taken before the intervention (pre-test) and after the intervention (post-test) for both the intervention and control groups, in order to control for any baseline differences between the two groups.

Lorimer and Jowett (2010) used an experimental design to research the effect of feedback on sport coaches' empathic accuracy (being able to accurately perceive another's thoughts, feelings, moods in the moment; see Box 5.2).

Box 5.2 Experimental Design Example—The Effect of
Feedback on the Empathic Accuracy of
Badminton Coaches

Lorimer and Jowett (2010) studied changes in the empathic accuracy of sport coaches in relation to feedback. Sixty badminton coaches were assigned to either an experimental or a control group, with 30 participants in each group. Participants were shown a video of a training session between a badminton coach and a female athlete. The video was divided into 10 segments, with an 80-second pause between each. During the pauses, participants wrote down what they thought the athlete had been thinking and feeling. After each pause, those in the experimental group were given corrective feedback (through the video giving information on what the athlete had actually been thinking and feeling in the previous segment) (IV). Those in the control group did not get this feedback.

Each participant's empathic accuracy (DV) for each segment was rated by three independent researchers on a three-point scale. These were then added up for each participant to give scores for the first five segments, the latter five segments, and the total score.

A mixed ANOVA statistical test, explained later in the chapter, showed that both groups improved in empathic accuracy with exposure to the athlete (an increase from the first five to the latter five segments), but the group who had received feedback on their performance improved significantly more than the control group. They concluded that coaches asking questions of, and receiving feedback from, athletes will help coaches to accurately understand them.

Although experimental designs do allow us to infer causality, there are some disadvantages, particularly in terms of the limited number of variables that can be investigated, and the lack of ecological validity (i.e., experiments do not often reflect a training environment). A design that would provide a high level of ecological validity is an ethnographic design.

Ethnographic Designs

Ethnographic research is a qualitative approach where the researcher studies a specific group by being immersed in the group's setting. This allows the research to authentically capture the perspectives of group members. It is usually conducted over a substantial period, in order to develop trust with those being studied and to gain an understanding of what is happening within the group. Ethnographic research generally involves the use of observation, particularly participant observation, although data may also be collected through in-depth interviews and artefacts from the setting (e.g., documents, emails, and diaries). It is important that the researcher recognises the impact of their own characteristics (e.g., age, gender, sporting background) on all aspects of the research, including their choice of setting and participants, relationships with the group members, the data collected, and the analysis of that data.

In athletic development research, Devaney et al. (2018) used an ethnographic design to study how elite youth cricketers adapt to life as a full-time athlete (see Box 5.3).

Box 5.3 Ethnography Design Example—Lifestyle Support of Elite Youth Cricketers

Devaney et al.'s (2018) research aimed to understand the lifestyle concerns of elite youth cricketers and the meaning they ascribe to them, and to understand how athlete lifestyle support should be positioned at this stage of young cricketers' journeys.

The study involved 20 players, aged 15 to 19, within two squads on a talent development programme and 14 support staff (including coaches, physiotherapists, a performance analyst, and a psychologist). The researcher was able to access the setting as a Personal Development and Welfare (PDW) practitioner, which involved individual and group support.

Over 15 months, data was collected through observations (daily practice, day-to-day lives), informal conversations with players and staff, and formal conversations within the PDW role. Notable moments were noted as soon as possible and then written about more fully in a daily research log. These were supported by reflective diary entries, where the researcher made sense of the observations and conservations.

The data analysis identified five themes:

- players appreciating lifestyle support;
- adapting to the new environment;
- managing competing demands;
- educational choices and professional contracts; and
- identity negotiation in critical moments.

The researchers concluded that counselling approaches and strong practitioner-player relationships may contribute to wellbeing and impact cricket performance.

Although ethnographic research can give us a rich insight into the perspectives of a specific group within a particular context, there are some difficulties with using this design. As well as demanding a huge amount of the researcher's time, an ethnography also requires the researcher to gain access to the group, which can be extremely problematic for an outsider. So, what other designs can provide us with in-depth data within a shorter time scale? One option would be to utilise a case study design.

Case Study Designs

Case studies are comprehensive investigations of one or more individuals (e.g., an athlete/coach, a team, a school, an organisation, an event), which aim to present an in-depth analysis of them within their natural environment. Case studies are particularly useful in unique or rare situations, and in areas where there is a lack of in-depth investigations. Despite not being generalisable to the wider population, case studies can enhance our understanding of the experiences of the individual.

As the focus of case studies is on depth, rather than breadth, they involve only small samples, sometimes with the participation of just one individual. Although case studies primarily take a qualitative approach, they may involve the collection of qualitative (e.g., interviews, observations, diaries, personal notes, medical/clinical notes, archival records) and quantitative (e.g., psychometric tests) data. A case study of an athlete may be enhanced using interviews with coaches, teammates, sport psychologists, physiotherapists, and parents, as well as the athlete him/herself. The information collected may include retrospective material, providing an alternative to a time-consuming longitudinal study (discussed in the following section).

So, how may a case study approach be implemented as a research method in athletic development? If a researcher wants to investigate how elite fencers deal with transitions during their sporting career, but does not have the timescale or resources to conduct an ethnographic or longitudinal study (discussed in the following section), they may decide to carry out a retrospective case study with fencers approaching their retirement from the sport. Such a study was carried out by Debois et al., in 2012, with an elite female fencer at the end of her career (see Box 5.4).

Box 5.4 Design Example—Career Transitions of an Elite Female Fencer

Debois et al. (2012) conducted a case study to explore how an elite female fencer dealt with key events and transitions during her career. The participant (who was given the anonymous alias 'Francine') had begun foil fencing at the age of 8, was selected for the World Championships at 19, changed to sabre fencing at 22, won the European title at 26, took part in the Olympic Games at 28 but failed to qualify at the next games at 32, at which point she retired.

The researchers collected qualitative data from a retrospective in-depth interview at the end of Francine's career recounting the main stages and key transitions of her life, and notes from sport psychologist interviews over the previous 14 years. The interview text was independently coded by two researchers to identify meaningful information for each stage, which was then grouped into categories according to common features.

Francine identified three life stages and 11 transitions (nine related to sport, one to education, and one to her personal life). The analysis revealed that her path to excellence included both positive and crisis transitions, supporting the usefulness of regular psychological interviews to help athletes negotiate transitions.

Although case studies can provide valuable, detailed accounts they are subjective, which means there are limitations regarding which aspects are included, and are difficult to replicate. Furthermore, the collection of retrospective data, as in the previous example, may be problematic as it is dependent on the memory of the participants and the availability of information from their athletic career. Instead of collecting retrospective data, a prospective longitudinal design could be considered.

Longitudinal Designs

The majority of studies within the field of athletic development involve the collection of data at one point in time, such as in cross-sectional designs. However, as stated by Cobley and Till (2017), these "cannot detect development change, causal effects, interactions between variables or identify variables associated with onward learning or improvement" (p. 251). For this reason, they propose the use of longitudinal designs, being conducted over short (six months to two years) or longer time periods, with a minimum of three repeated observations of the same participants. Longitudinal designs may involve the collection of quantitative and/or qualitative data.

For example, Adie et al. (2012) wanted to investigate the relationship between perceived autonomy supportive coaching and the wellbeing of elite youth soccer players. The authors noted that much of the previous research in this field came from cross-sectional studies, which could not demonstrate the relationship between changes in motivational process and changes in wellbeing over time. Adie et al. (2012) addressed this by conducting a longitudinal study, which is outlined in Box 5.5.

Box 5.5 Longitudinal Design Example—Perceived Coach-Autonomy Support, Basic Need Satisfaction and Well- and Illbeing of Elite Youth Soccer Players

Adie et al. (2012) investigated 91 male soccer players (aged 11–18) from a School of Excellence in the UK, although 37 didn't complete the study as they had left the team or been injured, resulting in a final sample of 54 participants.

The participants completed a quantitative Likert questionnaire at the beginning, middle, and end of two consecutive competitive seasons, measuring:

- perceived coach-autonomy support (e.g., 'I feel that my coach provides me with choices and options');
- basic need satisfaction: autonomy need (e.g., 'My choices express who I really am'); competence need (e.g., 'I think I am pretty good at soccer'); and relatedness need (e.g., 'On this team, I feel supported'); and
- well-/illbeing: subjective vitality (e.g., 'I feel alive and full of energy'); and emotional and physical exhaustion (e.g., 'I feel so tired from soccer training that I have trouble finding energy to do other things').

The results showed that perceptions of coach-autonomy support positively predicted changes in basic need satisfaction and wellbeing over time. A key message from the findings was that players who perceived the coach to be more autonomy supportive across the study experienced higher levels of satisfaction with autonomy, competence, and relatedness needs and more subjective vitality.

So, if longitudinal studies are considered an exemplary design for researching athletic development, why are they not used more widely? The main difficulties are that they require a lot of time and resources, the results may be affected by confounding variables, and there is a high level of attrition. Indeed, in Adie et al.'s (2012) study, 40% of the original sample dropped out over the two competitive seasons of being studied. This is a reasonably short time period for a longitudinal study—for longer studies, attrition rates may be even higher.

RESEARCH INSTRUMENTS

Researchers use a variety of instruments, which are the *specific tools* used to collect data. The main instruments are outlined in the following text, and you will have seen how these are used within various research designs in the previous section.

Interviews

An interview is a conversation between a researcher and a participant, designed to elicit certain information related to the research question. Normally, interviews are recorded, and a text transcript created for analysis. Interviews may be:

- structured (where the questions and question order are fully specified in advance);
- semi-structured (where a list of open-ended questions is specified, but it allows for additional questions to be asked and areas to be explored in more depth); and
- unstructured (where there are no predetermined questions and it is more participant-led).

For example, Debois et al. (2012) used an interview in their case study of an elite female fencer in order to explore the key events and transitions during her career (see Box 5.4).

Focus Groups

A focus group is a form of interview that takes place with several participants (usually four to eight) at the same time, which allows for interaction between the participants and provides a more in-depth discussion than a one-to-one interview. The researcher's task is to keep the group on-topic and ensure that everyone is given the opportunity to contribute. The discussion is recorded and transcribed, as with interviews.

Observations

Observation involves the researcher observing and recording (e.g., using audio, video, or observation sheets) the behaviour of the participant(s). This may take one of two forms:

- non-participant observation (where the researcher observes from the outside and does not engage with the participant(s)/activity) or
- participant observation (where the researcher takes part in the activity and engages with the participant[s])

For example, Devaney et al. (2018) used participant observation in their ethnographic research of the lifestyle concerns of elite youth cricketers (see Box 5.3).

Questionnaires

A questionnaire is a series of questions presented to participants either on paper, online, face-to-face, or via telephone. Questionnaires may be used to collect either quantitative (e.g., through the inclusion of Likert scales and rankings) or qualitative (e.g., through the inclusion of open questions) data. For example, Adie et al. (2012) used a questionnaire in their study of perceived autonomy supportive coaching and wellbeing in elite youth soccer players (see Box 5.5).

Psychometric Tests

A psychometric test is a measurement of a specific psychological characteristic, such as anxiety or confidence. Such a measure is likely to have been standardised using an appropriate normative group so that a participant's score can be compared to a similar population group. A psychometric test must be shown to be both valid (i.e., that it measures what it claims to measure) and reliable (i.e., that it is consistent over time or when used by different testers). For example, Sanders and Stevinson (2017) used psychometric tests in their study of risk factors for mental health difficulties following retirement in professional footballers (see Box 5.1).

Strengths and Limitations

Researchers may use more than one type of research instrument within their study, selecting those instruments that are most appropriate for collecting the data required to answer the research question. Some of the main strengths and limitations of each instrument are shown in Table 5.2.

TABLE 5.2 Strengths and limitations of different research instruments

Instrument	Strengths	Limitations
Interviews	In-depth information; allows for clarification; may pick up on non-verbal cues from participants	Very time-consuming/expensive; small samples; requires trained interviewers; responses may be affected by presence of interviewer; results may be hard to analyse
Focus groups	Can interview several people efficiently; allows for clarification; participants stimulate each other	Lack of confidentiality/anonymity; some participants may dominate discussions; moderately time-consuming/expensive; results may be hard to analyse
Observations	Natural setting; high ecological validity	Requires skilled observer; participants may respond differently if aware of observer; difficult with large groups; lack of control over environment; difficult to generalise results
Questionnaires	Can use with large samples; quick and easy; can easily be analysed statistically; allows for group comparisons	Lacks in-depth data; cannot gauge participants' understanding of the question
Psychometric tests	Allows you to compare scores to a norm group; allows for statistical analysis; allows for group comparisons	Lacks in-depth data; may require trained tester (dependent on the test); cannot be adapted (without invalidating norms)

HOW IS DATA ANALYSED?

The first part of this chapter explored some of the choices that researchers make about their research approach. When researchers publish this in a journal article, their approach is typically headed the 'method' section or similar. In addition to collecting data, researchers also need to be clear about how they will analyse it. Published research will often explain how the researchers analysed their data towards the end of a method section; this leads into a section on 'results' and then 'discussion/analysis' or similar.

This latter part of the chapter will outline some of the data analysis processes used within both quantitative and qualitative research approaches. Data analysis is a process of gathering, organising, and synthesising data, with the goal being to highlight useful information (Smith, 2010).

Quantitative Data Analysis

If you are new to quantitative data analysis, the statistical terminology can be quite off-putting. The aim of this section is to introduce you to the most common statistical terms that you are likely to come across in your reading.

Descriptive Statistics

Descriptive statistics allow researchers to summarise and illustrate their data set (through measures of central tendency and dispersion which are explained in the following text) using tables and graphs. For example, one of the very basic abbreviations that you are likely to see in such tables is n or N, which simply refers to the *number* of cases within the sample (e.g., n = 347).

Measures of central tendency provide information about the typical value for a distribution of scores, with the most commonly used being the mean, median, and mode. The *mean* is the arithmetical average of the set of scores, calculated by summing all the scores and dividing by the number of scores in the set. The *median* is the middle score in the set when placed in numerical order, so 50% of scores fall at or below the median, and 50% fall at or above it. Finally, the *mode* is the most frequently occurring score(s). For example, a study may include 10 athletes with the following ages: 15, 20, 22, 23, 23, 24, 25, 26, 28, and 31. This set of data has a mean of 23.7, a median of 23.5, and a mode of 23.

Measures of dispersion provide information about the spread of scores around the mean (or median/mode), with the most commonly used being range and standard deviation. The *range* is simply the difference between the highest and lowest values in a set of scores, which provides a rather crude measure of dispersion (e.g., in the previous example, the range is 15 years [16 to 31]). The *standard deviation (SD)* is an estimate of the average amount by which the scores in a set of scores vary from the mean of the scores. For example, a study may report that the mean age of the male athletes was 23.4 years (SD 6.3 years), and the mean age of the female athletes was 24.0 years (SD 1.6 years). This tells us that the female athletes were more clustered together in age compared to the male athletes.

Testing for Associations: Correlation

In addition to the measures of central tendency and dispersion, there are tests that allow researchers to start to test associations between, or draw conclusions from, their quantitative data rather than just describing it. Correlation tells us the relationship between two variables—how changes in one variable are associated with changes in the other variable. This is represented numerically by a correlation coefficient, which ranges from -1 to $+1$. There are various kinds of correlations, with the most commonly used being Pearson's correlation coefficient (r), although you may also come across Spearman's correlation. These tests essentially do the same thing but are based on different mathematical equations depending on the type of data a researcher has collected.

The sign in the coefficient illustrates whether it is a positive $(+)$ or negative $(-)$ correlation. In a positive correlation, as one variable increases, the other also increases; whereas in a negative correlation, as one variable increases, the other decreases. The value of the coefficient (ranging from 0 to 1) represents the strength of the relationship between the variables, so a coefficient that is close to 0 indicates little or no relationship between the two variables, whereas a coefficient that is close to $+/-1$ indicates a strong relationship.

It is important to appreciate that correlation doesn't imply causality—it shows that the variables are related but not that one is the cause of the other. For example, there may be a strong positive correlation between level of sport participation and academic performance in adolescents. This doesn't mean that taking part in sport leads to the attainment of higher exam grades, or that doing well academically leads to higher levels of sport participation. Instead, there may be other factors (e.g., motivation) that cause the change in both variables.

Testing for Differences

Tests of difference are used where two or more samples or conditions are tested to see if they statistically differ on a DV. For example, do males and females (IV) differ in their beliefs about sport (DV)? A researcher's selection of a statistical test will depend on the number of IVs, the number of groups, and the nature of the different groups. There are various statistical tests for measuring differences, with those most commonly used being shown in Table 5.3.

TABLE 5.3 Commonly used tests for differences

Test	Statistical Abbreviation	Description
Chi-square	χ^2	Used for nominal (categorical) data: the frequency obtained for each category is compared with the frequency expected by chance. For example, comparing male and female (IV) athletes on their selection of a preferred coaching style (DV).
Independent samples t-test	t	Determines whether the means of two unrelated groups are significantly different from each other. For example, comparing male and female (IV) scores on a mental toughness scale (DV).
Paired samples t-test	t	Determines whether the means of one group (or matched pairs) on two occasions are significantly different from each other. For example, comparing a group's mental toughness scores (DV) before and after a resilience intervention (IV).

(Continued)

TABLE 5.3 (Continued)

Test	Statistical Abbreviation	Description
One-way Analysis of Variance (ANOVA)	F	Determines whether the means of two or more unrelated groups (grouped on one IV) are significantly different from each other. For example, comparing rugby players', tennis players', and gymnasts' (IV) scores on a mental toughness scale (DV).
Factorial ANOVA	F	Determines whether the means of unrelated groups (grouped on two or more IVs) are significantly different from each other. For example, comparing male and female (IV1) rugby players', tennis players', and gymnasts' (IV2) scores on a mental toughness scale (DV).
Repeated measures ANOVA	F	Determines whether the means of a group tested on two or more occasions are significantly different. For example, comparing a group's mental toughness scores (DV) before, immediately after, and six months after a resilience intervention (IV).
Mixed ANOVA	F	This is similar to a factorial ANOVA, but whilst one IV uses independent (unrelated) groups, the other IV uses repeated measures. For example, comparing male and female (IV) scores on a mental toughness scale (DV) before and after a resilience intervention (repeated measures IV).

When researchers report the results of a statistical test, they will usually state the p-value, which indicates the statistical significance of the result. This is a critical element of understanding quantitative research findings, and is, therefore, focused on in the spotlight box.

Spotlight On: P-Values

A p-value is the *probability* of a statistical outcome as extreme as the one that has been observed in our sample data, if there is no actual effect (i.e., no association or difference) in the population. So, a small p-value suggests that the observed outcome is less likely to be due to chance and there is more likely to be an actual effect (i.e., a genuine association or difference).

But at what level can we be confident enough that the effect is genuine? The generally accepted threshold is that when there is less than a 5% chance (.05 probability) of getting the data we have if no effect exists, then we are confident enough to accept that the effect is genuine. So, researchers will generally reject the null hypothesis (that there is no effect) when they have a p-value of less than .05, which is shown in the statistical notation as 'p < .05'. This is regarded as a 'significant' effect.

You may also see reported p-values of $p < .01$ (which means that there is less than a 1% chance of getting the data we have if no effect exists) or even $p < 0.001$ (which means that there is less than a 1/1000 chance of getting the data we have if no effect exists).

For example, in Lorimer and Jowett's (2010) study, they found that both groups improved in empathic accuracy from the first five to the latter five segments ($p < .01$), and that the feedback group improved more than the control group ($p < 0.01$), which are both highly statistically significant results.

Qualitative Data Analysis

Data collection using a qualitative approach often produces extensive audio or video recordings (e.g., from interviews and observations) which are transcribed into text, resulting in huge amounts of written material, which need to be organised and interpreted. For example, in their ethnographic study, Devaney et al. (2018) collected a mass of data from observations and conversations with players and staff, which were recorded in notes, research logs, and diary entries.

Once the data is transcribed, it needs to be reduced by organising it into categories or themes, through a coding process. Codes may be developed deductively (i.e., based on the theory being explored) or inductively (based on the data itself), or through a mix of both. In order to code the data effectively, the researcher needs to be immersed within it. After the initial coding, the researcher will then consider how the codes fit together to form broader themes, from which the researcher can develop conclusions related to their research question.

There is no one set procedure for analysing qualitative data. Within published research, you may come across several methods, such as thematic analysis (as was used by Devaney et al., 2018), grounded theory, and interpretative phenomenological analysis. Although these methods of qualitative analysis take slightly different approaches, there are some clear similarities, with elements that will form part of most qualitative analysis methods, including:

- transcription of any audio/video recordings into written text;
- familiarising oneself with the data through reading and re-reading it;
- coding/identifying interesting areas;
- grouping these areas into broader themes/categories;
- labelling and defining themes;
- producing a map/table of themes; and
- relating the themes back to the data, with the possible use of quotes from the transcription.

CLOSING THOUGHTS

This chapter has demonstrated that there is no optimal design for research in athletic development, as all the varied research designs have their strengths and limitations. A researcher's choice of design will be based on their methodological approach and the research question that they are trying to answer. Ultimately, investigating any sort of development over time is complex, as the expansive longitudinal design that would be desirable is extremely time-consuming, but there are also limitations to research carried out at one moment in time, and issues with memory recall for retrospective studies. Furthermore, finding a sample of athletes who have successfully progressed and developed in sport means that the people who have dropped out or struggled are often missing from samples. Therefore, the skill of interpreting athletic development research is to appreciate some of the limitations but also to recognise the diverse ways in which people progress in sport. After reading this chapter, you are more likely to have the necessary knowledge to make sense of the research studies that you come across.

REFERENCES

Adie, W. J., Duda, J. L., & Ntoumanis, N. (2012). Perceived coach-autonomy support, basic need satisfaction and the well- and ill-being of elite youth soccer players: A longitudinal investigation. *Psychology of Sport and Exercise, 13*(1), 51–59. https://doi.org/10.1016/j.psychsport.2011.07.008

Cobley, S., & Till, K. (2017). Longitudinal studies of athlete development. In J. Baker, S. Cobley, J. Schorer, & N. Wattie (Eds.), *Routledge handbook of talent identification and development in sport* (pp. 250–268). Routledge.

Debois, N., Ledon, A., Argiolas, C., & Rosnet, E. (2012). A lifespan perspective on transitions during a top sports career: A case of an elite female fencer. *Psychology of Sport and Exercise, 13*(5), 660–668. https://doi.org/10.1016/j.psychsport.2012.04.010

Devaney, D. J., Nesti, M. S., Ronkainen, N. J., Littlewood, M., & Richardson, D. (2018). Athlete lifestyle support of elite youth cricketers: An ethnography of player concerns within a national talent development program. *Journal of Applied Sport Psychology, 30*(3), 300–320. https://doi.org/10.1080/10413200.2017.1386247

Jones, I. (2015). *Research methods for sports studies* (3rd ed.). Routledge.

Lorimer, R., & Jowett, S. (2010). Feedback of information in the empathic accuracy of sport coaches. *Psychology of Sport and Exercise, 11*(1), 12–17. https://doi.org/10.1016/j.psychsport.2009.03.006

Sanders, G., & Stevinson, C. (2017). Associations between retirement reasons, chronic pain, athletic identity, and depressive symptoms among former professional footballers. *European Journal of Sport Science, 17*(10), 1311–1318. https://doi.org/10.1080/17461391.2017.1371795

Smith, M. (2010). *Research methods in sport*. Learning Matters.

SECTION II

Social Influences on the Athlete's Journey

Nichola Kentzer

An athlete does not develop in isolation—their sporting journey can be shaped by those around them (Hogg & Vaughan, 2018). Indeed, the importance of an athlete's social environment is a feature in all the main psychological perspectives of athletic development outlined in Chapter 2. For example, Côté et al. (2009) discuss choices (sampling vs specialisation) and opportunities in childhood which are arguably influenced heavily by a young person's family. Examples of high-profile family support can be seen in the sport of tennis with Venus and Serena Williams' father, and Andy and Jamie Murray's mother—who have both been identified as key influences in their children's development.

Other athletes have followed parents into their chosen sport, such as Jacques (and Gilles) Villeneuve and Damon (and Graham) Hill (Formula One), and Eilish (and Liz) McColgan (athletics). Moreover, siblings can influence choice and ongoing support in their sport, with Alistair and Jonny Brownlee (triathlon), Giannis and Thanasis Antetokounmpo (basketball), and Becky and Ellie Downie (gymnastics) as examples. It can also be the case that family members coach their children, as in the case of Eilish McColgan who is coached by her mother at elite level. This, however, is not the norm and consequently the relationship an athlete builds with their coach can be key to their development as an athlete and to performance success (Jowett & Shanmugam, 2016). The athlete is joined by not only family and coaches on their athletic development journey, however, but by other individuals that can influence their sporting experiences, including physical education (PE) teachers. Indeed, PE and school sport is often the first experience of organised sport for children.

Each athlete experiences a unique journey and it is important to highlight, and understand, the uniqueness of the different social influences. To study these experiences, it can be helpful to examine the complexity of the social environment which surrounds the athlete, and the key individuals they interact with, by viewing it through a visual medium. One framework that achieves this is Henriksen et al.'s (2010) athletic talent development environment (ATDE) working model which draws on an approach where athletic development results from daily interactions between the athlete and their environment (see Figure 2.1 in Chapter 2).

This section of the book aims to examine the social influences on an athlete's developmental journey, which include a number of the features in Henriksen and colleagues' model, starting with the influence of the coach. In Chapter 6, *Coach-Athlete Relationships: The Role of Ability, Intentions and Integrity*, Sophia Jowett and Katelynn Slade critically discuss traditional approaches to coaching and propose a combined coach-athlete-centred approach, one that values both parties in the dyad equally. The chapter considers the components of a quality coach-athlete relationship and examines coach philosophy and the core values of ability, intentions, and integrity. There is a reflection on the darker side of coaching before concluding with an example of a practical tool that can be used to facilitate more effective coach-athlete relationships.

Communication in the coach-athlete relationship, described as the "fuel" for quality in the dyad (Jowett, 2018), can impact on the athlete experience. In Chapter 7, *Towards Mutual Understanding: Communication and Conflict in Coaching*, Lauren R. Tufton introduces types of communication and considers our use of language. The chapter examines the importance of communication in coaching and offers strategies for effective communication. The chapter moves on to a critical discussion of conflict within the coach-athlete relationship before concluding with a consideration of management strategies and the use of third-party interventions to support conflict resolution.

Having considered the relationship between the athlete and the coach, in Chapter 8, *Creating an Optimal Motivational Climate for Effective Coaching*, Iain Greenlees presents a critical overview of the coach's influence on athlete motivation. The chapter examines two key theories of motivation: self-determination theory and achievement goal theory, and how each can be applied to help us to understand the influence of the coach. This theoretical content is drawn on to consider how a coach can develop an empowering and effective motivational climate. The chapter concludes with a feature that examines other individuals who can impact on the motivational climate.

It is not only the coach that has an influence on the athletic development journey. In Chapter 9, *The Family Behind the Athlete*, Jessica Pinchbeck examines how parents and siblings can influence the sporting choices and opportunities available to a young athlete impacting on their long-term sporting journey. The chapter critically examines how levels, and types, of parental involvement can influence individuals, drawing on key theoretical content. The chapter concludes with an overview of attachment and how this can help us to understand familial relationships in sport.

In the final chapter of the section, Chapter 10, *How Does the School Setting Influence Athletic Development?*, Nichola Kentzer explores the role of educational settings in the introduction, and facilitation, of PE and school sport to young people and how this can be influential in athletic development. The chapter considers the impact of attending educational establishments which focus their efforts on the development of talented prospective elite athletes, and how key individuals, such as the PE teacher, can influence a young person's sporting experience. The chapter concludes with a practical consideration of how the PE teacher could promote an optimal environment for athletic development.

The five chapters in this section of the book demonstrate the complexity of the social influences that can impact on the athletic journey and attempt to inform the practice of coaches, sport psychologists, and other practitioners to support athletes' wellbeing and performance.

REFERENCES

Côté, J., Lidor, R., & Hackfort, D. (2009). ISSP position stand: To sample or to specialize? Seven postulates about youth sport activities that lead to continued participation and elite performance. *International Journal of Sport and Exercise Psychology*, *7*(1), 7–17.

Henriksen, K., Stambulova, N., & Roessler, K. K. (2010). Holistic approach to athletic talent development environments: A successful sailing milieu. *Psychology of Sport and Exercise*, *11*(3), 212–222.

Hogg, M. A., & Vaughan, G. M. (2018). *Social psychology* (8th ed.). Pearson Education Limited.

Jowett, S. (2018, February 19). Communication: The fuel of effective and successful coach-athlete relationships. *UK Coaching*. https://community.ukcoaching.org/spaces/10/welcome-and-general/blogs/general/11878/communication-the-fuel-of-effective-and-successful-coach-athlete-relationships

Jowett, S., & Shanmugam, V. (2016). Relational coaching in sport: Its psychological underpinnings and practical effectiveness. In R. J. Schinke, K. R. McGannon, & B. Smith (Eds.), *Routledge international handbook of sport psychology*. Taylor and Francis Ltd., pp. 471–484.

CHAPTER 6

Coach-Athlete Relationships

The Role of Ability, Intentions, and Integrity

Sophia Jowett and Katelynn Slade

There are many examples of high-profile coaches who have embraced and applied the notion of the "relational coaching environment" (Jowett & Shanmugam, 2016, p. 471) at the heart of which lies building good quality relationships. Coaches who have achieved the highest sport accolades with their athletes all over the world have talked openly about the role and significance of the coach-athlete relationship. They include Pep Guardiola (football), Mike Krzyzewski (basketball), Lisa Alexander (netball), Marcus Wiese and Danny Kerry (hockey), Aimee Boorman (gymnastics), Ans Botha (athletics), and Mel Marshall and Bob Bowman (swimming). It becomes immediately apparent that these coaches recognise the value of connecting with each athlete in their team signalling that they have nothing but their athletes' very best interests at heart. Such coaches become 'talent magnets' because athletes want to work with and for them.

Regardless of whether the sport environment emphasises performance or participation, it is undisputable that coaches' overarching aim is to support athletes to achieve their goals, meet their needs, support their development, and help them grow physiologically, socially, and psychologically. However, some coaches fall short. Some coaches may not fully understand the power of connecting, belonging, and relating with their athletes in the team or squad. These coaches may believe that by maintaining an impersonal approach they are fulfilling their role in a neutral and unbiased manner. Nonetheless, anecdotal and empirical evidence suggest that strong and healthy connections between coaches and athletes contribute to long-lasting and cumulative effects on coaches' and athletes' performances as well as mental health and wellbeing (e.g., Jowett et al., 2017). This chapter aims to discuss the role and significance of the coach-athlete relationship within the context of coaching while exploring ways to develop good quality, effective, and successful coach-athlete relationships.

COACH-ATHLETE RELATIONSHIP AND COACHING: WHAT IS THE LINK?

Over the years there has been a notable change to the process and practice of coaching. The way coaching is practised at this present time is somewhat different from the way it was practised 10 or so years ago. For example, Kidman (2005) highlighted a shift from a coach-centred to an athlete-centred approach to coaching and yet another shift was more recently observed where these two

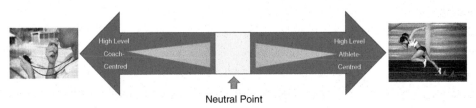

High Level
Coach-
Centred

Neutral Point

High Level
Athlete-
Centred

Neither Coach- nor Athlete-Centred Coaching

FIGURE 6.1 The diametrically opposite approaches to coaching: coach-centred and athlete-centred

approaches were combined (Jowett, 2017). In the *coach-centred approach*, the coach is the focus and is at the centre of coaching. In this approach the coach imparts and transmits knowledge and skills to the athletes. The coach has the biggest role to play by commanding and leading. As a result, the athlete has very little choice and s/he plays a passive role in the coaching process (see e.g., Evans, 2014). In the *athlete-centred approach*, the athlete is the focus and is at the centre of coaching. The athlete has the biggest role to play as s/he directs learning, asks questions, and even designs and completes tasks independently and in association with fellow athletes. As a result, the athlete is faced with a great deal of choice to fulfil their needs and wants and s/he plays an active role in the coaching process (Bowles & O'Dwyer, 2019; Headley-Cooper, 2010). These two approaches are portrayed *at the opposite ends of a continuum* (see Figure 6.1).

As Kidman (2005) explained, the opposite of athlete-centred coaching is coach-centred coaching and thus as a coach you can apply either approach. However, an over-emphasis on either the coach or on the athlete can lead to rigidity or can hamper flexibility. In a sport environment, like every achievement-orientated environment (e.g., school, work) where unpredictability and complexity are potent and common characteristics (cf. Edmondson, 2018), coaches and athletes are required to demonstrate adaptability or agility (e.g., Ritchie & Allen, 2015) in order to successfully deal with numerous circumstances that are presented to them including poor or inconsistent performances, selection versus deselection, injury, burnout, and other personal events outside sport (e.g., school, work).

In addition, a complete focus on either the coach or the athlete would seem unreasonable. For example, an athlete-centred approach neglects the coach's role in the same way a coach-centred approach neglects the athlete's role. With the emphasis shifting from the coach to the athlete in recent years, there is an obvious play down of the coach's role in the coaching process. A coach as an authority figure who has (or should have) the capacity in terms of the knowledge and experience, as well as skills and competence to influence, instruct, and guide the athlete/s is somewhat lost within the athlete-centred approach (Bowles & O'Dwyer, 2019). Coaches as much as athletes have an important role to play and need to be equally recognised and valued within the process and practice of coaching. Moreover, both approaches seem to pay inadequate attention to the central role the coach-athlete relationship plays within coaching. Coaches and athletes develop and maintain a relationship that can be characterised as either good, bad, or indifferent at any given time over the course of their sporting journey. However, neither approach provides a clear basis for togetherness or connection between the athlete and the coach. Instead, both approaches place emphasis on a single individual (coach or athlete) and sit diametrically opposite in the continuum of coaching. While Kidman (2005) within the athlete-centred approach and more recently Cooper and Allen (2018) within the coach-centred approach made references

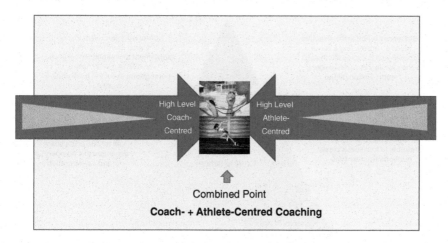

FIGURE 6.2 The combined coach-athlete approach to coaching

to relationship aspects such as trust and collaboration, such references are conceptually and by extension operationally confusing.

To address some of the shortcomings of the coach-centred and athlete-centred approaches to coaching, a *combined coach-athlete-centred approach* to coaching is proposed which has the coach-athlete relationship at its heart. This alternative approach not only provides a reconciliation of two diametrically opposing coaching approaches but also an opportunity to unravel the confusion and offer clarity. This approach values the coach and the athlete equally and considers their joint contributions. The combined approach embraces 'the give and take' that exists between coaches and athletes. Thus, the reciprocity that exists in coach-athlete interactions is key to genuine connection and provides a basis for growth, development, and progress. It allows for both freedom and choice (as per the athlete-centred) but also for structure and instruction (as per the coach-centred) within the coaching process and practice (see e.g., Côté & Gilbert, 2009). This approach underlines that coaching is an interpersonal affair where neither the coach nor the athlete can do it alone, neither of them has all the answers; they need one another for maximal effect (i.e., challenge and support). The interrelating between the coach and athlete is the focus of this combined approach and purposeful coach-athlete relationships are at the centre of coaching (see Figure 6.2).

The relationship between coaches and athletes has long been acknowledged as an important factor to coaching by psychologists (e.g., Greenleaf et al., 2001), pedagogists, and sociologists (e.g., Cushion, 2007). More recently, Jowett (2017) proposed that the quality of the relationship can serve as a measure of the effectiveness and success of coaching. The next section defines and describes good quality coach-athlete relationships.

WHAT DOES A GOOD QUALITY COACH-ATHLETE RELATIONSHIP LOOK LIKE?

It is neither random nor coincidental that high profile coaches such as Jurgen Klopp (Liverpool FC), Marcus Weise (former German Olympic Hockey Coach), Mel Marshall (GB Olympic Swimming Coach), Lisa Alexander (former Australian Netball Coach), and athletes such

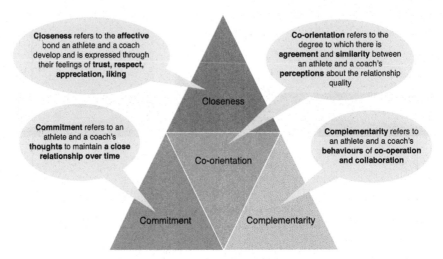

FIGURE 6.3 The 3+1Cs model of quality coach-athlete relationships

as Michael Phelps (USA, Olympic Champion), Jessica Ennis-Hill (GB, Olympic Champion), Wayde van Niekerk (SA, Olympic Champion), and Michael Jordan and Kobe Bryant (NBA legends) refer to the important role the coach-athlete relationship played in their sustained performance success and personal satisfaction in sport. It takes deliberate and systematic effort to develop coach-athlete relationships of the highest quality that are both effective and successful (see Jowett, 2007, for definitions as these relate to *effective* and *successful* relationships). However, what does a good quality coach-athlete relationship look like? How can we describe the relationship or connection coaches and athletes develop over the course of their sporting partnership? Can we differentiate between good- versus not-so-good-quality relationships? Can we objectively and tangibly capture such an elusive and complex phenomenon? The content and nature of coach-athlete relationships has been the focus of research for over 20 years. Jowett and colleagues have collected data (both qualitative and quantitative) from thousands of athletes and coaches over the years and found that the quality of the coach-athlete relationship can be summarised utilising the following four interpersonal constructs known as the 3+1Cs: closeness, commitment, complementarity, and co-orientation (see Figure 6.3). Brief descriptions of the 3+1Cs follow.

Closeness

The construct of closeness captures coaches' and athletes' interpersonal feelings or the affective tone of the relationship. Closeness contains four key relational properties: trust, respect, appreciation, and interpersonal liking. Trust is placing confidence in your coach/athlete and respect is treating each other well while appreciation is showing that you value your coach/athlete. Feelings of trust, respect, and appreciation are characteristics of reciprocal liking between the coach and the athlete. Liking signals that these two individuals have something in common and, importantly, a degree of understanding for one another.

Commitment

The construct of commitment captures coaches' and athletes' interpersonal thoughts, motivations, and willingness to maintain close ties over time. These thoughts suggest longevity, prospect, and prosper of the relationship. Commitment is the glue that unites two individuals through ups and downs, though good times (e.g., success) and not-so-good times (e.g., failures). Coaches'/athletes' commitment is tested and becomes extremely important especially during difficult and challenging times such as deselection, injury, burnout, or some other personal disruption.

Complementarity

The construct of complementarity is synonymous to co-operation and captures coaches' and athletes' co-operative acts of interaction. Co-operation includes such interpersonal behaviours as being responsive to each other's efforts; being receptive, open, approachable, and friendly (as opposed to distant, cold, and hostile); and being relaxed and comfortable in each other's presence (as opposed to tensed and stressed). Complementarity also captures the specific roles coaches and athletes assume in the relationship. Coaches are the leaders, instructors, and orchestrators and athletes are the executors, makers, and doers.

Co-orientation

The construct of co-orientation simply captures the degree to which there is shared knowledge and understanding between the coach and the athlete (e.g., how much do each know and understand the other?) reflecting their perceptual consensus or common ground. The existence of a common ground is important because it promotes better and more positive coach-athlete interactions and supports the discussion and resolution of conflict if/when it occurs.

The 3+1Cs provide a conceptual description of the coach-athlete relationship and offer a framework to assess the relationship quality. Since the conception of the 3+1Cs in addition to the corresponding measures being developed and validated (see Jowett, 2009; Jowett & Ntoumanis, 2004), quantitative research has investigated the correlates of the coach-athlete relationship quality, such as personality and gender (individual characteristics), level of participation and type of sport (social-cultural), length and type of relationship (relationship-based), and outcomes such as motivation and confidence (intrapersonal), satisfaction, and conflict (interpersonal), as well as collective efficacy and team cohesion (group-based; see Figure 6.4).

This research has shown that good quality coach-athlete relationships are likely to experience low levels of perceived conflict (Wachsmuth et al., 2018b), fear of failure (Sagar & Jowett, 2015), burnout (Davis et al., 2019), exhaustion (Davis et al., 2018), and threat and stress appraisal (Nicholls et al., 2016). Moreover, good quality coach-athlete relationships are likely to experience high levels of motivation (Adie & Jowett, 2010), positive coach behaviours (Jowett et al., 2017), team cohesion (e.g., Jowett et al., 2012), and collective efficacy (Roberto et al., 2019). Importantly, good quality relationships are associated with high levels of both performance and wellbeing, including high levels of life satisfaction, self-actualisation, and positive affect (e.g., Davis & Jowett, 2014). Subsequently, coaches and athletes who want to thrive through their sport should focus on creating an environment that is based on the combined coach-athlete approach where the relationship is at the heart of coaching.

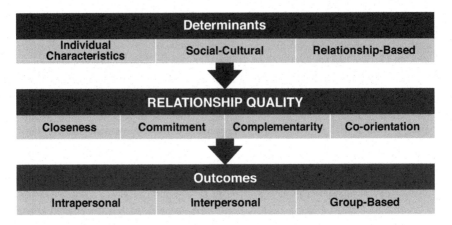

FIGURE 6.4 Determinants and outcomes of the coach-athlete relationship quality

APPLIED CASE STUDIES

The quality of the relationship depends on coaches' and athletes' make-up including their memories, perceptions, feelings, and past interactions as well as expectations and hopes for the future (e.g., Davis et al., 2013). The two case studies that follow provide information about the nature and content of the coach-athlete relationship as well as other cues related to different individual, environmental, and temporal characteristics that impact the relationship quality and in turn the effectiveness of interactions. An understanding of the interplay of these characteristics is key in fully appreciating the past, present, and future of relationships.

CASE STUDY 6.1

Empowering the Relationship and Empowering Both the Athlete and the Coach

Ella (coach) starts the season with a new team of players. She is enthusiastic, organised, and energised (and somewhat anxious)—her initial aim is to get to know each player in the team. While Ella is not the most outgoing or extraverted coach, she values human connection and feels that players need to be understood. She wants to find out through one-to-one conversations about her players' goals, aspirations, motivations, likes, dislikes, and preferences; she also wants to know a little bit about their personal background (e.g., family, school, work). The creation of an environment where there are open channels of communication is one of Ella's main priorities and something that she wants to sustain for as long as she works with this team of players. Ella has been coaching for a while; however, she has little experience as a player herself. She loves coaching and is passionate about sport and all that it offers. Ella appreciates other aspects of life like travelling, listening to music, and rock climbing. She also has a family and her dogs are very much part of it. Her two children often come to training and watch their mum coach and Ella hardly ever misses the opportunity to talk about her children and her dogs to her players. The team of players seem to be welcoming Ella's coaching approach and there is a sense of anticipation and excitement at the start of each session. Ella uses autonomous supportive coaching behaviours; she allows choice, asks questions, listens, and praises players. She made sure to clarify at the job interview that there is no room in her coaching for punishment, control, and intimidation. It was also clear in the interview that she leads by example with humility. Her autonomous supportive style of coaching is coupled with creating a task-involving climate where emphasis is placed on self/athlete-improvement, learning, co-operation, and individual effort. Ella has, however, made clear to her players that she is a competitive coach and as a result she wants to create a competitive team. She also wants to focus on creating a positive environment where there is structure—a clear framework within which players operate. Moreover, there is no room for favouritism and Ella wants to work to eradicate any sense of bias or unfairness; she wants all players to feel they are treated well and fairly. Ella had a couple of team meetings discussing and clarifying with the players the mission, purpose, and goals. The players seem to be satisfied with the levels of support, instruction, and leadership they are provided thus far and have enjoyed spending time on a one-to-one basis with the coach. They are clear about their individual and team goals, what they need to do to be selected in competition, and the expectations in training and competition. They reported that this level of clarity has helped them feel less stressed and less threatened. Athletes commented that because Ella is making every effort to get to know them all well, she is able to tailor the training to meet their needs not only physically (technical and tactical) but also psychosocially. She knows which 'chord to strike' to motivate them and to give them the confidence they need without making them feel undervalued or misunderstood. They look forward to the competitive season starting soon, following several weeks of preparation and building connections. Ella so far seems to have conveyed to her players messages of trust, respect, appreciation, commitment, responsibility, and cooperation—all of which contribute to the development of good quality coach-athlete relationships.

CASE STUDY 6.2

Disempowering the Relationship and Immobilising Both the Athlete and the Coach

Robert is the new coach of a programme that has been struggling in recent years. Robert is looking forward to forging a new path and pushing his players to get results, no matter the cost. Robert is a coach with an accomplished track record and truly believes in his coaching philosophy and approach. Robert values performance, goal attainment, and obedience which he makes clear to the team at the start of the season. Robert spends little effort engaging with his players outside of training and prefers to stick to conversations around sport and performance. The players have feelings of apprehension at Robert's approach as there is very little input on their part, but they initially believe in him as Robert reassures them that his approach can be successful if they stick with it. At the beginning of the season, the team is performing the best it ever has with Robert as the coach. The players and Robert feel they have a connection and while training is unforgiving and relentless, the success in competition provides the comfort they need. However, after a poor performance by the team resulting in the first loss of the season, Robert becomes frustrated and angry with his team, singling out and placing blame on a few players for the loss. The singled-out players felt humiliated in front of the team and the players who were not affected directly felt deflated and uninspired. The next day at the training practice, Robert uses excessive physical training as a punishment for the poor performance. Team and individual confidence decrease as a result of Robert's handling of the team's first loss. The players start to question their commitment to their coach and the programme. The team's performance continues to decline. Robert's frustration and anger grows, and he increasingly begins to belittle and humiliate players for making mistakes. Robert also starts to 'kick' players out of drills or training sessions who are not performing up to standard as "those players are wasting everyone's time". Continuing an impersonal and authoritarian (lacking support and motivation) approach, a number of players decide to voice their feelings to the team captain. The team captain holds a one-to-one meeting with Robert to discuss the concerns of the players. Robert doesn't listen to the team captain and players' concerns because his way has "always worked in the past and no one has complained before". Robert continues to use excessive physical training as punishment and belittlement as means to motivate the players. The team reports that after voicing their concerns and needs multiple times to Robert, he refuses to engage with the team to work on a new approach. The athletes no longer trust Robert as a coach and question his intentions; the realisation that he does not care about their needs or perspectives and that he is not prepared to work with/for them fills them with dissatisfaction. The majority of the players are now convinced that this environment is far from ideal; fear and intimidation have affected their motivation, confidence, and wellbeing. Robert is not the coach they needed or wanted and so the team are considering their next move.

WHAT DOES THE DARK SIDE OF THE COACH-ATHLETE RELATIONSHIP LOOK LIKE?

A poor quality coach-athlete relationship can be just as impactful as a good quality relationship built upon mutual trust, respect, commitment, and cooperation. High-profile stories from athletes who have experienced the dark side of the coach-athlete relationship have been told by athletes such as Mary Cain (USA, runner) and Laurie Hernandez (USA, Olympic gymnast). Mary released her story in the *New York Times* in 2019 detailing her experience while training under Alberto Salazar at Nike (Cain, 2019). Mary reported being subjected to psychological abuse and weight control by her coach. Salazar was described as exerting controlling and intrusive behaviour, affecting her emotionally and physically. Laurie's story recounted instances of being called "weak, lazy or messed up in the head" by her coach that left her at times frozen and crying in the training gym when she was just an adolescent (Macur, 2020, para 2).

The sexual, psychological, and physical abuse, and neglect of athletes by their coaches has been brought to the forefront of current sport safeguarding concerns and athlete protection and wellbeing (see Chapter 14). The sexual exploitation and abuse of athletes has received much-needed attention in research as athletes have narrated experiences of coaches *using, taking advantage of, and manipulating* their position of trust for personal gain (Hartill, 2014) that has left athletes with lasting effects such as guilt, shame, decreased confidence, disordered eating, and other mental health issues (Brackenridge, 2001; Kerr et al., 2019). Non-sexual forms of abuse, such as psychological, physical, and neglect, are also experienced by athletes in sport from their coaches with psychological abuse experienced the most (Kerr et al., 2019; McPherson et al., 2017). Belittlement, scapegoating, humiliation, excessive physical training, and denial of attention and support can have impactful and lasting effects much like sexual exploitation and abuse (Stirling & Kerr, 2013). Notably, sexual, psychological, and physical abuse have been found to be experienced at a higher prevalence in elite sport because typically the only measure of success is winning and winning at all costs (e.g., Vertommen et al., 2016).

Accounts of damaging and psychologically abusive coach-athlete relationships are not new in the literature (see Stirling & Kerr, 2009). However, while the coach-athlete relationship may provide the context or situation within which inappropriate and unacceptable acts take place, the same type of relationship also provides the context or situation where two people genuinely connect to achieve their goals and aspirations (see Jowett & Wachsmuth, 2020). What differentiates one relationship from another is the degree to which their relationship is an authentic and genuine one. An authentic and purposeful, good quality relationship (defined as having high levels of 3+1Cs) provides a sound platform from which relationship members act in ways that value each other as well as the opportunity to grow and develop separately and together. In this relationship, the athlete and the coach support and challenge one another because they want to be the best they can be, not only for oneself but for each other. Subsequently, in such relationships power is shared between the coach and athlete—power is a characteristic that serves the relationship and not the individual in the relationship. If power becomes a characteristic that serves one person in the relationship (e.g., power that is controlled and harboured by the coach), it is inevitable that the other would feel powerless and so the lack of power is likely to hold them back (e.g., the athlete feels disempowered and trapped). As Jowett and Wachsmuth (2020) explained, viewing power as something that both coaches and athletes have and hold may help prevent abuse in sport and in coaching more specifically.

Conflict and negative feelings associated with it can exist even when the coach-athlete relationship is characterised by high levels of trust, respect, commitment, and co-operation (i.e., high levels of 3+1Cs) because of the high stakes within the sporting environment (Wachsmuth et al., 2017). Conflict is likely to be dealt with very differently when coach-athlete relationships are damaged or broken such as when there is abuse and exploitation in interactions. For example, when potential conflictual situations arise, such as a disagreement or expressed dissatisfaction about selection or conversations surrounding body weight, they are managed with an imbalance of power and control rather than with mutual care, appreciation, respect, and responsiveness. Managing these challenging situations with disproportionate power and control harboured by the coach not only exacerbates existing psychological abuse but also creates the potential for psychological abuse between coaches and athletes who had no previous history of abuse by tipping the balance of power one way and destabilising or undermining a previously high quality coach-athlete relationship. The effects of this breakdown can cause feelings of being mistreated, insulted, or exploited and can consequently lead to decreased motivation and enjoyment, anger, anxiety, and performance decrements in athletes (Stirling & Kerr, 2013). Athletes who find themselves in such circumstances may feel powerless and defenceless which signals that the relationship with the coach is no longer purposeful and authentic, compromising the quality of the relationship.

WHAT HAS THE COACHING PHILOSOPHY GOT TO DO WITH AUTHENTIC COACH-ATHLETE RELATIONSHIPS?

Quality coach-athlete relationships characterised by high levels of trust, respect, appreciation and liking (closeness), intentions to maintain a close relationship over time through ups and downs (commitment), responsiveness, receptiveness, friendliness, and easiness (complementarity), as well as common ground (shared knowledge and understanding) underpin *connections* that are purposeful and productive for both coaches and athletes. In a good quality relationship, athletes gain a great deal of satisfaction because these relationships provide the platform for their improvement, learning, and growth within their chosen sport (see e.g., Mageau & Vallerand, 2003). Therefore, coaches want to know *how to best achieve performance improvements for their athletes*. While not an easy question to answer, one plausible answer in maximising performance is unlocking athletes' *potential*. Here coaching focusses more on athletes' future possibilities rather than current performance. If coaches don't believe that their athletes have hidden capacity waiting to be released, then they won't try hard enough to help them release it. Hockey coach Marcus Weise said in an interview, "When you coach you need to find a door that enables you to get access to the player" highlighting that coaches can only get the best out of their athletes if they reach out to, and connect with, them at a deeper level (see also Wachsmuth et al., 2020).

It is also common that athletes exceed their own expectations and those of their coach (see self- and coach-fulfilling prophecy; e.g., Solomon, 2010) suggesting that we simply don't know what athletes are hiding and thus it is a coach's job is to keep trying to find ways to untap the resource and turn it into performance. Coaches are not alone in this endeavour; athletes can play a key role in exploring and discovering with their coaches what works and what doesn't. Coach Mike Spracklen (1988 Olympic gold medallist [rowing]) said "I taught them all that I know technically . . . but this opens up the possibility of going further, for they can feel things that I can't see" (Fieldhouse, 2014). Essentially, effective coaching can and should take athletes beyond the limitation of coaches' own knowledge. Coaches can work with their athletes' knowledge, experience, and perceptions over and beyond their own. This may become increasingly important as the athletes develop and grow. Overall, coaching delivers results in large measure often due to the ways coaches and athletes relate, interact, and communicate.

Researchers (e.g., Chan & Mallett, 2011) acknowledge that interpersonal knowledge and social skills can help coaches interact effectively with their athletes. For coaches to fully integrate the coach-athlete relationship in the process and practice of their coaching or the combined coach-athlete approach to coaching, they will need to make this key relationship an integral part of their coaching philosophy. A coaching philosophy captures one's core values as well as guides actions—for example, what goals will be selected—and helps with how to achieve them. It allows coaches to improve their practice and better understand and meet the needs of their athletes (Nash et al., 2008). *Ability, intentions,* and *integrity* are core values attached to good quality relationships and positive interpersonal behaviours emerging from our research (e.g., Jowett & Cockerill, 2003) and from other researchers (e.g., Lara-Bercial & Mallett, 2016). It is proposed that making these core values part of one's coaching philosophy, not only would support coaches to navigate authentic and purposeful relationships with athletes but would also help coaches to make significant investments in their athletes. Such investments are likely to pay dividends in both the short and long run and contribute to athletes and coaches achieving both personal and interpersonal goals. The following sections describe the three core values.

Ability as a Coach

A primary responsibility for a coach is to perform the job with distinction and responsibility. Knowing one's sport (e.g., x's and o's, technical and tactical) or becoming a master of one's sport is a critical aspect because this knowledge fills athletes with the confidence that the coach has the capacity to teach and help them to reach their goals. At whatever level coaches operate and regardless of their skills, experiences, and qualifications, there is always room for further improvement. Athletes want to count on their coaches for information and want to view their coaches as competent and well-informed with the courage to make tough decisions and take risks, too. If a coach talks with the necessary competence, conviction, and sincerity, then s/he has space to focus on genuinely caring for their athletes. As football coach Jurgen Klopp said:

> I try everything to be as successful as possible . . . confidence is very important for a leader. . . . If I expect from myself that I know everything and I am the best at everything, I couldn't have confidence. I know I am good at a couple of things, really good at a few things . . . I need experts around me, having strong people around you with better knowledge in different departments than yourself. . . . That's leadership.
>
> (Shaw, 2019)

Coaches need to have the desire and passion to continually learn and, of importance, fill their athletes with confidence that they are capable to challenge and support them to achieve their goals.

Intentions as a Coach

Athletes want to be treated fairly and directly by their coaches and want to know that their coaches have their best interests at heart. In sport, there is no room for manipulation, intimidation, bullying, hostility, or exploitation. Such situations are unacceptable and damaging for the coaches and for the athletes. When athletes enter a new coach-athlete relationship, they might like to ask their new coaches the following questions: What are your intentions towards me? Are you going to treat me the best possible way? Athletes want coaches who are reliable and responsible; they want to have coaches who would help them achieve their short- and long-term goals while treating them fairly. For that reason, it is important that coaches spell out their positive intentions while ensuring that athletes know and understand them. In addition, coaches would need to frequently check whether their good intentions align with their coaching practices and leadership behaviours. Alignment of a coach's intentions and actions contributes to coaching that is both effective and successful. As coach Mike Krzyzewski explained, "In my relationships, I want you to believe me when I tell you that you are great *and* I want you to believe me when I tell you that you are not working hard enough" (UC Santa Barbara, n.d.). Athletes need to have faith in their coaches and coaches need to instill confidence in their athletes. This gives the coach-athlete relationship the potential to become stronger and last longer.

Integrity as a Coach

Integrity is more than honesty; it is about coaches knowing and understanding their athletes including their values, strengths, ambitions, weaknesses, and fears. Equipped with this knowledge and understanding, coaches can speak and act in ways that make their athletes feel valued, motivated, and inspired. Honesty is important and often encompassed within coaches' integrity. However, while coaches are honest by acting in line with what they said they will do, what they actually say and do may be in direct contrast to what athletes believe and value. This is often due to coaches not knowing and understanding their athletes; these coaches fail to view the world though their athletes' eyes. This discrepancy in perspectives, beliefs, and values can cause distrust. Distrust fuels a lot of problems in the coach-athlete relationship. For example, an athlete who says, "I distrust my coach" and "I avoid you and don't hear you because ultimately you are in it for self-serving reasons and not for me". Distrust is closely associated with respect, appreciation, and liking. The more the distrust, the less the openness in relationships. To avoid a situation like this, coaches need to listen and learn their athletes' values so that coaches can speak and act in ways they value. Coaches need to continuously ask themselves, "Do I know my athletes' values and what they stand for?" Being able to communicate with your athletes is the first step towards building shared knowledge. Shared knowledge eases interactions between coaches and athletes. Coach Lisa Alexander said,

> My job is all about communicating. . . . Saying the right thing at the right time can really motivate someone to deliver a performance that is very special. . . . There's always a line in the sand around how you are behaving toward the people you are caring for.
>
> (Gray, 2018)

Ability, intentions, and *integrity* are three core values that drive coaches' interpersonal behaviours and the formation of purposeful and productive coach-athlete relationships (e.g., Jowett & Cockerill, 2003; Lara-Bercial & Mallett, 2016). Such a value system is centred on viewing coaching practice and process as an interpersonal, social, or relational affair involving both the coach and the athlete. It provides a solid base of operation that should be flexible enough to embrace the individual athlete in a team or squad however small or large (Gould et al., 2017). Athletes who are entering a new sport environment including a new relationship with a coach will do well to ask about their coach's coaching philosophy and note whether ability, intentions, and integrity form part of it.

WHAT CAN ATHLETES AND COACHES DO TO DEVELOP BETTER RELATIONSHIPS WITH ONE ANOTHER?

Jowett et al. (2020), taking a long-term view on athletic development, suggested that building good quality relationships would require *both* the coach and the athlete to care for one another. It was put forward that care is a reciprocal concept within the coach-athlete relationship and thus not only the coach but also the athlete has a role to play (Jowett et al., 2020); it was further acknowledged that acts of care are squashed in poor quality relationships where distrust, hostility, and selfishness dominate (see Cronin & Armour, 2018). In good quality relationships, caring is manifested through expressing one's interest, concern, and attention for the other, leading to coaches adapting a more personalised, individualised, relational approach or applying a combined coach-athlete-centred approach to coaching (Jowett, 2017). In 2002, Gould and colleagues found that coaches of Olympic champions took time to individualise programmes, provide individual attention, meet individual needs, and understand his/her athlete as a person. To do so, a coach and an athlete have a mutual responsibility to develop and maintain good quality coach-athlete relationships. Ultimately, the relationship becomes a unique interpersonal space for transformation to occur just like the ones described by Gould and colleagues, and others (e.g., Lara-Bercial & Mallet, 2016).

To provide a medium to support coach development drawing on the latest research, the Coach-Athlete Relationship Empowerment (CARE), an online educational programme, was developed with financial support from the Olympic Centre Studies of the International Olympic Committee. The programme is detailed in the spotlight box that follows.

Spotlight On: Developing *Care* in the Coach-Athlete Relationship

CARE was developed to support athletes in gaining knowledge and understanding about the role and significance of the coach-athlete relationship. CARE aims to raise awareness by appealing to athletes to play an active role in building good quality relationships. Jowett et al. (2020) explained that the rationale for placing the athlete at the centre of this programme, was that coaches are likely to receive similar information through other means (e.g., courses, mentors, coach developers, alternative online offerings). CARE revolves around three well-researched themes: relationship quality (e.g., Jowett & Shanmugam, 2016), interpersonal conflict (e.g., Wachsmuth et al., 2018a), and communication (Rhind & Jowett, 2012). Jowett et al.'s (2020) intervention highlighted that CARE helps athletes know and understand

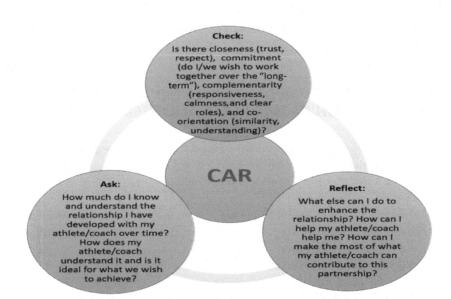

FIGURE 6.5 CAR: Check (self-check), Ask (other check), Reflect (feedback and feedforward)

the significance and purpose of good quality relationships. The online CARE educational programme can serve as a medium to empower athletes with knowledge and skills that they can readily use to build and/or maintain better working coach-athlete partnerships. CARE can be accessed here: https://vimeo.com/254342826 (preview) and http://bit.ly/care-course "Empowering the Athlete: The Coach-Athlete Partnership" (free on-line course).

CARE highlights that the relationship is an important vehicle in making coaches and athletes' sporting journeys meaningful and rewarding experiences. Relationships are dynamic; they change and evolve over time, so both coaches and athletes need to monitor the coach-athlete relationship. A simple way to ensure the relationship is taken care of is to utilise: Check, Ask, and Reflect (CAR; see Figure 6.5). To do this, three questions should be asked: (1) What do I think about the relationship? (this is a self-check against the 3+1Cs), (2) What does the other person (coach/athlete) in the relationship think about it? (this is another check and an opportunity to discuss how each person views the relationship [employing the 3+1Cs]) and (3) How can I/we based on what I/we know make this relationship better and stronger? (this is about using the feedback [past experiences, interactions, assessments] to feedforward and thus plan for further relationship improvements).

CAR is a simple way to assess the quality of the relationship and ensure that it is a healthy and harmonious one. The coach-athlete relationship is a phenomenon that concerns two people and thus both are required to make an effort and invest time and energy in making the relationship effective and successful—as the old saying has it: "It takes two to tango".

CLOSING THOUGHTS

Coaching has evolved over the past decades. A shift has been noted from coach-centred coaching to athlete-centred coaching to, more recently, a combined coach-athlete-centred approach. Coaching as a process and a practice, involving both the coach and athlete, provides more opportunities for growth and development where each of them support and challenge the other. The combined coach-athlete-centred coaching approach places the relationship these two people develop at the heart of coaching. A good quality relationship revolves around the 3+1Cs: closeness, commitment, complementarity, and co-orientation. Coaches and athletes have an important role to play in developing and maintaining good quality coach-athlete relationships. The integration of such core values as ability, intentions, and integrity in the coaching philosophy may support coaches in developing better working relationships with their athletes and in safeguarding against poor quality coach-athlete relationships. Even when coaches and athletes experience difficult and complex circumstances (e.g., poor performances, deselection, ill-health), coaches' core values can help navigate interactions. More research to understand the links between coach and athlete value systems, philosophies, practices, and athlete (and coach) satisfaction, wellbeing, mental health, and performance is warranted (e.g., Cassidy et al., 2009).

A focus on the coach-athlete relationship signals a new era for coaching, where coaching is a shared activity and responsibility. Coaches and athletes who make a conscious and deliberate effort to invest in their relationships can pay dividends in both the short and long term. Relationships are evolving as much as the people comprising them and are in need of continuous revitalisation. Subsequently, coaches and athletes need to have their finger on the *relationship* 'pulse' and make every effort to regularly communicate their interests, values, opinions, attitudes, and character. Ultimately, a good quality relationship creates an effective coaching situation where both the coach and the athlete feel safe and valued, and their interactions are sincere and honest, instead of restrained and shallow. Importantly, a good quality coach-athlete relationship is paramount because it has the capacity to become an important vehicle that takes the athlete and the coach on a journey of growth and development that is enjoyable and its destination worth pursuing.

REFERENCES

Adie, J. W., & Jowett, S. (2010). Meta-perceptions of the coach–athlete relationship, achievement goals, and intrinsic motivation among sport participants. *Journal of Applied Social Psychology*, *40*(11), 2750–2773.

Bowles, R., & O'Dwyer, A. (2019). Athlete-centred coaching: Perspectives from the sideline. *Sports Coaching Review*, 1–22.

Brackenridge, C. H. (2001). *Spoilsports: Understanding and preventing sexual exploitation in sport*. Routledge.

Cain, M. (2019, November 7). I was the fastest girl in America, until I joined Nike. *The New York Times*. www.nytimes.com/2019/11/07/opinion/nike-running-mary-cain.html

Cassidy, T., Jones, R., & Potrac, P. (2009). *Understanding sports coaching: The social, cultural and pedagogical foundations of coaching practice* (2nd ed.). Routledge.

Chan, J. T., & Mallett, C. J. (2011). The value of emotional intelligence for high performance coaching. *International Journal of Sports Science & Coaching, 6*(1), 315–328.

Cooper, D., & Allen, J. B. (2018). The coaching process of the expert coach: A coach led approach. *Sports Coaching Review, 7*(2), 142–170.

Côté, J., & Gilbert, W. (2009). An integrative definition of coaching effectiveness and expertise. *International Journal of Sports Science and Coaching, 4*(3), 307–323.

Cronin, C., & Armour, K. (2018). *Care in sport coaching: Pedagogical cases.* Routledge.

Cushion, C. (2007). Modelling the complexity of the coaching process. *International Journal of Sports Science & Coaching, 2*(4), 395–401.

Davis, L., & Jowett, S. (2014). Coach–athlete attachment and the quality of the coach–athlete relationship: Implications for athlete's well-being. *Journal of Sports Sciences, 32*(15), 1454–1464.

Davis, L., Appleby, R., Davis, P., Wetherell, M., & Gustafsson, H. (2018). The role of coach-athlete relationship quality in team sport athletes' psychophysiological exhaustion: Implications for physical and cognitive performance. *Journal of Sports Sciences, 36*(17), 1985–1992.

Davis, L., Jowett, S., & Lafraniere, MA. (2013). An attachment theory perspective in the examination of relational processes associated with coach-athlete dyads. *Journal of Sport and Exercise Psychology, 35*, 156–167.

Davis, L., Stenling, A., Gustafsson, H., Appleby, R., & Davis, P. (2019). Reducing the risk of athlete burnout: Psychosocial, sociocultural, and individual considerations for coaches. *International Journal of Sports Science & Coaching, 14*(4), 444–452.

Edmondson, A. C. (2018). *The fearless organization: Creating psychological safety in the workplace for learning, innovation, and growth.* John Wiley & Sons.

Evans, J. (2014). The nature and importance of coach-player relationships in the uptake of game sense by elite rugby coaches in Australia and New Zealand. In R. Light, J. Quay, S. Harvey, & A. Mooney (Eds.), *Contemporary developments in games teaching* (pp. 133–146). Routledge.

Fieldhouse, P. (2014). *How to maximise your teams performance through coaching.* www.legal-island.com/articles/uk/features/hr/2014/mar/how-to-maximise-your-teams-performance-through-coaching/

Gould, D., Dieffenbach, K., & Moffett, A. (2002). Psychological characteristics and their development in Olympic champions. *Journal of Applied Sport Psychology, 14*(3), 172–204.

Gould, D., Pierce, S. M., Cowburn, I. H. J., & Driska, A. (2017). How coaching philosophy drives coaching action: A case study of renowned wrestling coach J Robinson. *International Sport Coaching Journal/ISCJ, 4*(1), 13–37. https://doi.org/10.1123/iscj.2016-0052

Gray, I. (2018). *Why Lisa Alexander wants our next prime minister to be a netball player.* https://mbs.edu/news/why-lisa-alexander-wants-our-next-prime-minister-to-be-a-netball-player

Greenleaf, C. A., Gould, D., & Dieffenbach, K. (2001). Factors influencing Olympic performance: Interviews with Atlanta and Nagano U.S. Olympians. *Journal of Applied Sport Psychology, 13*, 179–209.

Hartill, M. (2014). Exploring narratives of boyhood sexual subjection in Male-sport. *Sociology of Sport Journal, 31*(1), 23–43.

Headley-Cooper, K. (2010). *Coaches' perspectives on athlete-centred coaching* [Master of Science]. Toronto: University of Toronto.

Jowett, S. (2007). Interdependence analysis and the 3 + 1Cs in the coach-athlete relationship. In S. Jowett & D. Lavallee (Eds.), *Social psychology in sport* (pp. 15–27). Human Kinetics.

Jowett, S. (2009). Validating coach-athlete relationship measures with the nomological network. *Measurement in Physical Education and Exercise Science, 13,* 1–18.

Jowett, S. (2017). Coaching effectiveness: The coach–athlete relationship at its heart. *Current Opinion in Psychology, 16,* 154–158.

Jowett, S., Adie, J. W., Bartholomew, K. J., Yang, S. X., Gustafsson, H., & Lopez-Jiménez, A. (2017). Motivational processes in the coach-athlete relationship: A multi-cultural self-determination approach. *Psychology of Sport and Exercise, 32,* 143–152.

Jowett, S., & Cockerill, I. M. (2003). Olympic medallists' perspective of the athlete–coach relationship. *Psychology of Sport and Exercise, 4,* 313–331.

Jowett, S., Nicolas, M., & Yang, S. (2017). Unravelling the links between coach behaviours and coach-athlete relationships. *European Journal of Sports & Exercise Science, 5*(3), 10–19.

Jowett, S., & Ntoumanis, N. (2004). The Coach–Athlete Relationship Questionnaire (CART–Q): Development and initial validation. *Scandinavian Journal of Medicine and Science in Sports, 14,* 245–257.

Jowett, S., & Shanmugam, V. (2016). Relational coaching in sport: Its psychological underpinnings and practical effectiveness. In R. Schinke, K. R. McGannon, & B. Smith (Eds.), *Routledge international handbook of sport psychology* (pp. 471–484). Routledge.

Jowett, S., Shanmugam, V., & Caccoulis, S. (2012). Collective efficacy as a mediator of the association between interpersonal relationships and athlete satisfaction in team sports. *International Journal of Sport and Exercise Psychology, 10*(1), 66–78.

Jowett, S., & Wachsmuth, S. (2020). Power in coach-athlete relationships: The case of the women's artistic gymnastics. In R. Kerr, N. Barker-Ruchti, C. Stewart, & G. Kerr (Eds.), *Women's artistic gymnastics: Socio-cultural perspectives.* Routledge.

Jowett, S., Wachsmuth, S., Shanmugam-Felton, V., Zhong, X., & Harwood, C. (2020). Coach-Athlete Relationship Empowerment (CARE): An online educational programme. Manuscript under review.

Kerr, G. A., Willson, E., & Stirling, A. E. (2019). *Prevalence of maltreatment among current and former national team athletes.* https://athletescan.com/sites/default/files/images/prevalence_of_maltreatment_reporteng.pdf

Kidman, L. (2005). *Athlete-centred coaching: Developing inspired and inspiring people.* Innovative Print Communications.

Lara-Bercial, S., & Mallett, C. J. (2016). The practices and developmental pathways of professional and Olympic serial winning coaches. *International Sport Coaching Journal, 3*(3), 221–239.

Macur, J. (2020, May 1). Olympic gymnast recalls emotional abuse "so twisted that I thought it couldn't be real". *The New York Times.* www.nytimes.com/2020/05/01/sports/maggie-haney-gymnastics-abuse.html?auth=login-google

Mageau, G. A., & Vallerand, R. J. (2003). The coach-athlete relationship: A motivational model. *Journal of Sports Science, 21*(11), 663–904.

McPherson, L., Long, M., Nicholson, M., Cameron, N., Atkins, P., & Morris, M. E. (2017). Children's experience of sport in Australia. *International Review for the Sociology of Sport, 52*(5), 551–569.

Nash, C. S., Sproule, J., & Horton, P. (2008). Sport coaches' perceived role frames and philosophies. *International Journal of Sports Science & Coaching, 3*(4), 539–554.

Nicholls, A. R., Levy, A. R., Jones, L., Meir, R., Radcliffe, J. N., & Perry, J. L. (2016). Committed relationships and enhanced threat levels: Perceptions of coach behavior, the coach–athlete relationship, stress appraisals, and coping among athletes. *International Journal of Sports Science & Coaching, 11*(1), 16–26.

Rhind, D. J. A., & Jowett, S. (2012). Development of the coach-athlete relationship maintenance questionnaire (CARM-Q). *International Journal of Sports Science & Coaching, 7*(1), 121–137.

Ritchie, D., & Allen, J. (2015). 'Let them get on with it': Coaches' perceptions of their roles and coaching practices during Olympic and Paralympic games. *International Sport Coaching Journal, 2,* 108–124.

Roberto, A. N. Junior, J., Fiorese, L., Luiz, L. Vieira, J., Ferreira, L., . . . & Vissoci, J. R. (2019). Coach-athlete relationship and collective efficacy in volleyball: Is the association explained by athletes' goal orientations? *Motricidade, 15,* 1–11. http://doi.org/10.6063/motricidade.14147

Sagar, S. S., & Jowett, S. (2015). Fear of failure and self-control in the context of coach-athlete relationship quality. *International Journal of Coaching Science, 9*(2).

Shaw, C. (2019). *Jürgen Klopp explains his approach to leadership.* www.liverpoolfc.com/news/first-team/351529-jurgen-klopp-leadership-interview-liverpool

Solomon, G. B. (2010). The influence of coach expectations on athlete development. *Journal of Sport Psychology in Action, 1*(2), 76–85.

Stirling, A. E., & Kerr, G. A. (2009). Abused athletes' perceptions of the coach-athlete relationship. *Sport in Society, 12*(2), 227–239.

Stirling, A. E., & Kerr, G. A. (2013). The perceived effects of elite athletes' experiences of emotional abuse in the coach-athlete relationship. *International Journal of Sport and Exercise Psychology, 11*(1), 87–100.

UC Santa Barbara. (n.d.). *Trust by Mike Krzyzewski.* https://sites.cs.ucsb.edu/~mikec/cs48/misc/quotes/trust.html

Vertommen, T., Veldhoven, N. S., Wouters, K., Kampen, J. K., Brackenridge, C. H., Rhind, D. J. A., Neels, K., & Van Den Eede, F. (2016). Interpersonal violence against children in sport in the Netherlands and Belgium. *Child Abuse & Neglect, 51,* 223–236.

Wachsmuth, S., Jowett, S., & Harwood, C. G. (2017). Conflict among athletes and their coaches: What is the theory and research so far? *International Review of Sport and Exercise Psychology, 10*(1), 84–107.

Wachsmuth, S., Jowett, S., & Harwood, C. G. (2018a). Managing conflict in coach–athlete relationships. *Sport, Exercise, and Performance Psychology, 7*(4), 371.

Wachsmuth, S., Jowett, S., & Harwood, C. G. (2018b). On understanding the nature of interpersonal conflict between coaches and athletes. *Journal of Sports Sciences, 36*(17), 1955–1962.

Wachsmuth, S., Weise, M., Jowett, S., & Höner, O. (2020). Die Trainer-Athlet Beziehung: Grundstein zum Erfolg? [The coach-athlete relationship: A cornerstone for success?] *Sportwissenschaft.*

CHAPTER 7

Towards Mutual Understanding
Communication and Conflict in Coaching

Lauren R. Tufton

Effective communication is an essential part of interaction in sport, and it is particularly pertinent to the success of the coach-athlete relationship. For example, through verbal and non-verbal communication, during a competition a long jumper might look up to the stands to receive pointers from their coach. This also occurs every time a ball is passed from player to player on a football pitch, where information is offered and received about the passer's intention to pass, the weight and angle of the pass, and the receiver's readiness to take the ball. In both instances, effective communication is the key to success as intended messages to one another can easily get 'lost in translation'. The long jump coach in the previous example has seconds to convey their message, which is often done with hand signals. Thus we see the challenges that might be faced in getting communication 'right'. Indeed, it is important to consider how we convey our thoughts, feelings, and behaviours in order to facilitate our interdependent goals and in turn generate positive relationships (Knowles et al., 2015), which are crucial to coach-athlete interactions. Understanding effective communication, often cited as a mitigating factor in the breakdown of relationships (Weinberg & Gould, 2019), is essential particularly as our ego often prevents us from considering, appreciating, or sometimes even hearing another individual's point of view (Bartholomew, 2017).

This chapter explores the nature of our communication, the skills associated with quality communication, and the contextual factors within sport which influence the development of strong working relationships, which are only achieved through clear communication strategies (Gordon, 2009). Furthermore, the challenges and opportunities presented by interpersonal conflict in coaching environments are discussed.

COMMUNICATION: THE ESSENCE OF SOCIAL INTERACTION

At any given moment via both verbal and non-verbal channels, whether intentional or not, we reveal information about who we are, how we see the world, how we feel, and what we are thinking (Hogg & Vaughan, 2018). Communication put simply is the encoding, transmission, and decoding of information (Martens, 1987). However, it is also a social construct, and its purpose may vary; for example, a coach may need to inform and encourage an athlete during a performance, or wish to convey their thoughts and feelings about the team scoring or conceding a point,

TABLE 7.1 Types of communication

Communication Behaviour		Definition
Linguistic (Verbal)	Verbal	The actual words used in speech
	Paralinguistic	Other aspects of speech i.e., stress, pitch, tone, pace, pauses/silences, volume
Non-linguistic (Non-verbal)	Tacesics	Bodily contact, touch
	Proxemics	Interpersonal distance, orientation, territoriality
	Kinesics	Body motion i.e., facial expression, gesture, eye-contact, posture, head movements

Source: Adapted from Hargie & Marshall, 1986, p. 36

or athletes may want to show their intentions to work hard and equally share their expectations of their teammates' efforts (Niculescu & Sabăn, 2018). Communication is best understood through a socioecological lens where the influence of individuals' varying demographics, values and beliefs, self-regulation skills, and their communicative limitations and aptitudes can be seen (Cherubini, 2019). Critically, for the individual to be perceived as genuine and authentic by the recipient, with the message being accurately received, there must be a consistency between the verbal and non-verbal information exhibited by the sender (Rogers, 1961). Table 7.1 provides a summary of the varying forms of verbal (linguistic) and non-verbal (non-linguistic) communication.

Now that we have distinguished between verbal and non-verbal forms of communication, we explore each in turn.

Verbal and Written Communication

The linguistic aspect of communication delineates both *what* is spoken or written, but also *how* it is spoken or written, through paralanguage and grammatical intonation respectively (Hogg & Vaughan, 2018). There are several factors which contribute to the micro-decisions about how one might speak in any given situation. Perspectives from speech accommodation theory (Giles, 1984) propose that an individual's speech style may be modified according to context (i.e., listener, situation). For example, consider how differently a pre-competition talk from a coach might be delivered compared to a one-to-one intimate conversation with a friend. Elements of paralanguage are used to convey the thoughts and emotions behind the words: these play a vital role in fostering the desired response from the listener.

More and more frequently in the digital age, we are communicating via the written word, be it through text messages, emails, or social media. Digital communication has for better or worse changed our social environment, bringing individuals greater immediacy and a more constant connection to people and information. However, one of the challenges for the written word is the lack of non-verbal elements of communication, which can lead to misinterpretation by the reader. Hence, the advent of the emoji designed to provide the recipient with a partial electronic characterisation of our related emotions. Whilst emojis are considered a modern invention, reflective of a digital age, creating symbols to convey meaning is one of the oldest forms of literacy (Fane, 2017), yet they are still vulnerable to misinterpretation and misuse. This may lead us to consider the cautionary challenges of using electronic messages within coach-athlete communications, for example a coach providing an athlete with feedback on their performance, may be best delivered in person rather than solely via text message. We will now explore the varying facets of non-verbal communication.

Non-verbal Communication

The non-verbal aspects of communication (see Table 7.1), often referred to as cues, encapsulate a wide range of elements such as gestures, touch and body positioning, physical appearance and posture, and facial expressions (Weinberg & Gould, 2019). Gestures can quickly and often inadvertently reveal a great deal about how someone is feeling during an interaction. For example, if an athlete crosses their arms or turns away, they may be perceived to be, or perhaps actually are, feeling defensive or unreceptive to a coach's feedback at that time. Similarly, an individual's facial expressions are crucial to connecting with others; a warm smile from a coach knows no language barrier and brings connection for everyone, in contrast a steely glare or shake of the head may illicit a different response from the athlete(s).

Touch and body positioning—for example, to calm or comfort another person—whilst effective in many ways, must be conducted in a respectful manner. Posture and physical appearance can also contribute significantly to the impression formed by others. For example, competition situations pose an important opportunity for the coach to communicate to the athlete or team their unconditional positive regard towards them and their efforts, irrespective of the result, for example shaking their hands and giving them a pat on the back. Additionally, an individual's physical appearance such as a coach or athlete wearing a uniform or team colours speaks volumes about their sense of identity, and their beliefs and values (Hogg & Vaughan, 2018) within the team or organisation.

COMMUNICATION WITHIN THE COACHING ENVIRONMENT

The ability to understand how others identify with and interpret the world assists us in understanding their actions; therefore, the skilled development of what some researchers term 'interpersonal constructs' is critical to facilitating learning within any coaching environment. Initially proposed by Delia (1977), the constructivist approach to interpersonal communication has been widely supported throughout a range of contexts including close relationships (Burleson et al., 2000), education (Applegate, 1980), and intercultural interaction (Applegate & Sypher, 1988). Most significantly however, its application within the context of sport reflects functional communication, defined as "the ability to generate and process messages in ways that enable people to accomplish their goals efficiently and effectively" (Burleson & Rack, 2008, p. 52). It offers the broad assumption that all individuals interpret the world differently and seek to create meaningful understanding of their interactions.

The development of interpersonal constructs is something that all individuals develop 'schemas' for over time (Burleson & Rack, 2008). These schemas are formulated information gained via verbal and non-verbal avenues of communication. Therefore, how we construe another individual is shaped by our predictions and interpretation of their behaviours, attitudes, appearance, traits, and dispositions (Kelly, 1955). According to Burleson and Caplan (1998) those individuals with a strong aptitude for accurately interpreting and understanding other people are thought to have highly attuned construing systems for interpersonal cognitive complexity.

The constructivist viewpoint of an individual's experience also asserts that it is embedded within the sociocultural and historical context within which they find themselves. Therefore, the environmental context can both influence and constrain how the individual interprets and finds meaning in their interaction with those around them (Burleson & Rack, 2008). A significant influence upon an athlete's experience within the coaching environment is that of a coach's philosophy of practice, which we will now explore in more depth.

The Influence and Application of a Coaching Philosophy

A coach's philosophy of practice is reflective of their intrinsic values and beliefs and is often shaped by their own previous experiences of being coached themselves, particularly if their experience was positive (Cherubini, 2019). This is typically translated through their coaching style (i.e., democratic, autocratic, holistic, laissez-faire) and in turn can significantly influence athletes' emotional, cognitive, and behavioural responses, not to mention their motivation (Amorose & Anderson-Butcher, 2015). It is important that a coach's communication behaviour aligns with their philosophy of practice (e.g., Yukelson, 2015). Therefore, time taken by a coach to understand their own beliefs, values, motivations, and intentions is a good starting point and opens the door for developing awareness of how their coaching philosophy will impact on their relationship with athletes and other stakeholders.

Côté and Gilbert (2009) proposed that the coaching process is "the consistent application of integrated professional, interpersonal, and intrapersonal knowledge to improve athletes' competence, confidence, connection and character in specific coaching contexts" (p. 316). This widely cited definition recognises the importance of acknowledging both content and relatability (Cherubini, 2019) in the coaching process. A coach can possess all the knowledge in the world about their sport, but if they cannot translate that knowledge to their athletes, they will not be effective (Kidman & Hanrahan, 2011).

The *professional* knowledge described by Côté and Gilbert (2009) refers to the technical and tactical knowledge of the sport. In American football, a technical aspect of a coach's knowledge might be training an athlete to develop specific skills such as the quarterback's passing technique. Whereas a tactical aspect in the same sport might be a coach's knowledge of specific plays to run at the appropriate moment in a game. Fry (2015) observed that whilst having knowledge of the rules of a particular sport is important, a coach's "self-knowledge, insight into particular individuals with whom the coach interacts, and awareness of what human beings, and in some cases, nonhuman animals, are in general like" (p. 387) is even more critical, as it will determine when, and more importantly how, this information is imparted to their athletes. This emphasises that the "power of effective communication in shaping human attitudes, emotions and performance, is fundamental to successful sports coaching" (Cherubini, 2019, p. 451), and this is where the *intrapersonal* and *interpersonal* knowledge in coaching is applied (Côté & Gilbert, 2009). Indeed, the coach's "ability to transmit knowledge to athletes" (Fry, 2015, p. 387) is essential. However, moving away from this more traditional view of coaching, the dominant discourse of current coaching psychology research is the recognition of a more reciprocal communication strategy, facilitating greater understanding between coach and athlete (Jowett & Shanmugam, 2016).

STRATEGIES FOR EFFECTIVE COMMUNICATION IN SPORT

The single biggest problem in communication is the illusion that it has taken place.
George Bernard Shaw, playwright

Success in sport is largely determined by a coach's competency in effectively communicating to their athletes the required support—be it technical, tactical, motivational, or emotional—to help turn their aspirations into reality (Sagar & Jowett, 2012). However, this can only be achieved through effective communication strategies (Anshel, 2012) and coach-athlete mutual knowledge and understanding (Lorimer & Jowett, 2013).

Developing Emotional Intelligence as a Coach

Emotional intelligence is the culmination of the awareness of oneself and empathic understanding of others and is defined as:

> the ability to accurately perceive, appraise, and express emotion; the ability to access and/ or generate feelings when they facilitate thought; the ability to understand emotions and emotional knowledge; and the ability to regulate emotions to promote emotional and intellectual growth.
>
> (Mayer & Salovey, 1997, p. 10)

During the communication process, individuals' personalities, needs, and expectations have a strong influence on their behaviour and the subsequent outcome of the interaction (Niculescu & Sabǎn, 2018). Therefore, time and energy invested in developing an accurate understanding of both themselves (Côté & Gilbert, 2009) and each individual athlete is essential to effective coaching practice and positive coach-athlete relationships (Ehrmann, 2011). As described in the previous chapter, a substantial body of research evidence suggests that a quality coach-athlete relationship comprises the 3+1Cs; closeness, commitment, complementarity, and co-orientation. Communication is cited within the 3+1Cs framework as the fuel of the relationship (Jowett & Shanmugam, 2016).

The construct of co-orientation comprises two interdependent elements; empathic understanding and empathic accuracy. Whilst empathic understanding can be defined as a non-judgemental and comprehensive knowledge of the athlete as a whole person, empathic accuracy is more the perceptually intuitive capacity to understand and respond appropriately to the thoughts, feelings, and intentions of the athlete on a moment-to-moment basis (Burleson & Caplan, 1998). An important facet of empathy is the capacity to understand, without judgement, the other person's thoughts, feelings, or behaviours; to accept that "all feelings are legitimate: the positive, the negative, and the ambivalent" (Ginott et al., 2003, pp. 26–27). This reflects the constructivist approach to interpersonal communication discussed earlier in this chapter, acknowledging that a person could feel or think differently about a situation at any given moment. Individuals' thoughts, feelings, and behaviours are not perceived as right or wrong. However, the proposal that they are malleable and can change over time offers scope for the coach, through empathically accurate feedback, to encourage the athlete towards a more optimal perceptual state, generating in turn a positive impact on performance and the coach-athlete relationship (Jowett & Clark-Carter, 2006).

The two elements of empathic understanding and empathic accuracy have been described here in terms of the coach's knowledge and understanding of the athlete. However, the 3+1Cs model also recognises that in order to generate a quality relationship, both parties must consciously work towards developing a shared understanding of each other, thus reflecting a more balanced and reciprocal relationship (Jowett & Shanmugam, 2016). In Case Study 7.1, we explore an example of how elite athletes perceive their interactions with their coach, and its implications for their thoughts, feelings, and behaviours in training and performance.

CASE STUDY 7.1

Olympic Archers' Experiences of Coach-Athlete Interaction

Kim and Park's (2020) case study investigation explored athletes' perceptions of the effects of communication with their coach during significant moments in training and performance environments. Eight Korean Olympic archers took part in the study. In the semi-structured interviews, the researchers divided the interviews into three sections: athlete background and experience, positive and negative elements of coach communication during performance, and positive and negative elements of coach communication during training. An analysis revealed a number of main themes and sub-themes. The athletes' responses suggested that they perceived communication with their coach to be important during training and performance, and additionally when they were experiencing psychological crises. The main themes and respective sub-themes are outlined here:

Training: "My coach is a really good communicator. . . . I feel that he is a good storyteller" (p. 8).

Autonomy support—when arranging training schedules, athletes felt a stronger sense of responsibility and commitment if the coach engaged with the athletes' opinions.
Motivation—the athletes offered positive and negative examples of how coach-athlete communication could directly affect their motivation levels during training.
Skill and equipment—due to the intricacies of technique and equipment selection in archery, coach-athlete communication around this topic was particularly significant for positive and negative implications for the athletes during training.

Performance: "He wanted me to focus on what I usually think and feel when I am performing to the best of my abilities" (p. 6).

Self-awareness—coach communication was acutely impactful on their self-awareness, especially during a performance crisis.

Positive encouragement—following a decrease in performance levels, athletes reported feelings of uncertainty which affected decision-making and focus, therefore supportive coach behaviour was of value to help regain performance levels.

Psychological Crises: "When I am psychologically agitated, I tend to pay attention to my coach's verbal and non-verbal expressions" (p. 7).

Self-confidence—a coach's reactions and behaviour towards the athlete during times of crisis play a significant role in the athlete's confidence levels.

Anxiety—athletes reported that conversations with their coach during periods of anxiety can have a powerful impact on their anxiety levels.

The study identified that "communication can have both functional and dysfunctional effects on the athletes' performances and psychological conditions, depending on the verbal and nonverbal messages of the coach" (p. 9). Most significantly, athletes conveyed the importance of individualised communication from their coaches, emphasising the need to recognise the uniqueness of each individual athlete.

Navigating the Communication Climate

The findings in Case Study 7.1 are in keeping with the constructivist approach to studying interpersonal communication (Delia, 1977). This recognises that there is no 'one size fits all' solution to coach communication, that athletes' and coaches' perceptions, actions, and reactions can change across contexts, and are highly influenced by the perceptions, actions, and reactions of those around them (Cranmer & Brann, 2015). Within the coaching environment, interactions between coaches and athletes can take place in a multitude of contexts (Yukelson, 2015); for example, on a training ground, at a competition, in a locker room, or in a coach's office. Therefore, consideration must be made about the timing, appropriateness, and content of communication or feedback in any given situation (Millar et al., 2011). Indeed, interference to communication exchanges can take many shapes and forms, and it can be challenging for an individual to process multiple cues at once (Ehrmann, 2011). For example, in a performance environment, both the coach and the parent may be communicating conflicting instructions from the touchline with limited or no impact. Indeed, delaying feedback often provides the athlete with the opportunity to self-regulate themselves either in terms of emotional control or performance mastery (Millar et al., 2011).

Also notice how the dynamics of feedback in the coach-athlete relationship may change over time, particularly as the athlete becomes more competent. For example, with an experienced athlete the feedback may become more relational (emotional, motivational) from the coach as opposed to instructional, whereas the athlete themselves may also provide more verbal informational feedback. In contrast, a coach with a younger athlete may provide more instructional feedback and gain non-verbal behavioural feedback from the young athlete. However, Gould et al. (2012, p. 86) also asserted that "kids don't care what you know until they know you care",

TABLE 7.2 Coach reflections for self-awareness and empathic accuracy

Reflections to Improve Self-Awareness	Reflections to Improve Empathic Accuracy
Do my emotions affect how I treat people? If so, when? How?	Do I allow my athletes to express their feelings?
How do I react when I am stressed? Tired? Feel under attack?	Did I consider my athlete's perspective?
How is that reaction different from when I am relaxed? Comfortable? At ease?	Can I describe the look on my athlete's face during our talk?

Source: Adapted from VanSickle et al., 2010, pp. 31–32

therefore suggesting that coaches should prioritise the emotional needs of young athletes and adapt their own feedback accordingly.

An accurate understanding of athletes' needs and perceptions is critical to effective coaching. Research by VanSickle et al. (2010) suggested that there are often some discrepancies between the perceptions of coaches' emotional intelligence by the coach and athlete and propose a couple of reflective "checking in exercises" (p. 31) for coaches to improve their self-awareness and empathic accuracy. Table 7.2 offers some questions that a coach may wish to reflect upon in order to improve their coach communication.

The Reciprocity of Feedback

The assumption that the provision of feedback lies solely in the coach's domain is outdated, and the importance of a coach's receptivity to athlete feedback cannot be understated (Cassidy et al., 2016). This feedback can take many forms, verbal and non-verbal, and may reflect an athlete's attitude, emotion, clarity of understanding, and motivational needs (Cherubini, 2019). In fact, this feedback is the communication the coach is seeking from athletes through empathic accuracy to inform and therefore improve the effectiveness of their next communication to the athlete—be it informational, esteem, or emotional support (Cranmer et al., 2016). One highly effective mechanism for gaining meaningful feedback from athletes is active listening. The spotlight explores the key ingredients of developing this fundamental coaching skillset.

Spotlight On: Active Listening Skills

Active listening can be defined as offering one's undivided attention to the speaker's total communication (Weinberg & Gould, 2019), and using verbal and non-verbal communication cues to show the speaker that they have not only been heard but also understood (Katz & Hemmings, 2009). In a fast-paced environment like sport, the thoughts and feelings behind a coach and athlete's communications can easily go unheard or unsaid (Cherubini, 2019), therefore the measured use of active listening skills can be critical in maintaining mutual understanding. Importantly, active listening should be facilitated in a non-judgemental way allowing individuals the freedom to articulate their perceptions of experiences and share their associated thoughts and feelings. The purpose of active listening and associated skill elements of active listening are outlined here.

Factual Listening

The purpose is to seek clarity of gaining a full understanding of the content of the information shared in a communication exchange. There are three active listening skills which can be used to help achieve this.

> *Summarising*—is the process of collating the information provided by the speaker and succinctly presenting it back to them for confirmation, therefore ensuring mutual understanding.
> *Paraphrasing*—is re-expressing some of the salient information that the speaker has shared back to them in a purposefully reorganised manner. This provides the speaker with the opportunity to glean new or greater understanding of their own perspective.
> *Clarifying*—is asking specific questions of the speaker about what they have said to clarify that both parties have the same understanding of what has been described.

Emotional Listening

The purpose is to gain empathic understanding about how the speaker feels emotionally about the information being discussed. This provides the listener with an appreciation of the speaker's experiences and associated thoughts, feelings, and behaviours, and is typically facilitated through:

> *Reflecting*—is expressing back to the speaker the feelings that they have shared, implied, or exhibited. The listener needs to clarify their interpretation of these associated emotions ahead of any reflective response or feedback.

Source: Adapted from Katz & Hemmings, 2009, pp. 22–24, 33–35

The success or failure of a communication can be largely determined by the congruence, or lack thereof, across the interpretation and selective meaning each individual ascribes to the interaction. Luhmann's (1995) social systems theory suggests that communication is a selection process comprising three elements: information, utterance, and understanding. Consistent with the constructivist viewpoint, Luhmann's theory recognises the complexity of communication, and explores the levels of internal and external influences that may affect the individual's subjective interpretation of the interaction. Understanding coach-athlete communication through this socioecological lens (Cherubini, 2019) presents a greater opportunity to contextualise coach-athlete communication at a personal level (i.e., respective personalities, sex, age, cultural background) and the systemic team, organisational, sporting culture, and societal levels within which it is embedded (Borggrefe & Cachay, 2013). We will now explore the communication challenges posed by some of these factors at an interpersonal and organisational level.

Parents, Stakeholders, and Organisational Influences

In addition to developing clear communication strategies with their athlete(s), coaches should also consider the influence of other key stakeholders, such as parents, other coaches and support staff, the policy makers of their organisation, sponsors, and particularly their employer, upon coach-athlete communication (Stoszkowski & Collins, 2014). For example, a parent may have strong opinions about when and at what level their child should compete, or a sponsor's financial contribution may be determinant upon performances being maintained at a certain level. The extent to which each of these stakeholders can or will influence coach-athlete communication will vary. However, there is consistent evidence from coaches of all levels and sports that stresses the associated pressures and importance of fostering productive working relationships with athletes, sporting organisations, and their wider support team (Cassidy et al., 2016).

Team Culture and Its Influence on Coach-Athlete Communication

Whether it is grassroots participation at the local leisure centre or professional competitive sport, sport brings people together from diverse ethnic, sociocultural, and religious backgrounds. This can create communicational challenges of not only a potential variety of spoken languages but also "culturally specific behaviours and attitudes" (Borggrefe & Cachay, 2013, p. 17), which may influence the individual's subjective experience and understanding of teammates and the coach's intended communications. Research conducted by Morgan et al. (2019, pp. 4–7) on the conscious processes of high-performance teams suggests some constructive ways to collectively develop a shared vision and understanding of a positive team culture:

- inspiring, motivating, and challenging team members to achieve performance excellence;
- developing a team ethos based upon ownership and responsibility;
- cultivating a team identity and togetherness based upon a selfless culture;
- exposing the team to challenging training and unexpected/difficult situations; and
- promoting enjoyment and keeping a positive outlook during stressful periods.

These openly communicated strategies highlight that identifying roles and responsibilities, establishing cultural values, norms, and protocols, and recognising the team's collective efficacy and shared goals, enhances a sense of "confidence, competence, connection and character" (Côté & Gilbert, 2009, p. 316); there is, therefore, a heightened collective sense of self-efficacy in the athletes and coaches. It is in this unity that challenges like interpersonal conflict, which we will discuss later in this chapter, can be met with positive regard (Vealey, 2017).

The Subjectivity of Understanding and Response

On a personal level, successful mutual understanding of a given communication is subject to both the coach and athlete deriving the same meaning from the information. Borggrefe and Cachay (2013) asserted that "achieving understanding is a highly self-referential process; the meaning of a message will always be constructed based on system-specific structures and criteria of relevance" (p. 13), and challenges may occur when there is disparity between the coach's and the athlete's intentions and/or motivations. Respective interpretation can be influenced by internal factors such as residual feelings about previous interactions or other prior unrelated experiences, personality, age, sex, and cultural backgrounds. It can also be affected by situational factors within the context of the communication, for example whether or not teammates are present during an altercation between a coach and athlete, or even be influenced by personal responsibilities outside of the confines of sport such as family issues or work commitments (Borggrefe & Cachay, 2013).

Mutual understanding alone, however, is not sufficient for successful communication. An individual's response behaviour is indicative of whether the communication has been effective, and where communication is not successful this could lead to conflict within the coach-athlete relationship, the management of which we shall now explore in more detail.

INTERPERSONAL CONFLICT WITHIN THE COACH-ATHLETE RELATIONSHIP

Interpersonal conflict in sport has been defined as "a situation in which relationship partners perceive a disagreement about, for example, values, needs, opinions or objectives that is manifested through negative, cognitive, affective and behavioural reactions" (Wachsmuth et al., 2017, p. 5). It has been described as orientating either a specific task (training/performance aspect) or social issue (relational/personal); the latter having more challenging long-term implications for the relationship itself (Jehn, 1997). Conflict can easily occur in the coach-athlete relationship, be it through unmet expectations, lack of effort, training schedule disagreements, or more personal issues. Yet whether it has a detrimental or constructive effect on performance and the relationship and/or individuals' well-being will be greatly determined by the coach and athlete's communicative approach to the situation. This section will explore the determinants and consequences of conflict, strategies to prevent and manage conflict, and the incorporation, where necessary, of third-party interventions.

The Determinants and Consequences of Conflict

In 2013, Mellalieu et al.'s study explored conflict during competitions and revealed that it was primarily a result of communication breakdowns and a jostle for power in the relationship. However, the reported outcomes of conflict reflected a broad continuum of positive–neutral–negative impacts in terms of performance outcome and emotional reactions. Wachsmuth et al.'s (2017) subsequent critical review proposed an exploratory conceptual framework for understanding interpersonal conflict (see Figure 7.1), both in the coach-athlete relationship and within peer groups (e.g., teams). The framework identifies determinants and consequences which reflect conflict as a layered and multidimensional construct. As explained

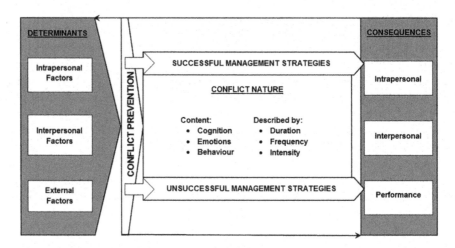

FIGURE 7.1 Conceptual framework of interpersonal conflict in sport

Source: Wachsmuth et al., 2017, p. 3

by Wachsmuth et al. (2017), on the left-hand side of the framework are the *determinants* such as intrapersonal (e.g., personality experience), interpersonal (e.g., poor communication), and external factors (e.g., the situation) which can cause, or influence, conflict. The central section of the framework presents the *cognitive, emotional,* and *behavioural processes* associated with conflict (including initial reactions and management behaviours) that can influence the use of *conflict prevention* and *management strategies*. The right-hand side of the framework highlights the *consequences* of conflict be it intrapersonal (e.g., well-being), interpersonal (e.g., cohesion), or performance (e.g. competition placing).

Using this conceptual framework, Wachsmuth et al. (2018a) sought to further understand the nature of coach-athlete conflict, through interviewing twenty-two coaches and athletes. The research proposed several mitigating factors which could contribute to individuals' perceptions and interpretations of any conflict episode. The findings identified five factors involved in interpersonal conflict: characteristics (e.g., frequency, timing), topics (e.g., lifestyle, misconduct, sport), cognition (e.g., appraisal, uncertainty), emotion (e.g., positive, negative, neutral), and behaviour (e.g., escalation, communication strategies). Practical implications of the research findings include the importance of increasing coach and athlete self-awareness of the consequences of conflict by adopting a "more problem-oriented, caring approach connected with a sense of calmness and relief [which] potentially facilitates coping and conflict management" (Wachsmuth et al., 2018a, p. 1960).

Managing Conflict in the Coach-Athlete Relationship

Rhind and Jowett (2010) proposed the COMPASS model of coach-athlete communication (see Figure 7.2), which offered seven strategies to promote and maintain high-quality coach-athlete communication. The strategy of 'conflict management' suggested that endeavouring to identify potential conflict(s) in advance and creating an open dialogue of communication to either resolve

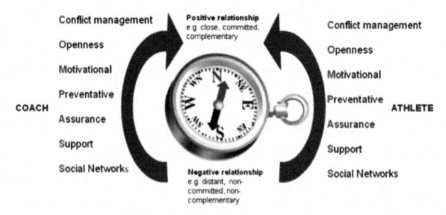

COACH		ATHLETE
Conflict management	Positive relationship e.g. close, committed, complementary	Conflict management
Openness		Openness
Motivational		Motivational
Preventative		Preventative
Assurance		Assurance
Support		Support
Social Networks	Negative relationship e.g. distant, non- committed, non- complementary	Social Networks

FIGURE 7.2 The COMPASS model of coach-athlete communication

Source: Rhind & Jowett, 2010, p. 118

or monitor these issues would assist coaches and athletes in either preventing conflict or settling the conflict with a more positive outcome.

Whilst this sounds like a very logical and proactive approach, other researchers have noted that in reality, conflict avoidance is actually a common strategy for athletes (e.g., Mellalieu et al., 2013), particularly when there is a significant imbalance of power in the relationship (Predoiu & Radu, 2013). Indeed, one previous investigation has cited coaches using controlling behaviour or punishment to overpower athletes during altercations (d'Arripe-Longueville et al., 1998), whereas other research has suggested that some athletes thrive on aggressively motivated behaviour from their coaches (Sagar & Jowett, 2012). In the spotlight that follows, some preventative measures and conflict management strategies for coach-athlete communication are outlined.

Spotlight On: Conflict Management Strategies

Wachsmuth et al. (2018b) explored strategies used by coaches and athletes to "minimise dysfunctional and maximise functional outcomes of interpersonal conflict" (p. 371). Coaches and athletes were found to use both intra- and interpersonal strategies to *prevent* conflict:

Implicit Conflict Prevention—efforts to maintain and enhance the quality of the coach-athlete relationship through closeness, commitment, and complementarity, which in turn generates an optimal performance environment.

Explicit Conflict Prevention—the use of self-regulation to manage their own thoughts, feelings, and behaviours and engaging in empathic accuracy to understand others' perceptions and intentions, and then responding appropriately.

The study also identified five strategies to *manage* conflict:

Role Responsibilities—engaging in and adopting appropriate roles to begin the process to work towards conflict resolution and taking ownership of their personal role responsibilities.

Intrapersonal—regulating emotions prior to engaging with a conflict partner, enabling a priori reappraisal and reassessment of the situation.

Interpersonal—the process must include both parties using open lines of communication and with invested engagement in collaboration and compromise, acknowledging each other's points of view.

External Support—often sought from friends, family, or teammates, although it is difficult to find an independent third party.

Conflict Management Barriers—acknowledging and managing the potential for an unwillingness to work together towards resolution due to poor relationship quality, obliviousness to conflict, and lack of follow-through on the agreed process.

The findings of this study suggest that with the implications of conflict behaviour in the coach-athlete relationship, there is the potential for both dysfunctional and functional outcomes. On an intrapersonal level in terms of individuals' well-being; on a performance level in terms of commitment, motivation, and satisfaction; and on an interpersonal level in terms of the strength of the relationship and the ability to move forward. The research also highlighted that implicit conflict prevention strategies were not sufficient in isolation, and should be supported by explicit conflict prevention strategies and, where necessary, independent mediation.

Third-Party Interventions

Beyond the world of sport, in other social and professional domains, mediation has been cited as an effective strategy for resolving challenging conflict situations (Kressel, 2014). Wachsmuth et al. (2018b) highlighted that when engaging a third party in coach-athlete scenarios it can be difficult to find someone who can remain impartial, let alone be equipped to mediate difficult conversations. The role is skilled, requiring the capacity to provide a safe space for both parties to speak freely, to act as an interpreter, and to identify the root cause of the problem, rather than "treating the symptoms" (Rhind & Jowett, 2012, p. 236) as well as to assist parties in working towards a mutually agreeable solution. This unenviable task often falls to a sport psychologist either operating independently or already working within the organisation.

Wachsmuth et al. (2020) explored what the perceived challenges might be for the sport psychologist when adopting the role of mediator in the coach-athlete relationship. This research identified several roles that sport psychologists already adopt: educator, consultant, analyst, action planner, counsellor, facilitator, and protector. The perceived challenges reported by the interviewed sport psychologists on mediation reflected concerns about procedural factors, their own role within the organisation, the ability to remain objective, coping with inflexible parties, and their own negative perceptions of their self-efficacy as a mediator. The researchers also acknowledged that in order to provide an effective intervention, the sport psychologist would need to have considerable contextual knowledge of the conflict and knowledge of the individuals involved, therefore necessitating both individual and dyadic sessions. However, negotiating the "(micro) political landscape" (Wachsmuth et al., p. 22) of the sporting organisation was perceived to impose a very significant influence on the likelihood of a successful intervention for the sport psychologists. Indeed, the impact of sporting organisations' socioecological and cultural climates on the personal and professional well-being of individuals within their environment is increasingly being scrutinised (e.g., Rowley et al., 2018). This highlights the profound impact of the social systems (Luhmann, 1995) within the organisation not only upon the coach-athlete relationship but also upon the ability of other individuals to successfully facilitate positive change.

Whilst it has been established that conflict is indeed inevitable, efforts made to create an environment where coaches and athletes perceive conflict as valuable for personal growth and developing resilience, and share a willingness to seek out opportunities for resolution, can only be beneficial (Wachsmuth et al., 2018b).

CLOSING THOUGHTS

What brings a coach and athlete together is an interdependent goal, born from a passion for sport. We have established that such passion can present challenges in terms of communication and conflict. However, these challenges can be met positively when efforts are made by the coach and athlete to create a working relationship with a strong sense of authenticity, self-awareness, and empathic accuracy. Through fervent reciprocity of trust, respect, and appreciation, coaches and athletes can develop the skills for open communication from a foundation of psychological safety, acknowledging without prejudice the other person's perspective and the legitimacy of their associated emotions. It is this mutually perceived strength in the coach-athlete relationship that will underpin a proactive and positive approach to conflicts, as they inevitably arise, which will ultimately foster the harmonious passion for facilitating constructive resolutions. Moreover, steps taken to foresee and plan for potential conflict issues in advance, whilst exercising positive communication strategies, can only be beneficial and would likely ensure greater receptivity to solution-focused communication orientation. Most pertinent to the success of the coach-athlete relationship, however, is the clear message that effective communication is not in what you say but in what the listener takes away.

REFERENCES

Amorose, A. J., & Anderson-Butcher, D. (2015). Exploring the independent and interactive effects of autonomy: Supportive and controlling coaching behaviours on adolescent athletes' motivation for sport. *Sport, Exercise and Performance Psychology, 4*(3), 206–218. https://doi.org/10.1037/spy0000038

Anshel, M. H. (2012). *Sport psychology: From theory to practice* (5th ed.). Benjamin Cummings.

Applegate, J. L. (1980). Adaptive communication in educational contexts: A study of teachers' communicative strategies. *Communication Education, 29*, 158–170.

Applegate, J. L., & Sypher, H. E. (1988). Constructivist theory and intercultural communication research. In Y. Kim & W. Gudykunst (Eds.), *Theoretical perspectives in intercultural communication* (pp. 41–65). Sage.

Bartholomew, B. (2017). *Conscious coaching: The art and science of building buy-in.* Bartholomew Strength LLC.

Borggrefe, C., & Cachay, K. (2013). Communicative challenges of coaches in an elite level sports system. Theoretical reflections on successful coaching strategies. *European Journal for Sport and Society, 10*(1), 7–29. https://doi.org/10.1080/16138171.2013.11687908

Burleson, B. R., & Caplan, S. E. (1998). Cognitive complexity. In J. C. McCroskey, J. A. Daly, M. M. Martin, & M. J. Beatty (Eds.), *Communication and personality: Trait perspectives* (pp. 233–286). Hampton.

Burleson, B. R., Metts, S., & Kirch, M. W. (2000). Communication in close relationships. In C. Hendrick & S. Hendrick (Eds.), *Close relationships: A sourcebook* (pp. 245–258). Sage.

Burleson, B. R., & Rack, J. J. (2008). Constructivism theory: Explaining individual differences in communication skill. In L. A. Baxter & D. O. Braithwaite (Eds.), *Engaging theories in interpersonal communication: Multiple perspectives* (pp. 51–62). Sage.

Cassidy, T., Jones, R. L., & Potrac, P. (2016). *Understanding sports coaching: The pedagogical, social and cultural foundations of coaching practice* (3rd ed.). Routledge.

Cherubini, J. (2019). Strategies and communication skills in sports coaching. In M. H. Anshel, T. A. Petrie & J. A. Steinfeldt (Eds.), *APA handbook of sport and exercise psychology, Vol. 1, Sport psychology* (pp. 451–467). American Psychological Association.

Côté, J., & Gilbert, W. (2009). An integrative definition of coaching effectiveness and expertise. *International Journal of Sports Science & Coaching, 4*(3), 307–323.

Cranmer, G. A., Anzur, C. K., & Sollitto, M. (2016). Memorable messages of social support that former high school athletes received from their head coaches. *Communication & Sport, 5*, 604–621. http://doi.org/10.1177/2167479516641934

Cranmer, G. A., & Brann, M. (2015). "It makes me feel like I am a part of this team": An exploratory study of coach confirmation. *International Journal of Sport Communication, 8*, 193–211.

d'Arripe-Longueville, F., Fournier, J. F., & Dubois, A. (1998). The perceived effectiveness of interactions between expert French judo coaches and elite female athletes. *The Sport Psychologist, 12*, 317–332. http://doi.org/10.1123/tsp.12.3.317

Delia, J. G. (1977). Constructivism and the study of human communication. *Quarterly Journal of Speech, 63*, 66–83. https://doi.org/10.1080/00335637709383368

Ehrmann, J. (2011). *InSideOut coaching: How sports can transform lives.* Simon & Schuster.

Fane, J. (2017, April 6). Why I use emoji in research and teaching. *The Conversation.* https://theconversation.com/why-i-use-emoji-in-research-and-teaching-75399

Fry, J. P. (2015). Philosophical approaches to coaching. In M. McNamee & W. Morgan (Eds.), *Routledge handbook of the philosophy of sport* (pp. 383–400). Routledge.

Giles, H. (1984). The dynamics of speech accommodation theory. *International Journal of the Sociology of Language, 46*, whole issue.

Ginott, H. G., Ginott, A., & Goddard, H. W. (2003). *Between parent and child.* Three Rivers Press.

Gordon, D. (2009). *Coaching science.* Learning Matters Ltd.

Gould, D., Flett, R., & Lauer, L. (2012). The relationship between psychosocial developmental and the sports climate experienced by underserved youth. *Psychology of Sport and Exercise, 13*, 80–87. http://doi.org/10.1016/j.psychsport.2011.07.005

Hargie, O., & Marshall, P. (1986). Interpersonal communication: A theoretical framework. In O. Hargie (Ed.), *A handbook of communication skills* (pp. 22–56). Routledge.

Hogg, M. A., & Vaughan, G. M. (2018). *Social psychology* (8th ed.). Pearson Education Ltd.

Jehn, K. A. (1997). A qualitative analysis of conflict types and dimensions in organizational groups. *Administrative Science Quarterly, 42*(3), 530–557.

Jowett, S., & Clark-Carter, D. (2006). Perceptions of empathic accuracy and assumed similarity in the coach–athlete relationship. *British Journal of Social Psychology, 45,* 617–637. http://doi.org/10.1348/014466605X58609

Jowett, S., & Shanmugam, V. (2016). Relational coaching in sport: Its psychological underpinnings and practical effectiveness. In R. Schinke, K. R. McGannon, & B. Smith (Eds.). *Routledge international handbook of sport psychology* (pp. 471–484). Routledge.

Katz, J., & Hemmings, B. (2009). *Counselling skills handbook for the sport psychologist.* The British Psychological Society.

Kelly, G. A. (1955). *A theory of personality: The psychology of personal constructs.* W. W. Norton & Company.

Kidman, L., & Hanrahan, S. J. (2011). *The coaching process: A practical guide to becoming an effective sports coach* (3rd ed.). Routledge.

Kim, Y., & Park, I. (2020). "Coach really knew what I needed and understood me well as a person": Effective communication acts in coach-athlete interactions among Korean Olympic archers. *International Journal of Environmental Research and Public Health, 17*(3101). https://doi.org/10.3390/ijerph17093101

Knowles, A. M., Shanmugam, V., & Lorimer, R. (2015). *Social psychology in sport & exercise: Linking theory to practice.* Palgrave Macmillan.

Kressel, K. (2014). The mediation of conflict: Context, cognition, and practice. In P. T. Coleman, M. Deutsch, & E. C. Marcus (Eds.), *The handbook of conflict resolution: Theory and practice* (3rd ed., pp. 817–848). John Wiley & Sons, Inc.

Lorimer, R., & Jowett, S. (2013). Empathic understanding and accuracy in the coach-athlete relationship. In P. Potrac, W. Gilbert & J. Denison (Eds.). *Routledge handbook of sports coaching* (pp. 321–332). Routledge.

Luhmann, N. (1995). *Social systems.* Stanford University Press.

Martens, R. (1987). *Coaches guide to sport psychology.* Human Kinetics.

Mayer, J. D., & Salovey, P. (1997). What is emotional intelligence? In P. Salovey & D. J. Sluyter (Eds.), *Emotional development and emotional intelligence: Educational implications* (pp. 3–31). Basic Books.

Mellalieu, S., Shearer, D. A., & Shearer, C. (2013). A preliminary survey of interpersonal conflict at major games and championships. *The Sports Psychologist, 27,* 120–129.

Millar, S. K., Oldham, A. R. H., & Donovan, M. (2011). Coaches' self-awareness of timing, nature, and intent of verbal instructions to athletes. *International Journal of Sports Science & Coaching, 6,* 503–513. http://doi.org/10.1260/1747-9541.6.4.503

Morgan, P. B. C., Fletcher, D., & Sarkar, M. (2019). Developing team resilience: A season-long study of psychosocial enablers and strategies in a high-level sports team. *Psychology of Sport and Exercise, 45,* 1–11. https://doi.org/10.1016/j.psychsport.2019.101543

Niculescu, G., & Sabăn, E. (2018). Strategy communication in sport. *Journal of Sport and Kinetic Movement, 1*(31), 50–53.

Predoiu, R., & Radu, A. (2013). Study regarding communication and styles of approaching conflict in athletes. *Procedia: Social and Behavioural Sciences, 92,* 752–756. http://doi.org/10.1016/j.sbspro.2013.08.750

Rhind, D. J., & Jowett, S. (2010). Relationship maintenance strategies in the coach-athlete relationship: The development of the COMPASS model. *Journal of Applied Sport Psychology, 22*, 106–121. http://doi.org/10.1080/10413200903474472

Rhind, D. J., & Jowett, S. (2012). Working with coach-athlete relationships: Their quality and maintenance. In S. Mellalieu & S. Hanton (Eds.), *Professional practice in sport psychology: A review* (pp. 219–248). Routledge.

Rogers, C. R. (1961). *On becoming a person.* Constable.

Rowley, C., Potrac, P., Knowles, Z. R., & Nelson, L. (2018). More than meets the (rationalistic) eye: A neophyte sport psychology practitioner's reflections on the micropolitics of everyday life within a rugby league academy. *Journal of Applied Sport Psychology*, 1–19. https://doi.org/10.1080/10413200.2018.1491906

Sagar, S. S., & Jowett, S. (2012). Communicative acts in coach-athlete interactions: When losing competitions and when making mistakes in training. *Western Journal of Communication, 76*, 148–174. http://doi.org/10.1080/10570314.2011.651256

Stoszkowski, J., & Collins, D. (2014). Communities of practice, social learning and networks: Exploiting the social side of coach development. *Sport, Education and Society, 19*(6), 773–788. https://doi.org/10.1080/13573322.2012.692671

VanSickle, J. L., Hancher-Rauch, H., & Elliott, T. G. (2010). Athletes' perceptions of coaches' emotional intelligence competencies. *Journal of Coaching Education, 3*, 21–41. http://doi.org/10.1123/jce.3.1.21

Vealey, R. S. (2017). Conflict management and cultural reparation: Consulting "Below Zero" with a college basketball team. *Case Studies in Sport and Exercise Psychology, 1*(1), 83–93. https://doi.org/10.1123/cssep.2017–0008

Wachsmuth, S., Jowett, S., & Harwood, C. (2017). Conflict among athletes and their coaches: What is the theory and research so far? *International Review of Sport and Exercise Psychology, 10*(1), 1–24. http://doi.org/10.1080/1750984X.2016.1184698

Wachsmuth, S., Jowett, S., & Harwood, C. (2018a). On understanding the nature of interpersonal conflict between coaches and athletes. *Journal of Sport Sciences, 36*(17), 1955–1962. https://doi.org/10.1080/02640414.2018.1428882

Wachsmuth, S., Jowett, S., & Harwood, C. (2018b). Managing conflict in coach-athlete relationships. *Sport, Exercise & Performance Psychology, 7*(4), 371–391. http://doi.org/10.1037/spy0000129

Wachsmuth, S., Jowett, S., & Harwood, C. (2020). Third party interventions in coach-athlete conflict: Can sport psychology practitioners offer the necessary support? *Journal of Applied Sport Psychology*, 1–26. https://doi.org/10.1080/10413200.2020.1723737

Weinberg, R. S., & Gould, D. (2019). *Foundations of sport and exercise psychology* (7th ed.). Human Kinetics.

Yukelson, D. P. (2015). Communicating effectively. In J. M. Williams & V. Krane (Eds.), *Applied sport psychology: Personal growth to peak performance* (pp. 140–156). McGraw-Hill Education.

CHAPTER 8

Creating an Optimal Motivational Climate for Effective Coaching

Iain Greenlees

Motivation, defined as "the process of initiating, directing and sustaining behaviour" (Conroy et al., 2007, p. 182), is key to sporting success and long-term participation. Motivation is required to choose to take up a sport or a sporting challenge (initiating) and to select specific sporting targets and goals (directing) that may take years of effort and persistence (sustaining) to achieve. Coaches want individuals to be attracted to their sport and to decide to join the activities they run. They also want individuals to put in the required levels of effort to improve and develop their potential over a prolonged period of time.

In recent years it has become accepted that although motivation is determined in part by personality traits, the environment also plays a major role in shaping it (Gilchrist & Mallett, 2016). Thus, coaches are in a unique position to influence motivation (and hence performance, achievement, and health) of the people they coach by changing the situations they create. Sport psychologists use the slightly broader terms 'environment' or 'climate' to refer to the way in which the coach structures their coaching and the atmosphere that they create. In the remainder of this chapter, the term 'motivational climate' will be used to encompass situation and environment.

This chapter will explore how to create an optimal motivational climate for athletic development. It will consider the impact coaches can have on motivational climate and focus on how coach leadership can promote an effective motivational climate. In order to do this, the chapter will first explore theoretical ideas concerning what determines our motivation. Although there are hundreds of theories of motivation in existence, the chapter will focus on two that are most commonly applied to sport and exercise settings: Self-Determination Theory (Deci & Ryan, 1985; Ryan & Deci, 2000) and Achievement Goal Theory (Nicholls, 1989).

SELF-DETERMINATION THEORY—KEY PRINCIPLES

Self-Determination Theory (SDT; Deci & Ryan, 1985, Ryan & Deci, 2000) is a general theory of motivation designed to further our understanding of the determinants of human action and psychological functioning. It is centred on the idea that individuals will experience most satisfaction, well-being, achievement, and personal growth when they engage in activities that they freely

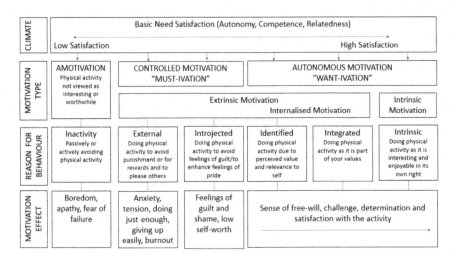

FIGURE 8.1 Schematic representation of key principles of Self-Determination Theory

Source: Adapted from Visser, 2017

choose—they are self-determined. The theory comprises four key propositions around this theme, all of which have received extensive research support across multiple life domains (e.g., sport, education, work, relationships), and across multiple populations (e.g., age, culture).

The first fundamental proposition of SDT (summarised in the second and third rows of Figure 8.1) is that rather than simply viewing motivation in terms of its quantity (seeing people as ranging from amotivation to high motivation), we also need to consider the quality, or types, of motivation people exhibit, as these will have very different consequences. Specifically, Ryan and Deci (2000) proposed that people differ in the primary reasons they choose to take up, invest effort, and persist in activities and these reasons can be classified according to how freely the activities are chosen— how self-determined/autonomous they are. People who engage in the activity primarily for the enjoyment and pleasure they derive from doing the activity (intrinsic motivation), because they see it as a central part of their identity and value system (integrated regulation), or because they value the activity for the benefits it will have for them (identified regulation) are said to possess more self-determined (or autonomous) motivation. These people participate in activities because they want to (termed "want-ivation" by Visser, 2017). Those people who participate in an activity due to external rewards, inducements, or coercion (extrinsic motivation) or those who participate in an activity simply to avoid feelings of guilt or to present themselves in a certain way (introjected regulation) are said to be non-self-determined or controlled. These people participate because they feel they have little choice in the matter (termed "must-ivation" by Visser, 2017).

The second, and central, fundamental proposition of SDT is that where an individual sits on the continuum from self-determined (autonomous) to non-self-determined (controlled) motivation will influence a large range of cognitive, emotional, and behavioural responses. This is summarised in the bottom row of Figure 8.1. Specifically, Ryan and Deci (2000) propose that the more an individual demonstrates self-determined forms of motivation, (i.e. the more intrinsically motivated they are), the more positive consequences will be derived from participation. This proposition has received a host of research evidence to support it, across many populations (e.g., ages, genders, cultures) and many life domains (e.g., education, sport, the workplace). Within sport and exercise settings, evidence has consistently supported the proposition that more self-determined forms of motivation are associated with variables such as effort investment, long-term persistence and skill development, lower performance anxiety and burnout, and better performance (Standage & Ryan, 2012). Crucially, research evidence has also demonstrated the link between self-determined forms of motivation and psychological health and well-being (Weiss & Amorose, 2008).

Given the potential benefits of moving people towards more self-determined motivation, the third fundamental proposition (summarised at the top of Figure 8.1) concerns the determinants of self-determined motivation. Here, Deci and Ryan (2008) proposed that the pleasure experienced from doing an activity in itself (intrinsic motivation) is determined by the extent to which three basic human needs are satisfied in doing that activity. These are the needs for competence (the need to feel as though we are good at an activity and able to accomplish challenges), autonomy (the need to feel in control of our choices and our development), and relatedness (the need to feel connected to others and to experience a sense of belonging to a group or collective). Again, extensive research evidence supports the view when these needs are satisfied and, when they are not thwarted, greater levels of self-determination are shown (Amorose & Anderson-Butcher, 2007).

This leads to the final fundamental proposition of the theory which asserts that it is the psychosocial environments, or climates (the top row in Figure 8.1), that we operate in, and the individuals who manage and create those environments, which will exert the strongest influence on whether needs are met or thwarted (Deci & Ryan, 2008). In sport, the central character is the coach or exercise leader as it is they who are in a position to provide clear, constructive performance-related feedback following performance (need for competence). They are also in a position to involve the athletes in the decision-making process and to provide them with strategies to improve (need for autonomy), and who may also be in the best position to create a positive team-climate that develops social, as well as task-related, relationships. Again, a range of research studies have demonstrated the power coaches have in supporting (or thwarting) autonomy, competence, or relatedness (Amorose & Anderson-Butcher, 2007).

ACHIEVEMENT GOAL THEORY—THE IMPORTANCE OF WHAT CONSTITUTES SUCCESS

Achievement Goal Theory (AGT; Nicholls, 1989) is a theory that shares similar ideas and premises with SDT and is also a popular way of understanding motivational climates (Duda, 2013). The fundamental premise of AGT is that individuals are motivated to demonstrate competence (and/or avoid demonstrating incompetence). Thus, individuals will choose activities and challenges in which they believe they can be successful and demonstrate competence, and avoid activities and challenges in which they may not succeed. This explains why, when given a choice of practice activities, athletes will tend to practice the skills they are good at and neglect the skills they are not so good at. However, pivotal to the theory is that there is more than one way in which competence and success can be demonstrated. Specifically, competence can be displayed by being better than others (what theorists such as Duda would term as being ego-involved) or it can be displayed by showing improvement relative to previous performances (being task-involved). Thus, someone who is ego-involved will judge their competence by what they have won or by their

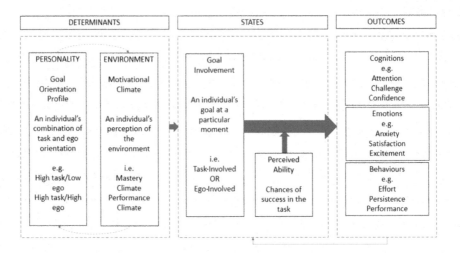

FIGURE 8.2 Schematic representation of key principles of Achievement Goal Theory

ranking whereas someone who is task-involved will judge their competence by how much they have improved (e.g., reduced personal best time). The theory proposes that, for any given activity, at any one moment an individual will be either task-involved or ego-involved but that this involvement can change rapidly. For instance, an athlete may start a performance focused purely on achieving the fastest time they can but, due to the goading of an opponent, switch to the sole objective of beating that opponent.

Achievement goal theorists argue that the goal (ego- vs task-involved) that an individual will focus on for a given activity will determine their cognitions, emotions, and behaviours (see Figure 8.2). Specifically, individuals who are task-involved are proposed to experience positive emotions and moods (confidence, calmness, enjoyment) and display productive behaviours (effort, persistence). Conversely, individuals who are ego-involved are predicted to display unproductive behaviours but only when they lack confidence in their ability to be successful (Duda & Treasure, 2015). When an individual who is ego-involved but has high levels of perceived ability—for example, Usain Bolt on the starting line of the men's 100m or Christiano Ronaldo standing over a vital free-kick—then positive motivation ensues. These predictions from AGT are borne out in research. For instance, Hall and Kerr (1997) found, in a sample of youth sports performers, that those who were more task-involved in a competition experienced less competitive anxiety. The more ego-involved the performer, the more anxiety they experienced, but only if they reported low perceived ability. Due to the methodological difficulties of measuring dynamic states, such as goal involvement, little research has been conducted further on the impacts of involvement.

Given the potential importance of goal involvement, the question then becomes what determines the goal-involvement of an individual in competition and training? AGT predicts that goal involvement is influenced by personality dispositions and by the environment one operates in (see the left-hand side of Figure 8.2 in the Determinants box). In terms of personality, the theory proposes that, due to early socialisation experiences in sport and other domains, individuals will differ in the frequency and extent to which they become task- and ego-involved. For example, think of those people you know who will find a way to turn any activity into a competition (habitually ego-involved) and compare them to people who are more focused on how to improve their performances regardless of how competent they are (habitually task-involved). Within AGT, this individual difference is termed 'goal orientation'. As individuals are not simply either task or ego oriented and can be any combination of high, low, or moderate in both of them (e.g., high ego and task, high ego and low task), they are considered to have a 'goal orientation profile'. An individual's 'goal orientation profile' will potentially exert a strong influence on the achievement goals an individual will adopt (e.g., someone high in ego orientation and low in task orientation is likely to adopt an ego-involved goal), their behaviours and their experience of sport. This is borne out in a range of research studies. For example, Smith et al. (2006) sampled 223 junior male soccer players, measuring their goal orientation profiles, quality of peer relationships, sport enjoyment and satisfaction. They found that sporting enjoyment, satisfaction, and quality of peer relationships were significantly lower for those who reported being high in ego orientation and low in task orientation than for any other group, including those people with high ego orientation and high task orientation. Two key take-home messages from this body of research are that, first, goal-orientation profiles do shape individuals' sporting experiences and, second, that being highly ego oriented is not necessarily a bad thing when it is accompanied by high levels of task orientation.

Whilst goal orientations do influence motivation, the environment that individuals operate in will also shape the goals they select (Duda & Treasure, 2015). Importantly for coaches, AGT predicts that the climate created by the coach, and the signals of competence that they emphasise and reward, will at least exert an equally important effect on achievement goals selected and, hence, motivational behaviours and cognitions. Specifically, coaches can generate an ego-involving, or performance, climate, which is where the coach values and praises winning and being better than others. Alternately, they can generate a task-involving, or mastery, climate, which is where the coach values and praises an individual's effort and improvements. The nature of the climate a coach creates has been shown to influence several aspects of the sporting experience. Research shows that individuals who perceive themselves as being coached in a task-involving climate experienced higher levels of enjoyment, positive mood and satisfaction, and displayed higher levels of effort, self-rated improvement, and self-confidence; lower levels of stress, anxiety, and burnout; more positive peer relationships; and greater levels of sportspersonship (Duda & Treasure, 2015). In short, task-involving climates are associated with many positive outcomes.

This positive view of task-involving climates has been supported in a great deal of research. In a 2015 review and meta-analysis of the literature in this area, Harwood et al. found several large associations between task-involving climates and positive outcomes (e.g., with intrinsic motivation). However, Harwood et al. (2015) did note several limitations with the current literature. First, research is limited in that it has focused on correlations between variables rather than using research designs that can examine whether the climate causes such positive outcomes. Second, the research is largely cross-sectional (conducted at one moment in time) rather than looking to explore the longer-term (longitudinal) consequences of climates. Third, research has tended to use college and school athletes, so it is still unclear if these results apply to elite level performers. Another noteworthy finding of Harwood et al.'s (2015) review was that correlations between ego-involved climates and negative outcomes were not substantial. This casts doubt on the view that ego-involved climates are universally negative, suggesting that such a climate may not impact certain individuals (e.g., elite athletes, athletes with high perceived ability). Overall, however, the review indicates the potential benefits that can be gained by creating a more task-involving motivational coaching climate.

DEVELOPING EFFECTIVE MOTIVATIONAL CLIMATES

Creating change in individuals may best be achieved by changing the situations or environments they operate in. This resonates with both theories (SDT and AGT) covered in this chapter that highlight the role of the environment in shaping motivation. Possibly one of the reasons for the enduring popularity of both AGT and SDT amongst sport psychology and coaching researchers and practitioners is that, rather than simply proposing that the environment is important, they provide some clear guidance on *how* motivating environments can be shaped. In the sections that follow, the chapter outlines specific coaching behaviours and actions that can create motivation according to each of the theories and then explore some of the research that has examined interventions that are inspired by the theories.

Needs Supportive Coaching

SDT, and the positive research it has produced, has inspired several interventions. In coaching settings, these tend to revolve around changing coaches' behaviours and the organisation of practices to ensure that the three basic needs—autonomy, competence, and relatedness—are met. A needs supportive approach refers to a style of coaching that considers the perspectives of their athletes, acknowledges their feelings, provides relevant information to athletes for them to improve, and offers opportunities for choice (Gilchrist & Mallett, 2016).

There are many ways in which coaches can support the needs of the athletes they coach so there is not one set protocol for delivering needs supportive coaching (Berntsen & Kristiansen, 2019). *Autonomy supportive coaching* is coaching that provides individuals with the sense that they are in control of the activities that they do. It involves giving more power to the group and individual members of the group to decide what they want to do and how they do it. *Relatedness supportive coaching* is coaching that encourages the group to develop and allows friendships to emerge so that the individual feels a connection to the other members. Here, the individual feels that the coach takes an interest in the participant's welfare, is helpful and trustworthy, and is genuinely interested in their development as a person. Finally, *competence supportive coaching* is coaching that provides individuals with the sense that they are competent, or can achieve competence with persistence, at the task at hand. Table 8.1 provides an overview of key behaviours to support each of the three needs.

How Effective Are Coaching Interventions Designed to Enhance Needs Supportive Behaviours?

Over the last 20 years, several writers (e.g., Mageau & Vallerand, 2003) have suggested specific skills and behaviours coaches/physical activity instructors can engage in. Recently, Berntsen and Kristiansen (2019) developed the Motivation Activation Programme in Sports (MAPS) for the Norwegian Ski Federation to develop the needs supportive behaviours of coaches. The targeted behaviours include enquiring about and acknowledging athletes' feelings, displaying trust in athletes' abilities, providing choice and rationales, allowing athletes to take initiative in sessions, providing positive feedback, and focusing on athlete improvement over performance attainments (mastery climate). Although this programme has not been experimentally evaluated, qualitative interviews with the coaches involved did show support for the effectiveness and importance of the

TABLE 8.1 Examples of coach needs supportive behaviours/activities (N.B. There may be substantial crossover in needs that are supported by these behaviours.)

Basic Need	Description	Strategies
RELATEDNESS	Feeling of belonging in a sport/group or activity	Getting to know each athlete as a person rather than just as an athlete
		Encouraging groupwork and sense of team
		Rotate groupings and encourage interaction through peer discussion, peer feedback, and peer coaching
		Empathises with athletes' difficulties
COMPETENCE	Feeling able to complete activities and to improve	Individualise practice drills to varied skill levels
		Design activities to ensure progression from simple to complex skills
		Encourage use of training and competition diaries to foster self-reflection
		Recap sessions with focus on athletes' achievements
		Wait for requests for help and feedback from athletes rather than correcting immediately
AUTONOMY	Feeling in some way in control of one's destiny and having a say in how things run	Providing choice on practice drills and activities
		Providing choice of team goals and challenges
		Involve athletes in setting rules for team/squad
		Explain why different activities are being included and discuss rationale
		Encourage initiative through athletes leading aspects of practice (e.g., warm-up)
		Avoiding use of punishments and controlling language ('you may want' to rather than 'because you have to')
		Asking for athletes' suggestions for the content of future sessions

MAPS intervention. However, the effectiveness of the intervention was felt by the coaches to be dependent on both the maturity of the athlete and having sufficient time to develop the strategies and to tailor them to the athlete.

In spite of a large body of evidence supporting the key tenets of SDT, intervention-based studies, which are studies that have sought to change coaching behaviours and monitor the effects of these changes over time, in the sport context are scarce (see Langan et al., 2013 for an overview). The research of Berntsen and Kristiansen (2019) demonstrates that such interventions are, within limits, palatable to coaches and perceived to be effective. Research also shows that they can be successful in changing coaching behaviours. For example, Langan et al. (2015) conducted a 12-week SDT-based intervention, consisting of a series of workshops designed to educate coaches on the importance of needs satisfaction and how to do it, with six Gaelic football coaches. Their results indicated that the intervention was successful in changing coaching behaviours (e.g., increasing levels of autonomy support). Similarly, Cheon et al. (2015) showed that a five-hour training programme was sufficient to change coaching behaviours of Paralympic coaches. However, the evidence of any impact on athletes is limited. Cheon et al. (2015) did show that the intervention enhanced athlete motivation but in Langan et al.'s (2015) study, whilst the intervention did reduce Gaelic footballers' burnout levels pre- to post-intervention, no changes in athlete motivation were seen. Clearly, further research that examines the long- and short-term impacts of such interventions in competitive sport is warranted.

Whilst the research mentioned previously does show support for coaching interventions based on SDT principles, what it does not always do so well is provide much information concerning how the interventions were conducted and the challenges that were faced by the coaches implementing the interventions. In the case study in Case Study 8.1, an article that set out to do just that is summarised.

CASE STUDY 8.1

Using SDT to Enhance the Performance of an Olympic Relay Team

In 2005, the sport psychologist and coach Clifford Mallett published a case study outlining the two-year-long SDT-inspired intervention he used with the 2004 Olympics Australian men's athletics relay teams (4x100m and 4x400m). Mallett discussed a number of needs-supportive strategies. These included:

Providing a rationale for activities and offering choice within boundaries: Athletes were provided some choice as team training schedules were discussed and negotiated rather than imposed. Additionally, prior to the finals, teams were informed of the selected athletes but were also given an extensive rationale for the decision. However, the athletes then decided the final running order. To support them, athletes were provided with information concerning the pros and cons of all potential orders. Mallett argued that this approach increased commitment to the decision but also enhanced perceived competence (as the rationales and group discussions provided athletes with information concerning why they were suited to each leg).

Acknowledging athletes' feelings and perspectives: Mallett discussed the importance of gathering athletes' suggestions and feedback concerning training. This included using an athlete-centred approach to feedback and video analysis. Specifically, rather than providing his evaluation of performances first, Mallett asked the athletes to view performances and discuss strategies to improve training and competition performances.

Providing opportunities for initiative-taking: Athletes were encouraged to work together to solve problems and develop strategies. For instance, in the development of baton exchanges, Mallett outlined a four-pronged approach to feedback that started with the runners providing feedback and offering solutions, then moved to other members of the team providing comments and then made use of video information to prompt further discussion. Only after this did Mallett provide feedback. This was designed to promote independence, develop relatedness through the team working together and enhance confidence in the teams' knowledge of their event.

Providing competence feedback and focusing on performance and process goals: Mallett provided detailed individualised and team feedback to the athletes. This included timings of specific elements of the race. Athletes were also set specific targets for elements of their performances. These targets, when met, enhanced perceptions of competence. When not met, athletes worked together to generate solutions. This aimed to build competence and relatedness.

Mallett argued that the approach was a success, pointing to improved performances that exceeded expectations (the 100m team were ranked 14th in the world prior to the games and finished 6th, and the 400m team finished with a silver medal) and the enhanced team-coach relationship and commitment of the athletes. However, no SDT variables (e.g., intrinsic motivation levels) were assessed at any point and no comparisons were made with other teams who did not receive the intervention (a control group). The article relied on anecdotal evidence and, since Mallett is not an objective observer, its value as academic knowledge can be questioned. However, the article does provide a fascinating insight into the meeting of the 'science' of self-determination theory with the 'art' of coaching and is well worth a read.

The information contained in Case Study 8.1 and the preceding section indicate the potential utility of SDT-informed coaching interventions across a range of sport settings. The aim of the next section is to review those parallel research efforts that have sought to examine the effects of interventions designed to create task-involving motivational climates.

Creating Task-Involving (Mastery) Motivational Climates

Given the impressive range of literature that supports the principles of AGT and the positive impact of creating a task-involving motivational climate, the question is: 'How can a coach create a task-involving motivational climate?' Fortunately, a taxonomy developed by Epstein (1989) in educational psychology has been refined for use by coaches by Ames (1992). Ames proposed the acronym TARGET (Task, Authority, Recognition, Grouping, Evaluation, and Timing; see Table 8.2) to summarise ways to promote task-involving climates. This provides suggestions concerning the organisation of coaching activities and drills (Task, Authority, Groupings, and Timing) and the way in which feedback, praise, and rewards are offered (Recognition and Evaluation). Currently, there is some debate (Kingston et al., 2020) as to whether all elements of TARGET need to be in place to create a mastery climate or whether deficits in one area may be compensated for by task-involving behaviours in other dimensions (e.g., rewards for effort and improvement).

TABLE 8.2 Example TARGET strategies

TARGET Dimension	Description	Strategies
TASK	The specific tasks and practices given to athletes	Structuring practices so that a range of flexible challenges and tasks are available for athletes to select a challenge that is relevant to them.
		Where possible, make challenges easily measurable/scorable so that individuals can see improvements/plateaus in performance and set self-referenced performance goals (e.g., improve by 10%).
		Consider the repeatability of challenges so that they can be completed outside of formal practice.
AUTHORITY	Extent of athlete participation in decision-making processes	Allow athlete involvement in the decision-making process.
		Encourage athletes to take ownership and leadership of practice (e.g., athlete-led warm-up, athletes developing their own).
		Make use of athlete feedback to consider their perspective.
RECOGNITION	What is recognised and praised by the coach and when?	Focus on recognising and praising individual progress, effort, and improvement.
		Where possible, provide private feedback that allows for discussion of individual progress.
		Praise and recognise (in private and in public) instances of executing controllable aspects of performance (e.g., "Great hustle" or "Good footwork" versus "Wow, you can't coach that!!").
GROUPING	How athletes are arranged in practice and competition	In practice mix group size and membership to ensure that no clear hierarchy is evident.
		Encourage peer feedback and support.
		Encourage group problem-solving.
EVALUATION	Standards used to evaluate learning and performance	Encourage athletes to self-evaluate through use of personal feedback and video analysis.
		Making training performance less ambiguous through the use of specific and measurable drills so that self-evaluation is easier.
		Focus evaluative comments on controllable aspects such as effort, strategy, and progress and improvements.
TIMING	Time demands placed on individuals to learn and allocation of coach time	Acknowledge different learning rates and trajectories.
		Provide, where possible, activities that athletes can practice independently at their own pace.

Source: Adapted from Duda & Balaguer, 2007, p. 129

How Effective Are Coaching Interventions Designed to Create Mastery Climates?

Whilst the TARGET guidance is intuitive and does reflect the principles of AGT well, researchers have sought to examine whether the guidelines can be used by coaches and how effective it is in producing positive motivational climates and outcomes for performers. In terms of the palatability and usability of TARGET guidelines, Kingston et al. (2020) showed that TARGET-consistent behaviours can be readily observed, and were being implemented, in the behaviours of football academy coaches. This indicates that producing task-involving climates is possible and practical. In terms of intervention research then, as with needs supportive coaching, only a limited number of studies have been conducted (e.g., Smith et al., 2007). However, Cecchini et al. (2014) did provide experimental evidence to support the efficacy of a TARGET-based intervention. The researchers recruited 40 football and basketball coaches who were coaching over 283 athletes between them. Half of the coaches received a 12-week intervention that consisted of 30 hours of theoretical and practical education concerning why and how to implement TARGET behaviours. The other coaches formed the control group and received no intervention. The researchers found that when comparing their ratings before and after the intervention, athletes of the coaches that received the intervention perceived a significant change in the coaching climate, reported significantly greater satisfaction of basic needs, and reported putting in more effort and persistence in training. Athletes of coaches in the control group did not show any such changes. More dramatically, when the authors collected follow-up data six months later they found the positive changes were still evident. This research clearly provides evidence to support coach education in task-involving climates.

The principles of AGT, and many of the research studies that have explored it, have always resonated with me as a performer and as a sport psychology consultant. In Case Study 8.2, I outline how I tried to integrate some of the principles of TARGET into my consultancy work.

CASE STUDY 8.2

Creating Mastery Climates for Junior Golfers

In the early 2000s I was employed by the English Golf Union, and a number of county associations, to provide sport psychology support to a range of development squads. Commonly, my work involved attending training weekends to provide coaching and sport science support to young golfers. In my early experiences with this system what often struck me was the general ineffectiveness of these sessions to inspire and motivate ALL of the golfers. Often, by the end of the weekend golfers' effort and focus during practice and on the course was low and many players left quickly, quietly and, on occasion, in tears.

In reflecting on what was happening, I (and a number of the coaches whom I spoke to) considered the coaching climate that had been generated. Specifically, the traditional approach that entailed many features of an ego-involving climate. Many training activities were organised as peer vs peer competitions (from a pitching practice that became a scored competition to the final round that included prizes for lowest overall score, fewest putts, etc.). Equally, coach-player discussions often centred on competition performances (who had won which junior competition), handicap reductions (who had the lowest handicap, who was reducing theirs the quickest) and feedback was often delivered very publicly. Reflecting further, this system worked well for the more able golfers who had good chances of winning most of the attention and rewards but for the younger, middle-group golfers the days could become a series of failures (not winning any of prizes or the attention of the organisers). To me, this was at the heart of the disengagement.

Although not all organisers were willing to enact changes, some coaches shared these reflections and tried to make changes. These changes included:

- Developing scorable skills tests that reflected on-course demands (e.g., playing a 70-yard shot to the green). Players practiced these during the training weekend and then used them in their own practice.
- Working with the golfers to develop self-referenced, improvement-related goals and to develop their own skills tests for these aspects.
- Balancing prizes awarded for competitive performance with awards and recognition for improvements and efforts made between and during the weekends.
- Mixing groups up more so that groupings were more balanced in terms of handicap, age, and abilities.
- Encouraging golfers to evaluate training and competition performance in terms of controllable performance- and process-related criteria.

Whilst I would love to say the changes were dramatic and that I meticulously collected data to show this, I did not. However, the situation did show me how motivational climates can exert a powerful impact on an athlete's experience of being coached and how small changes can make meaningful differences. The initial responses from the coaches and the golfers who were involved was positive. We felt the golfers worked more effectively on the tasks that they were set and showed signs of using what they learned from the weekends in their day-to-day practices.

Combining AGT and SDT—Empowering Coaching

The two theories (AGT and SDT) have clearly spawned a great deal of research attention, first to examine the tenets of the theories and second to explore the efficacy of interventions that have been inspired by the theories. What is clear from the preceding discussions are the similarities between the applied implications of the theories, for example, the importance of athlete-centred coaching, democracy in coaching, and the development of perceived competence. These similarities, and the strength of evidence for both approaches, have recently led to the development of a hybrid coaching system.

Duda (2013) argued for the need to integrate aspects of the motivational climate outlined by SDT and AGT. Drawing on these theories, Duda proposed that the key aspect of the motivational climate is the extent to which it is *empowering* or *disempowering* for the athletes. Specifically, the combination of needs supportive and task-involving climates produces an "empowering" climate (Duda, 2013, p. 311). An empowering motivational climate is one in which athletes feel respected and valued, connected to others, can exert some control of their training and competition decisions, and are encouraged to strive for goals such as increased effort and task mastery. Conversely, a disempowering motivation climate is highly ego-involving and controlling. The fundamental assumption of this approach is that coach-created climates which are more empowering (and are absent of disempowering behaviours) are those that create the most satisfied and motivated athletes and lay the most effective foundations for athletic development and persistence.

This approach to coaching has led to the development of a specific and trademarked training programme to develop empowering coaches (see https://empoweringcoaching.co.uk/ for more details) and has been at the centre of a European Union funded project designed to enhance physical activity amongst adolescents, the PAPA (Promoting Adolescent Physical Activity) Project (for more details on this programme, see www.projectpapa.org/). Currently, research evidence to support the efficacy of the training programme is limited but there is promising research to suggest that athlete perceptions of an empowering climate may be linked to important outcomes. For instance, Fenton et al. (2016) found a positive correlation between athletes' perceptions of an empowering coaching climate, self-determined forms of motivation and sports enjoyment. As enjoyment of sport was also associated with levels of physical activity and body fat (such that people who enjoy physical activity more tend to have lower body fat percentages) then this implicates empowering coaching climates in promoting health and well-being. Similarly, Appleton and Duda (2016) found that disempowering motivational climates were associated with indicators of burnout and physical ill-health but that this could be reversed if coaches displayed some elements of empowerment. However, the current research should be interpreted cautiously as it only indicates that empowering coaching climates may be correlated with key outcomes (e.g., sporting enjoyment, physical health, mental well-being) as opposed to showing that the climate causes these variables to change. For example, it could simply be that people who enjoy sport more are more likely to be treated in an empowering fashion by their coaches. Despite the limitations of this research it does provide some grounding for the further exploration of intervention strategies rooted in the empowering coaching approach.

Before concluding the chapter, we consider a final, fundamental question: Just how important are coaches in determining the motivation of athletes, especially youth athletes? Theorists and researchers, who are often coaches themselves, have largely taken for granted the idea that coaches are the primary determinant of motivation. But is this true? One research study, presented in the spotlight, questions this and considers other potential influences.

Spotlight On: To What Extent Do Coaches Influence Their Athletes' Motivation?

Atkins et al. (2015) from the University of North Texas completed a large-scale study (sampling 405 male youth sports performers between the ages of 12 and 15) that explored the extent to which coach-created, parent-created, and peer-created motivational climates influence the motivation of their athlete/child/peer. The rationale for this was that the behaviours and attitudes of family members and peers may exert just as powerful, or more powerful, an impact on key aspects of motivation as coaches due to the greater amount of time these groups are in contact with the athlete.

The participants completed measures that assessed their perceptions of the motivational climates created by coaches, parents, and peers and to assess their goal orientation, sporting enjoyment, perceived competence, satisfaction, and intention to continue with sport. The results indicated that parent- and peer-created motivational climates were stronger predictors of these variables than were coach-created motivational climates. Whilst influential to an extent, this research does show that, at least for youth performers, parents and peers may be more important to consider and that efforts on behalf of coaches to become more task-involving may not be as fruitful as was once thought.

This finding is consistent with my experiences of working with young performers, especially where coaches may have limited contact with their performers (e.g., a national-level coach of a development squad who only sees performers a few times a year). All the efforts to create a task-involving climate would soon be diminished when the players turned each skill test into a competition with each other (peer climate overwhelming the coach climate). Equally, and more sadly, our pains to stress the importance of development and improvement could disappear when a father asks, upon picking up the player: 'Did you win? You'll never make it if you can't beat this lot!'. This finding is also consistent with the recognition by many sporting organisations that vital work is needed to educate parents of sports performers.

CLOSING THOUGHTS

Regardless of the underpinning theory used to examine sporting climates, a large body of evidence now exists, across a range of populations and activities, to demonstrate the power of coach-created motivational climates on a whole range of important coaching outcomes (motivation, enjoyment, satisfaction, well-being, positive moods, learning, and performance). This knowledge has also informed the development of a series of guidelines and coaching programmes designed to teach coaches how to create the most effective environments for their athletes. Whilst the evidence for the effectiveness of these interventions is relatively sparse, it is growing and does show that a) task-involving/needs-supportive climates can be created relatively easily by coaches, and b) they do have a positive impact on the athletes that experience them. However, much further research into, and refining of, these coaching programmes is needed to increase support for them and to identify which elements of the climates are most essential and how they can be developed most effectively.

REFERENCES

Ames, C. (1992). Achievement goals, motivational climate, and motivational processes. In G. C. Roberts (Ed.), *Motivation in sport and exercise* (pp. 161–176). Human Kinetics.

Amorose, A. J., & Anderson-Butcher, D. (2007). Autonomy-supportive coaching and self-determined motivation in high school and college athletes: A test of self-determination theory. *Psychology of Sport and Exercise, 8,* 654–670. https://doi.org/10.1016/j.psychsport.2006.11.003

Appleton, P. R., & Duda, J. L. (2016). Examining the interactive effects of coach-created empowering and disempowering climate dimensions on athletes' health and functioning. *Psychology of Sport & Exercise, 26,* 61–70. https://doi.org/10.1016/j.psychsport.2016.06.007

Atkins, M. R., Johnson, D. M., Force, E. C., & Petrie, T. A. (2015). Peers, parents, and coaches, oh my! The relation of the motivational climate to boys' intention to continue in sport. *Psychology of Sport & Exercise, 16,* 170–180. https://doi.org/10.1016/j.psychsport.2014.10.008

Berntsen, H., & Kristiansen, E. (2019). Guidelines for need-supportive coach development: The Motivation Activation Program in Sports (MAPS). *International Sport Coaching Journal, 6,* 88–97. https://doi.org/10.1123/iscj.2018-0066

Cecchini, J. A., Fernandez-Rio, J., Mendez-Gimenez, A., Cecchini, C., & Martins, L. (2014). Epstein's TARGET framework and motivational climate in sport: Effects of a field-based, long-term intervention program. *International Journal of Sports Science & Coaching, 9*(6), 1325–1340. https://doi.org/10.1260/1747-9541.9.6.1325

Cheon, S. H., Reeve, J., Lee, J., & Lee, Y. (2015). Giving and receiving autonomy support in a high-stakes sport context: A field-based experiment during the 2012 London Paralympic Games. *Psychology of Sport and Exercise, 19,* 59–69. https://doi.org/10.1016/j.psychsport.2015.02.007

Conroy, D. E., Elliot, A. J., & Coatsworth, J. D. (2007). Competence motivation in sport and exercise: The hierarchical model of achievement motivation and self-determination theory. In M. S. Hagger & N. L. D. Chatzisarantis (Eds.), *Intrinsic motivation and self-determination in exercise and sport* (pp. 181–192). Human Kinetics.

Deci, E. L., & Ryan, R. M. (1985). *Intrinsic motivation and self-determination in human behavior.* Freeman.

Deci, E. L., & Ryan, R. M. (2008). Self-determination theory: A macrotheory of human motivation, development, and health. *Canadian Psychology/Psychologie Canadienne, 49*(3), 182–185. https://doi.org/10.1037/a0012801

Duda, J. L. (2013). The conceptual and empirical foundations of Empowering Coaching™: Setting the stage for the PAPA project. *International Journal of Sport and Exercise Psychology, 11*(4), 311–318. https://doi.org/10.1080/1612197X.2013.839414

Duda, J. L., & Balaguer, I. (2007). The coach-created motivational climate. In S. Jowett & D. Lavallee (Eds.), *Social psychology of sport* (pp. 117–130). Human Kinetics.

Duda, J. L., & Treasure, D. C. (2015). The motivational climate, athlete motivation, and implications for the quality of sport engagement. In J. M. Williams & V. Krane (Eds.). *Applied sport psychology: Personal growth to peak performance* (pp. 57–77). McGraw-Hill.

Epstein, J. (1989). Family structures and student motivation: A developmental perspective. In C. Ames & R. Ames (Eds.), *Research on motivation in education: Volume 3* (pp. 259–295). Academic Press.

Fenton, S. A., Duda, J. L., & Barrett, T. (2016). Optimising physical activity engagement during youth sport: A self-determination theory approach. *Journal of Sports Sciences, 34*(19), 1874–1884. https://doi.org/10.1080/02640414.2016.1142104

Gilchrist, M., & Mallett, C. J. (2016). The theory (SDT) behind effective coaching. In R. Thelwell, C. Harwood, & I. Greenlees (Eds.), *The psychology of sports coaching: Research and practice* (pp. 38–53). Routledge/Taylor and Francis.

Hall, H. K., & Kerr, A. W. (1997). Motivational antecedents of precompetitive anxiety in youth sport. *The Sport Psychologist, 11*(1), 24–42. https://doi.org/10.1123/tsp.11.1.24

Harwood, C. G., Keegan, R. J., Smith, J. M. J., & Raine, A. S. (2015). A systematic review of the intrapersonal correlates of motivational climate perceptions in sport and physical activity. *Psychology of Sport and Exercise, 18*, 9–25. https://doi.org/10.1016/j.psychsport.2014.11.005

Kingston, K., Wixey, D. J., & Morgan, K. (2020). Monitoring the climate: Exploring the psychological environment in an elite soccer academy. *Journal of Applied Sport Psychology, 32*(3), 297–314. https://doi.org/10.1080/10413200.2018.1481466

Langan, E., Blake, C., & Lonsdale, C. (2013). Systematic review of the effectiveness of interpersonal coach education interventions on athlete outcomes. *Psychology of Sport and Exercise, 14*(1), 37–49. https://doi.org/10.1016/j.psychsport.2012.06.007

Langan, E., Blake, C., Toner, J., & Lonsdale, C. (2015). Testing the effects of a self-determination theory-based intervention with youth Gaelic football coaches on athlete motivation and burnout. *The Sport Psychologist, 29(4)*, 293–301. https://doi.org/10.1123/tsp.2013-0107

Mageau, G. A., & Vallerand, R. J. (2003). The coach-athlete relationship: A motivational model. *Journal of Sports Sciences, 21*(11), 883–904. https://doi.org/10.1080/0264041031000140374

Mallett, C. J. (2005). Self-determination theory: A case study of evidence-based coaching. *The Sport Psychologist, 19*(4), 417–429. https://doi.org/10.1123/tsp.19.4.417

Nicholls, J. G. (1989). *The competitive ethos and democratic education.* Harvard University Press.

Ryan, R. M., & Deci, E. L. (2000). Self-determination theory and the facilitation of intrinsic motivation, social development, and well-being. *American Psychologist, 55*(1), 68–78. https://doi.org/10.1037/0003-066X.55.1.68

Smith, A. L., Balaguer, I., & Duda, J. L. (2006). Goal orientation profile differences on perceived motivational climate, perceived peer relationships, and motivation-related responses of youth athletes. *Journal of Sports Sciences, 24*(12), 1315–1327.

Smith, R. E., Smoll, F. L., & Cumming, S. P. (2007). Effects of a motivational climate intervention for coaches on young athletes' sport performance anxiety. *Journal of Sport & Exercise Psychology, 29*(1), 39–59. https://doi.org/10.1123/jsep.29.1.39

Standage, M., & Ryan, R. M. (2012). Self-determination theory and exercise motivation: Facilitating self-regulatory processes to support and maintain health and well-being. In G. C. Roberts & D. C. Treasure (Eds.), *Advances in motivation in sport and exercise* (pp. 233–270). Human Kinetics.

Visser, C. F. (2017). *The motivation continuum: Self-determination theory in one picture.* www.progressfocused.com/2017/12/the-motivation-continuum-self.html

Weiss, M. R., & Amorose, A. J. (2008). Motivational orientations and sport behavior. In T. S. Horn (Ed.), *Advances in sport psychology* (pp. 115–155). Human Kinetics.

CHAPTER 9

The Family Behind the Athlete

Jessica Pinchbeck

The family a child is born into and brought up in has been shown to have a profound impact on athletic development (e.g., Birchwood et al., 2008), and this is due to a combination of genetics as well as the social environment created by the family (Tucker & Collins, 2012). The family typically forms the key social interactions and main point of reference regarding physical activity and sport in early childhood. Therefore, parents and siblings can be important influencers. A child's sport participation can be influenced by two main factors. The first is observing behaviours, such as seeing their parents and siblings being physically active and taking part in sport. The second is through experiencing family attitudes and beliefs, specifically the value that the family places on sport and physical activity. This chapter explores a range of family influences from a psycho-social perspective, combining psychological factors and the social environment to explain thoughts and behaviours. This exploration starts with how and why parents create and support opportunities for their children to take part in sport, and once involved in sport how parental behaviours can impact a child's motivation and their sporting experience. As part of this discussion the chapter also looks at the way parental attachments may shape athletic development, the influence of siblings, and the changing requirements of parental and family influence throughout an athlete's journey through sport.

SOCIALISATION INTO SPORT

Socialisation into sport focuses on the influences that encourage a child to be initially attracted to sport, although this involves more than simply taking children to as many different activities as possible. Socialisation is "an active social process whereby values and norms are transmitted, taught, and hopefully adopted by the individuals being socialised" (Dixon et al., 2008, p. 539). As part of this socialisation process there are various socialising agents that act upon a child's decision to want to participate in sport and one of these is the family (Fredricks & Eccles, 2005). For most children the family is a primary socialisation factor into sport and society and is typically identified as underpinning the entire sport experience of young people (Bailey et al., 2010). When children are young it is usually the parents that organise, encourage, and support their child's sports participation. As such, the hallmark of successful socialisation generally involves "the transmission of positive values between parents and children" (Danioni et al., 2017, p. 75). Therefore, it is important to consider how parental values and beliefs regarding sport participation influence that of their child, and achievement and motivation theories can provide a framework through which to do so.

Expectancy Value Model

Eccles et al. (1983) expectancy-value model (EVM) considers motivational factors that affect an individual's decisions about various activities and achievement-related choices and how significant others influence these decisions. The model was initially related to school achievement, and in particular gender differences in mathematics beliefs and choices, but has since been applied to other domains including sport (e.g., Simpkins et al., 2012; Wang et al., 2017). In fact, data supported the model even more strongly in the sport domain than the academic domain. This is attributed to the model being a 'choice model' and sport containing more free choice than academic subjects (Eccles & Harold, 1991). Evidence supporting EVM is well established and it provides a useful lens through which to explore parental influence on children's motivation in sport and is consistent with the process of children's socialisation into sport as well as motivational theories based upon self-efficacy and perceived competence (Partridge et al., 2008).

The model proposes that the two most important factors that determine an individual's choice behaviours are their expectations for success and the value of the task (Eccles et al., 1983). Individuals are more likely to engage in a task that they think they will do well in and value its importance. When applied to children's sports participation, the model predicts that children who perceive themselves to have a high ability in the task will be more likely to participate than children who are less confident about their sporting ability. However, this is a very simplistic view; EVM offers further explanation of how a task is valued. Task value is formed by four factors:

- utility value (the extent to which a task relates to a child's current and future goals)
- intrinsic value (the enjoyment/satisfaction gained by the child by participating in the task)
- attainment value (importance of doing well at the task)
- relative cost (any perceived negative aspects of participating in the task)

(Fredricks & Eccles, 2005)

Therefore, a child will participate in sport more frequently if they enjoy the activity, believe it is important to their goals, believe that sports participation is central to their self, and there are low costs to their participation. However, a child's beliefs and expectations are shaped by many different factors including various 'socialisers' such as parents, teachers, and peers who influence a child's motivation through their own beliefs and behaviours (Fredricks & Eccles, 2004).

EVM proposes that, firstly, parents' beliefs about a domain (such as sport) influence their behaviours in endorsing their child's engagement in that domain. Secondly, parents' behaviours, in turn, influence children's self-concepts and task values (their motivational beliefs). Thirdly, the child's motivational beliefs shape the child's subsequent behaviours. EVM also discusses the relationship between parents' and children's beliefs and the influence they exert on one another as well as the influence of the child's gender within the process of forming parental beliefs and behaviours (Simpkins et al., 2012). To address parental influence further, Eccles (1993) developed the model of parents' socialisation of motivation (Figure 9.1). The model illustrates that parents act as providers of experience, interpreters of experience, and role models (Fredricks & Eccles, 2005) as shown in boxes E, F, and G.

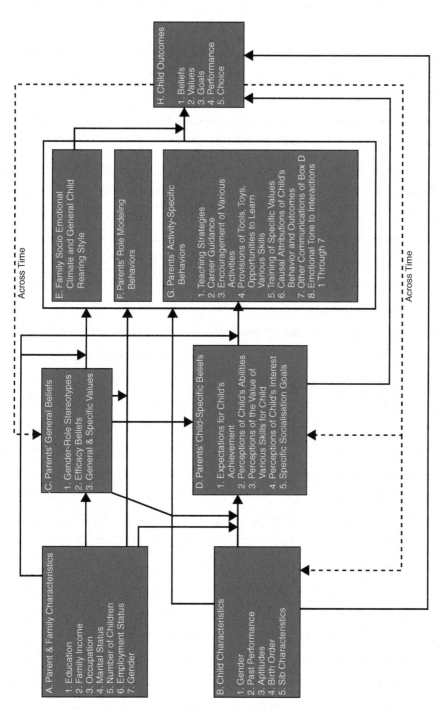

FIGURE 9.1 Eccles' 1993 model of parents' socialisation of motivation

Source: Eccles & Wigfield, 2020, p. 4

Parents as Providers of Experience

Parents provide experiences by enrolling in, paying for, and transporting their children to and from sporting activities. Parents provide or limit opportunities relative to what they feel are important and also what they feel the child will be successful in (Dixon et al., 2008). Different activity domains (such as art, sport, music) are viewed by parents to have very different values and these differences are determined by their own beliefs and experiences (Partridge et al., 2008). For example, if a parent values achievement in sport and perceives their child will experience success in a particular sport, they are more likely to provide greater encouragement in this activity. Parental beliefs and behaviours are also shaped by the social context. EVM includes many variables that influence a child's sporting activity including the characteristics of the family (social and demographic), personal characteristics of both the parent(s) and children, forming general and specific beliefs about each child within the family, emotional characteristics of the family, and parental roles and behaviours (Milošević & Vesković, 2013). These variables help to explain the differences in parental provision of opportunities and encouragement for siblings within the same family (Partridge et al., 2008) and are linked to parental ambition (Straub, 2019). For example, a study by Courtney et al. (2019) found that a child's weight may impact the opportunities a parent provides, with parents of overweight children providing greater support for physical activity only if they perceived their child as possessing a level of coordination greater than children of the same age and gender.

Parents as Interpreters of Experience

According to EVM, parents not only provide the opportunity for their child to participate in sport, but they also interpret the outcomes of the child's experiences. The extent to which parents are able to understand both their own and their child's emotions will influence the helpfulness of the interpretation of their child's sporting experience (Harwood & Knight, 2015). For example, how a parent reacts or behaves in response to their child's experiences may influence the child's interpretation of the experience as positive or negative. Parents provide emotional support and positive experiences for their child's sports involvement (Fredricks & Eccles, 2005) and in the initial years of sport involvement, parental feedback is the main source of information for children to assess their own competence (Fredricks & Eccles, 2004). Research has shown that children's participation in sport and their ability beliefs are related to their parents' beliefs about the child's abilities (Weiss, 2019). Parents' satisfaction with and interpretation of their children's sport experience are also key factors influencing continued participation (Brustad, 1993). This aspect of EVM underpins much of the research exploring parental influence and is discussed in greater detail throughout this chapter.

Parents as Role Models

In the context of sports participation parents serve as role models for their children, with children often copying their parents' behaviours. Children are thus more likely to be involved in sport when family members are also involved (Bailey et al., 2010). Parents can be role models for their children by participating in or coaching sport (Fredricks & Eccles, 2004), by simply enjoying sport (Dixon et al., 2008), and by behaving appropriately at their child's sports events (Harwood & Knight, 2015). Social learning theory (Bandura, 1986), which proposes that people learn from one another through observation, imitation, and modelling, provides a theoretical explanation for parental influence and role modelling. In the current climate where children spend much of their time on electronic devices, a study by Brzęk et al. (2018) found that the level of physical activity in younger children (aged 7–12 years) depended upon the children's relationship with their parents and the parents' level of activity. Findings by Eckelt et al. (2019) supported this notion by recommending that activities involving both parents and children are important in enhancing children's physical activity levels. However, other studies have shown that gender differences may be evident with parents' physical activity holding a greater influence for boys (e.g., Dozier et al., 2020), as well as cultural influences also playing a role (e.g., Johansson et al., 2016).

From an EVM perspective children's self-perceptions of ability and value towards achievement are also modelled by parents' attitudes and behaviours. For example, Brustad (1993) found that parents who expressed high levels of enjoyment of physical activity reported encouraging their children's physical activity more than parents who experienced less enjoyment. In turn this higher parental encouragement was also linked to greater perceived confidence for children. Similarly findings by Babkes and Weiss (1999) showed that children of parents who were physically active and enjoyed their activity reported greater enjoyment, perceived competence, and intrinsic motivation to play soccer. The importance of positive parental support for sport has also been linked to children's enjoyment of sport and physical activity (e.g., Sánchez-Miguel et al., 2013; Shen et al., 2018). Table 9.1, compiled by Harwood and Knight (2015), provides a useful application of the three roles parents fulfil in their child's athletic development.

TABLE 9.1 Roles of parents

Role	Examples of Role Fulfilment	
Providers	Providing tangible support	Signing children up for training Transporting children to competitions Paying for coaching and equipment
	Providing informational support	Talking to children about training and competitions Providing information regarding nutrition Seeking information regarding competition preparation
	Providing emotional support	Helping children after losses and during slumps Comforting children after disappointing or negative sporting experiences (e.g., opponents cheating) Supporting children while they are injured
Interpreters	Effort is more important than outcome	Positively reacting to wins and losses contingent on effort Providing feedback on child's performance Maintaining positive feedback throughout competitions Highlighting the importance of attitude and effort
	Valuing the range of benefits associated with sport	Discussing different outcomes associated with sport participation (e.g., improvement, fitness, friendships) Providing opportunities for social interactions Reinforcing life skills developed in sport
	Encouraging sportspersonship	Providing positive feedback for a good attitude Celebrating sporting behaviours Discussing the importance of sporting behaviours

(Continued)

TABLE 9.1 (Continued)		
Role	Examples of Role Fulfilment	
Role Models	Encouraging sport participation	Engaging in sport themselves Watching and reading about sport Having an active lifestyle
	Sporting behaviours	Maintaining composure at competitions Congratulating opponents for their performances
	Valuing effort over outcomes	Putting 100% effort into own sporting endeavours Reacting positively to their own losses

Source: Harwood & Knight, 2015, p. 29

Case Study 9.1 provides an applied example of how parents may act as providers, interpreters, and role models (highlighted in **bold**) in different ways and demonstrates sport socialisation in action.

CASE STUDY 9.1

The Ferguson Family

The Ferguson family comprises mum, dad, Grace (age 11), and Arthur (age 9).

Arthur has always been an athletic child. He loves being active and is naturally fast and strong, winning all of his races at school sports day and being picked for all of the sports teams at primary school. He is incredibly competitive and loves being adventurous such as climbing trees and trampolining. Dad, who is a big football fan and used to play football when he was younger, thinks Arthur has great potential as an athlete and encourages him to play football and rugby outside of school. Mum, who isn't sporty or active at all, enjoys seeing Arthur's success. Together both parents act as **providers of experience** and ensure he has all the latest kit needed and pay for him to take part in special tournaments and additional coaching sessions (**providing tangible support**). They take an active interest in his sport, watching most of his games, celebrating his achievements, and supporting him when things don't go well (**providing emotional support**). They also encourage his friendships and respect the coaches (acting as **interpreters of experience** and positive **role models**). Arthur loves playing rugby and enjoys the physical side of the game. He isn't too keen on football as the focus is all on winning and it is far more serious than rugby, but he knows his dad wants him to carry on as he has already been approached by several football development schemes.

Grace is not as physically capable or adventurous as Arthur. She was never seen as particularly 'sporty' at primary school and was rewarded more for her academic efforts. However, a combination of experiences, including watching Arthur play football, playing football with him in the garden, and experiencing secondary school physical education (PE) lessons, has led Grace to develop an interest in football and, encouraged by her PE teacher, she wants to join a local football team. Her parents consider her to have limited ability in football and feel that her time would be better spent on other activities that benefit her academically (**providers of experience**). They also feel adding another sports activity would put greater pressure on their already stretched time and financial resources taken up by Arthur's sports (**providing tangible support**). Grace loves Arthur but often finds it frustrating that the family's weekend revolves around his sport and she is only allowed to play football at school.

The situation of these siblings illustrates how different factors may influence parents as **providers of experience**. Arthur is seen to be 'sportier' and naturally gifted; therefore, his parents are willing to invest time and money in his athletic future as opposed to Grace who up until now has shown little interest or prowess in sport. With family resources limited, the parents have opted to distribute more time and money to develop Arthur's potential. This decision will be influenced by many factors (as shown in Figure 9.1). For example, Arthur's father values football for his son but doesn't see the same activity as important for his daughter. Mum is not active and therefore may not value physical activity, particularly for girls, indicating a gendered difference in parental beliefs and values. Although Grace's PE teacher is encouraging her to take up football, it is the parents that ultimately control Grace's participation in extracurricular activities as **providers of experience**, **interpreters of experience**, and **role models**.

SIBLING INFLUENCES

So far in this chapter we have focused on the role of parents, as does the majority of research. This has resulted in the marginalisation of siblings, when it is the sibling relationship that is often the longest relationship one shares and therefore has the potential to influence physical activity experiences from childhood throughout the life course (Blazo & Smith, 2018; Osai & Whiteman, 2017). Siblings are important socialising agents, as shown in Case Study 9.1, and should be considered in relation to an individual's sport socialisation. Sibling influences are reported to be most evident during sport in the early years and arise from shared sport experiences (both informal and organised sport), competition among siblings, and role modelling (Lundy et al., 2019).

Shared Experiences and Role Models

In a systematic review of siblings and physical activity experiences, Blazo and Smith (2018) concluded that having siblings compared to being an only child related to more physical activity. This contrasts with the view that increased family size reduces the amount of resources for each child and therefore less opportunities and provision of sport. However, studies suggest that a larger family provides greater opportunities to co-engage in physical activity among siblings (Blazo & Smith, 2018). This may be explained by the majority of research using Caucasian middle-class samples, and therefore differences in sibling influences may be found in different demographics. For example, McMinn et al. (2011) reported having siblings was associated with doing more physical activity for white European participants but not for South Asian participants. In addition, the sex composition of siblings within the family appears to mediate outcomes (Blazo & Smith, 2018) with some studies reporting that gender differences exist within sibling influence. For example, Davison (2004) found that for girls, support from a brother or sister was related to higher physical activity, whereas for boys, higher physical activity was only associated with support from a brother suggesting that boys are less likely to be influenced by the athletic prowess of a sister than a brother. In contrast, other studies show that younger siblings benefit, regardless of gender, from the exposure to their older sibling's sport experiences (e.g., Lundy et al., 2019). Such intricacies and contradictions require further investigation.

Positive and Negative Experiences

Research on siblings has largely focused on the positive and negative influences of the sibling-athlete relationship (Nelson & Strachan, 2017). Spanning across various sport experiences studies have reported siblings as positive sources of encouragement and support as well as negative sources of jealousy and rivalry (Blazo & Smith, 2018). For example, older siblings may have acted as socialising agents, whereby younger siblings observed their older siblings participating and imitated their behaviours, initiating their involvement in sport (Hopwood et al., 2015). Older siblings have also been shown to act as positive role models for work ethic. However, when an older sibling is successful in sport, younger siblings may experience bitterness and jealousy (Côté, 1999). In any family where one child is more talented than the other and the distribution of resources is uneven, with the talented child receiving more, resentment and tension between siblings may result (Côté & Hay, 2002), as demonstrated by the situation in Case Study 9.1 with Grace and Arthur.

Competition and rivalry between siblings have also been shown to have positive and negative effects. Positive experiences can be achieved through influencing motivation, whereby younger siblings aspire to be as good as or better than an older sibling (Lundy et al., 2019). In contrast younger siblings can experience negative effects by feeling overshadowed by older siblings (Lundy et al., 2019). Birth order has also been linked to athletic development, suggesting that later-born children are more likely to become elite athletes and therefore more successful in the sporting domain (Carette et al., 2011; Hopwood et al., 2015). One such explanation for this phenomenon is that firstborn children focus on their own development, and are typically measured against their own progress, whereas younger children compare themselves, and are often compared, to older siblings. Younger siblings constantly strive to perform better than older siblings who are typically bigger, stronger, and more powerful. This behaviour may result in firstborns possessing a desire to learn, as opposed to secondborns who may develop a greater motivation to win (Carette et al., 2011).

Research provides undoubtable evidence that, in addition to parents, siblings do influence one another's sport and physical activity involvement. However, more investigation is required to explore how siblings affect activity levels and experiences, particularly relating to gender, sport choices, and continued participation across the lifespan (Osai & Whiteman, 2017).

CREATING A POSITIVE MOTIVATIONAL CLIMATE

The benefits of sport participation are widely documented, although not all children and adolescents have positive experiences and their levels of participation and the enjoyment they gain from it will differ significantly (Quested & Duda, 2011). Parental involvement varies greatly when children are participating in organised sport and can have a significant impact on the quality of a child's sporting experience in a variety of ways, including motivational climate. The quality of the experience can influence whether a child enjoys the activity and therefore links this enjoyment to continued participation and athletic development (Bailey et al., 2015). For example, there is growing evidence to suggest that if the early experiences of children include participating in a variety of sports that are fun and enjoyable, they are likely to have greater positive experiences and increased developmental outcomes (Bridge & Toms, 2013). Motivation theories can help us to consider the reasons children participate in sport and their links to positive outcomes. Similar to the motivational climates created by coaches (see Chapter 8), parents can also generate either an ego-involving, or performance, climate (where the parent values and praises winning and out-performing others) or, a task-involving, or mastery, climate (where the parent values and praises their child's effort and improvements). This section revisits the motivational theory discussed in Chapter 8 with an emphasis on parental influence.

Self-Determination Theory

Children participate in sport for many reasons. For some children participation is driven by the fun and enjoyment of the activity, whereas other children may participate to please a parent or to gain a reward. It is these varied reasons for sports involvement that have been investigated by many researchers using the Self-Determination Theory (SDT; Deci & Ryan, 1985; Deci & Ryan, 2000). SDT asserts that an individual's motivation is determined by the degree to which the needs of competence (to achieve things), autonomy (to be in control of ourselves), and relatedness (to belong and feel accepted) are satisfied. The reason for a child's initial participation and their continued participation in sport and/or exercise are linked to how self-determined they deem the activity to be. Figure 9.2 explains SDT in context for youth sport participation.

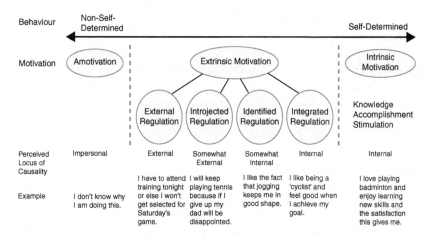

FIGURE 9.2 The motivation continuum

Source: Adapted from Deci & Ryan, 2000, p. 72

At the far left of the continuum is amotivation, defined as the absence of intrinsic and extrinsic motivation which arises when an individual feels the activity is no longer worthwhile and that they will never accomplish the desired outcomes (Deci & Ryan, 1985). Amotivation is linked to perceived high levels of incompetence and lack of control, and can result in withdrawal. Placed along the continuum with low to high self-determination levels are the four types of extrinsic motivation moving respectively from external regulation to integrated regulation. Integrated regulation, although a form of self-determined behaviour, is still considered an extrinsic motivation as it is performed to achieve personal goals rather than the pure appeal of the activity. This disregards the thinking that extrinsic motivation is synonymous with non-self-determined behaviour.

At the far right of the continuum lies intrinsic motivation, which has been further categorised by Vallerand and colleagues (1989) as intrinsic motivation to know (participating in an activity for the pleasure experienced while learning), intrinsic motivation to accomplish things (participating for the positive feelings experienced when striving to achieve a goal), and intrinsic motivation to experience stimulation (to encounter exciting emotions and feelings). SDT therefore lies at the heart of youth athletic development as intrinsically motivated children participate in sport for various reasons, such as enjoyment, interest, and satisfaction (Quested & Duda, 2011), with more self-determined behaviour linked to greater persistence in sport.

Cognitive Evaluation Theory

To help explain what factors threaten or enhance intrinsic motivation for the sport or activity, Cognitive Evaluation Theory (CET; Deci, 1975)—considered to be a sub theory of SDT—suggests that situational factors affect motivation by shaping people's perceptions of competence, autonomy, and relatedness (Ryan & Deci, 2019). If an individual engages in an activity for personal reasons and their involvement is chiefly self-determined, their perceived locus of causality (individuals' perceptions of the causes of their behaviour) will be internal (see Figure 9.2). Introducing more external motivators enhances an external perceived locus of causality and decreases intrinsic motivation, although the impact of extrinsic motivators depends on whether they are perceived to be controlling the individual's behaviour or providing information and positive feedback. In summary, motivators that an individual considers to provide information can enhance intrinsic motivation, whereas those perceived as controlling can diminish it (Ryan & Deci, 2019). For example, an athlete gaining a scholarship, seen as an extrinsic motivator, may reinforce the athlete's perceptions of competence and therefore be perceived as informational. In contrast, parental use of extrinsic motivators to incentivise performance, such as offering sweets or money for winning or achieving a high place, has been linked to increasing pressure and anxiety (Keegan et al., 2009) and dropout (Fraser-Thomas et al., 2008) when perceived as controlling. However, for some children such motivators acted as an increased incentive (Keegan et al., 2009), illustrating that it is the perception of such rewards and how they are perceived by the child that determine the influence on intrinsic motivation.

Childhood is the most important time to lay the foundations on which to encourage lifelong, intrinsically motivated sport participation (Côté & Hancock, 2016). For example, Arthur (from Case Study 9.1) cites intrinsic motives for playing rugby but reveals more extrinsic motives (such as pleasing his dad) for playing football and therefore is perhaps more likely to withdraw from football in the future even though he is talented. Considering the level of self-determined behaviour in a child provides a useful lens through which to view parental influence with parental support, praise, and understanding unequivocally linked with enhanced intrinsic motivation and enjoyment of sport (Ullrich-French & Smith, 2006).

Achievement Goal Theory

One of the ways that parents may influence their child's sports experience is through the goals that they set for their children to achieve. Achievement Goal Theory (AGT; Nicholls, 1989), introduced in Chapter 8, explains the behavioural outcomes that certain types of goals create. Goal orientations are said to be developed through socialisation that occurs in childhood, and therefore it can be assumed that parents play a major role in their development (Nicholls, 1989). In fact, it has been suggested that parents play a more significant role than coaches from an achievement goal perspective (O'Rourke et al., 2014). Parents, knowingly or unknowingly, create a motivational climate in sport for their child through either placing emphasis on results (ego-involving) or personal progress (task-involving). Parents' situational behaviours, goal orientation, values, attitudes, and beliefs influence their child's goal orientation, which in turn shapes their perceived competence. A child's perceived competence determines whether the child demonstrates an adaptive or maladaptive motivational pattern. For example, an ego involving climate has been linked to maladaptive motivation patterns whereby a child is unable to adjust satisfactorily to the environment or situation. In sport this can include experiencing feelings of pressure, engaging in antisocial behaviour, adopting the belief that ability determines success, and even withdrawing from sport (Ruiz et al., 2019). In contrast task-involving climates promote more adaptive motivations linked to intrinsic motivation and striving to achieve (Ruiz et al., 2019).

A child's experience of sport will also be shaped by the way in which their competence levels are measured. Whether initiated by parents or coaches, the literature exploring motivational climate in youth sport unambiguously expresses the benefits of a mastery climate (O'Rourke et al., 2014). The motivational climate, which is often determined by parents' supportive behaviours, is key for understanding children's psychological outcomes and intentions to remain involved in sports (Atkins et al., 2013). Parents should therefore strive to align with the principles of EVM, SDT, and AGT to consider how to create the most positive motivational climate for their own child(ren) (see Box 9.2).

Box 9.2 Creating a Positive Motivational Climate

General principles that parents can consider when creating a motivational climate for their child involve:

- consideration of whether their own beliefs and values influence the opportunities and experiences they provide for their child(ren)
- encouraging their children to participate in sport for reasons such as enjoyment, interest, and satisfaction
- setting task goals that align with the child's aims
- providing informational and supportive feedback placing emphasis on their child's personal progress rather than measuring their child against the performance of others
- avoiding the use of extrinsic motivators to encourage participation, instead focusing on intrinsic rewards

PARENTAL INVOLVEMENT: ENHANCING EXPERIENCES

Motivation- and achievement-related theories (such as those discussed in the chapter so far) have provided a solid foundation and furthered understanding of why specific parental attitudes, beliefs, and behaviours are formed. Such theories have also shown how parents may shape a child's motivation as well as contribute to the development of certain psychosocial outcomes (Knight, 2019). There are various ways that parental involvement may influence a child's psychosocial outcomes (e.g., motivation, self-perception, well-being) and these include parenting style, parenting practices in a range of contexts, and parental relationships and interactions with others in the sporting environment (Harwood et al., 2019). Research evidence has clearly established that some parental behaviours are associated with positive outcomes for young athletes and others are associated with more negative outcomes (Knight et al., 2017).

Levels of Parental Involvement

The extent to which parents are involved in their child's sport varies greatly and there are several models of parental involvement in sport that help explain such involvement. One of the most widely cited is Hellstedt's (1987) Parental Involvement Continuum, which defines parents as either underinvolved, moderately involved, or overinvolved (see Figure 9.3). The underinvolved parent is characterised by a lack of emotional, financial, and functional involvement; rarely attends events; is reluctant to volunteer their help; has little interest in interacting with the coach; and does not help their child set realistic goals. In contrast the overinvolved parent is classified as 'excessive' often satisfying their own needs through their child or hoping that their child's success will prove fruitful in some way. Overinvolved parents are unable to separate their own needs from those of their child. Located between these two extremes are the moderately involved parents, who provide direction to their child but do not overpower them, are firm but supportive, are willing to listen to the coach, and help set realistic goals for their child. Although receiving criticism for its lack of derision from research evidence, the model is widely used within the sports literature (e.g., Brackenridge, 2006; Danioni et al., 2017) and provides a useful starting point to consider parental involvement within sport with both ends of the continuum linked to negative consequences such as parental pressure and lack of support.

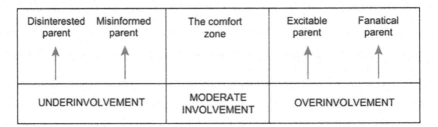

FIGURE 9.3 The parental involvement continuum

Source: Hellstedt, 1987; Brackenridge, 2006, p. 7

In their investigation of optimal parent involvement in tennis, Knight and Holt (2014) emphasised parents' understanding and enhancing their child's journey. This was underpinned by three categories: sharing and communicating goals, with parents and children adopting the same aims for the child's tennis involvement; developing an understanding emotional climate, where children perceive that parents understand their experiences; and engaging in enhancing parenting practices at competitions, including specific behaviours parents should display. Although specific to tennis, Knight and Holt (2014) surmise that optimal parenting is reached when parents make an effort to understand and enrich their children's experience over time as well as acknowledge that their child is an individual with unique needs.

Parental Behaviour

Specific parental behaviours in the sporting context and how parents interact with others in the sporting environment, such as coaches, other parents, and other young athletes, all have impact on a child's sport experience (Harwood et al., 2019). To extend parental behaviour research further, Knight and colleagues have conducted a range of research to address young athletes' preferences for parental behaviours. For example, in a study of 42 male and female 12- to 15-year-old tennis players, Knight et al. (2010) reported that players wanted their parents to be supportive without placing unnecessary pressure upon them. More specifically, players felt that parents should not give technical and tactical advice but that they should comment on effort and attitude, offer practical advice, follow tennis etiquette, and match nonverbal behaviours with supportive comments.

Research also indicates that parent-child interactions are different in team sports compared to individual sports. In a study of female adolescent athletes from team sports, Knight et al. (2011) found that although the results complemented previous findings on preferred behaviours in individual sports they also demonstrated specific behaviours related to the whole team. Findings indicated that prior to the competition the athletes wanted parents to help them to physically and mentally prepare, during competition they wanted parents to focus on effort rather than performance, interact positively with other athletes, and maintain control of their emotions. Explicit behaviours that were not welcomed included drawing attention to themselves and the athlete, coaching, and arguing with officials. Following competition athletes wanted positive and realistic feedback.

The Parenting Journey: A Developmental Approach

Throughout childhood into early adolescence, parents significantly influence their children's lives. However, the role of the parents and the type of support provided changes as the child enters late adolescence to allow for the child to have greater autonomy and involvement in decision-making. One of the most widely used models for investigating family involvement across an athlete's development is the Development Model of Sport Participation (DMSP; Côté, 1999), introduced in Chapter 2, which draws heavily on Bloom's (1985) work.

Côté's (1999) research resulted in the identification of three stages of participation: sampling, specialising, and investment years which provide a useful framework for viewing athletic development. During the sampling years (ages 6–13) parents encouraged their children to sample a range of fun and enjoyable sport activities. Between the ages of 13 and 15 years, the specialising years, the athlete made a commitment to one or two sports. Accompanying this, parents made a financial and time commitment to support their child as well as a growing interest in their child's sport; however, parents continued to emphasise school achievement as well as sport. In the investment years, athletes commit to one sport with the intention of making it as an elite sportsperson. Here parental roles were to increase the amount of tangible and emotional support—often making sacrifices themselves to do this—and supporting setbacks such as injury.

Since its conception the DMSP has been refined and researched culminating in an abundance of empirical supporting evidence (Côté & Vierimaa, 2014). One such study, by Huxley et al. (2018), of elite athletes during the specialising and investment stages of development found that parents were encouraging and firm during the specialising stage and provided authoritative guidance relating to the athletes' sporting experiences. During the investment stage, parental support shifted to encouraging greater autonomy and offering advice rather than giving direction. These findings support previous research (e.g., Côté, 1999) suggesting the need to adapt parenting styles to the stage of athletic development.

PARENTING EXPERTISE

Research and evidence on parental involvement and influence in a child's sporting experience was brought together in a position statement on parenting expertise in youth sport by Harwood and Knight (2015). The publication identified six key postulates of parenting expertise. These are illustrated along with their central concepts in Figure 9.4, and bring together the main theoretical stances discussed in this chapter including achievement and motivation theories, parental involvement, a developmental approach, and parental behaviours.

As illustrated by the six postulates parents have an important role to play in youth athletic development. However, attachment theorists propose that parental influence may begin long before the child engages in sport, as examined in the spotlight box.

Postulate no. 1: parents select the appropriate sporting opportunities for their child and provide necessary types of social support	• parents provide opportunities for their child to participate in a range of fun and enjoyable sporting activities with limited emphasis on competition and a focus on learning through play • parents and children have shared and communicated goals about what children want to achieve and parents provide the appropriate opportunities • parents provide appropriate tangible, emotional, and informational support relevant to the child's needs
Postulate no. 2: parents understand and apply an authoritative or autonomy-supportive parenting style	• parents create a healthy emotional climate for their child, through their application of specific parenting styles • parents work separately or together in applying an authoritative or autonomy-supportive style with their child

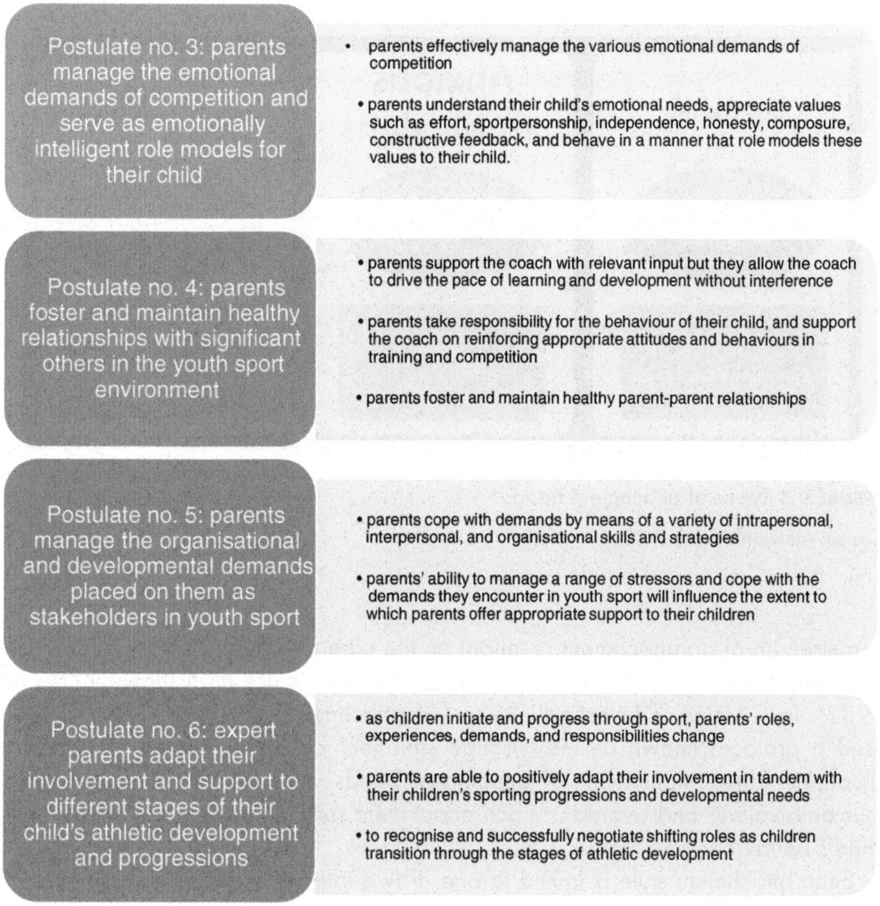

Postulate no. 3: parents manage the emotional demands of competition and serve as emotionally intelligent role models for their child	• parents effectively manage the various emotional demands of competition • parents understand their child's emotional needs, appreciate values such as effort, sportpersonship, independence, honesty, composure, constructive feedback, and behave in a manner that role models these values to their child.
Postulate no. 4: parents foster and maintain healthy relationships with significant others in the youth sport environment	• parents support the coach with relevant input but they allow the coach to drive the pace of learning and development without interference • parents take responsibility for the behaviour of their child, and support the coach on reinforcing appropriate attitudes and behaviours in training and competition • parents foster and maintain healthy parent-parent relationships
Postulate no. 5: parents manage the organisational and developmental demands placed on them as stakeholders in youth sport	• parents cope with demands by means of a variety of intrapersonal, interpersonal, and organisational skills and strategies • parents' ability to manage a range of stressors and cope with the demands they encounter in youth sport will influence the extent to which parents offer appropriate support to their children
Postulate no. 6: expert parents adapt their involvement and support to different stages of their child's athletic development and progressions	• as children initiate and progress through sport, parents' roles, experiences, demands, and responsibilities change • parents are able to positively adapt their involvement in tandem with their children's sporting progressions and developmental needs • to recognise and successfully negotiate shifting roles as children transition through the stages of athletic development

FIGURE 9.4 Six key postulates of parenting expertise

Source: Adapted from Harwood & Knight, 2015

Spotlight On: The Importance of Attachment

Attachment theory (Bowlby, 1973, 1982) has predominantly been applied to examine how adult romantic relationships are influenced by attachment styles formed in childhood, but it has more recently been applied to relationships in sporting contexts. In addition to a parent's values and beliefs, the attachment between parent and child is suggested to have implications for a child's development not only in infancy but also throughout their childhood and into adulthood. This is explained by the tenets of attachment theory which suggest that the type

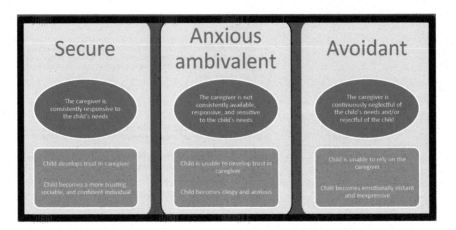

FIGURE 9.5 Types of attachment bonds

Source: Ainsworth et al., 1978

and strength of an attachment is reliant on the caregiver's availability, sensitivity, and responsiveness when the infant's proximity needs are high (Bowlby, 1973, 1982). In a series of investigations to test attachment, Ainsworth et al. (1978) used a protocol known as the 'strange situation' observing infants in different situations. Three main types of attachment bonds were identified: secure, anxious ambivalent, and avoidant. Each attachment style had specific effects on the child's behaviour (see Figure 9.5).

Each attachment style is linked to one of two internal working models (IWMs) that individuals develop: a model of self or a model of other (Bowlby, 1973). A model of self relates to how supported and loved one feels whereas a model of other links to the responsiveness and availability of the attachment figure or caregiver (Davis et al., 2013). If an individual has a secure attachment style and their interpersonal experiences involve consistent support, reassurance, and availability, they will have positive IWMs of both self and of others. In contrast if an individual has an insecure attachment style (anxious or avoidance) and their interpersonal experiences involve rejection or inconsistent support and availability, they are likely to have a negative IWM of themselves and their attachment figure. Building on Bowlby's work, Bartholomew (1990) developed a four category model of attachment (see Figure 9.6).

In a sporting context, athletes' avoidant and anxious styles of attachment were negatively linked to coach-athlete relationship satisfaction, sport satisfaction, and peer relationships (Davis & Jowett, 2010) and secure adolescent-parent attachments have been associated with positive sporting friendships (Carr & Fitzpatrick, 2011).

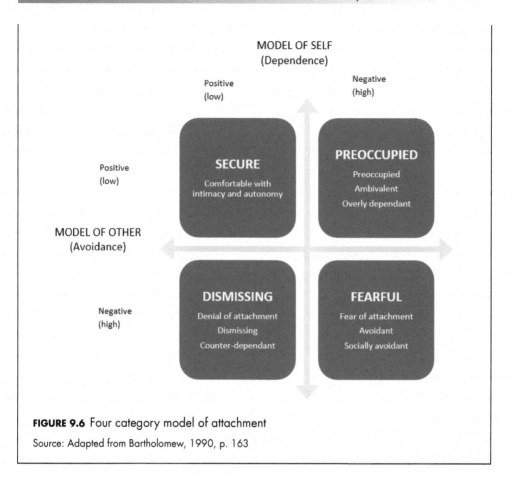

FIGURE 9.6 Four category model of attachment

Source: Adapted from Bartholomew, 1990, p. 163

CLOSING THOUGHTS

The research presented throughout this chapter undoubtedly demonstrates the profound impact of the family on youth athletic development. From attachments formed since birth to early childhood and initial socialisation experiences, sibling influences, and parental support provided throughout the stages of athletic development all contribute to shape an athlete. Initial research on family involvement focused very much on motivational theories such as EVM, SDT, and AGT. More recent research, by Knight and colleagues (e.g., 2017), expands this to include a wide range of qualitative studies to provide in-depth and rich data in a range of contexts to explore parental involvement and behaviour. Sibling relationships have received less attention, but from the research that has been conducted so far, variations and contradictions in the way that siblings seem to shape an individual's athletic development have been seen, with many areas requiring further investigation.

The empirical research into family influences presented in this chapter suggests that although general recommendations can be made in terms of how to create the most productive environment to develop young athletes, each child is unique and brings their own personality to the situation, not to mention the influence of significant others such as coaches, teachers, and peers. Therefore, parents should adopt an emotionally supportive approach to meet the individual needs of each young athlete, alongside the six postulates of parenting expertise generated from the research (Harwood & Knight, 2015).

REFERENCES

Ainsworth, M. D. S., Blehar, M. C., Waters, E., & Wall, S. (1978). *Patterns of attachment: A psychological study of the strange situation*. Lawrence Erlbaum Associates.

Atkins, M. R., Johnson, D. M., Force, E. C., & Petrie, T. A. (2013). "Do I still want to play?" Parents' and peers' influences on girls' continuation in sport. *Journal of Sport Behavior, 36*(4), 329–345.

Babkes, M. L., & Weiss, M. R. (1999). Parental influence on children's cognitive and affective responses to competitive soccer participation. *Pediatric Exercise Science, 11*, 44–62.

Bailey, R., Collins, D., Ford, P., MacNamara, Á., Toms, M., & Pearce, G. (2010). Participant development in sport: An academic review. *Sports Coach UK, 4*, 1–134.

Bailey, R., Cope, E., & Parnell, D. (2015). Realising the benefits of sports and physical activity: The human capital model. *Retos, 28*.

Bandura, A. (1986). *Social foundations of thought and action: A social cognitive theory*. Upper Saddle River, NJ: Prentice Hall.

Bartholomew, K. (1990). Avoidance of intimacy: An attachment perspective. *Journal of Social and Personal Relationships, 7*(2), 147–178.

Birchwood, D., Roberts, K., & Pollock, G. (2008). Explaining differences in sport participation rates among young adults: Evidence from the South Caucasus. *European Physical Education Review, 14*(3), 283–298.

Blazo, J. A., & Smith, A. L. (2018). A systematic review of siblings and physical activity experiences. *International Review of Sport and Exercise Psychology, 11*(1), 122–159.

Bloom, B. S. (Ed.), (1985). *Developing talent in young people*. New York: Ballantine.

Bowlby, J. (1973). Attachment and loss: Volume II: Separation, anxiety and anger. In *Attachment and loss: Volume II: Separation, anxiety and anger* (pp. 1–429). The Hogarth Press and the Institute of Psycho-Analysis.

Bowlby, J. (1982). Attachment and loss: Retrospect and prospect. *American Journal of Orthopsychiatry, 52*(4), 664.

Brackenridge, C. (2006, 10–13 March). *The parents' optimum zone: Measuring and optimising parental engagement in youth sport*. Commonwealth Games International Conference, Melbourne, Australia. http://bura.brunel.ac.uk/handle/2438/623

Bridge, M. W., & Toms, M. R. (2013). The specialising or sampling debate: A retrospective analysis of adolescent sports participation in the UK. *Journal of Sports Sciences, 31*(1), 87–96.

Brustad, R. J. (1993). Who will go out and play? Parental and psychological influences on children's attraction to physical activity. *Pediatric Exercise Science, 5*(3), 210–223.

Brzęk, A., Strauss, M., Przybylek, B., Dworrak, T., Dworrak, B., & Leischik, R. (2018). How does the activity level of the parents influence their children's activity? The contemporary life in a world ruled by electronic devices. *Archives of Medical Science: AMS, 14*(1), 190.

Carette, B., Anseel, F., & Van Yperen, N. W. (2011). Born to learn or born to win? Birth order effects on achievement goals. *Journal of Research in Personality, 45*(5), 500–503.

Carr, S., & Fitzpatrick, N. (2011). Experiences of dyadic sport friendships as a function of self and partner attachment characteristics. *Psychology of Sport and Exercise, 12*(4), 383–391.

Côté, J. (1999). The influence of the family in the development of talent in sport. *The Sport Psychologist, 13*(4), 395–417.

Côté, J., & Hancock, D. J. (2016). Evidence-based policies for youth sport programmes. *International Journal of Sport Policy and Politics, 8*(1), 51–65.

Côté, J., & Hay, J. (2002). Family influences on youth sport performance and participation. In J. M. Silva and D. E. Stevens (Eds.), *Psychological foundations of sport* (pp. 503–519). Allyn and Bacon Publishers.

Côté, J., & Vierimaa, M. (2014). The developmental model of sport participation: 15 years after its first conceptualization. *Science & Sports, 29*, S63–S69.

Courtney, J. B., Moss, H. E., Butki, B. D., & Li, K. (2019). Parent support, perceptions, and child attributes affect child activity. *American Journal of Health Behavior, 43*(2), 311–325.

Danioni, F., Barni, D., & Rosnati, R. (2017). Transmitting sport values: The importance of parental involvement in children's sport activity. *Europe's Journal of Psychology, 13*(1), 75.

Davis, L., & Jowett, S. (2010). Investigating the interpersonal dynamics between coaches and athletes based on fundamental principles of attachment. *Journal of Clinical Sport Psychology, 4*(2), 112–132.

Davis, L., Jowett, S., & Lafrenière, M.-A. K. (2013). An attachment theory perspective in the examination of relational processes associated with coach-athlete dyads. *Journal of Sport and Exercise Psychology, 35*(2), 156–167.

Davison, K. K. (2004). Activity-related support from parents, peers, and siblings and adolescents' physical activity: Are there gender differences? *Journal of Physical Activity and Health, 1*(4), 363–376.

Deci, E. L. (1975). *Intrinsic motivation.* Plenum Press.

Deci, E. L., & Ryan, R. M. (1985). *Intrinsic motivation and self-determination in human behavior.* Plenum.

Deci, E. L., & Ryan, R. M. (2000). The "what" and "why" of goal pursuits: Human needs and the self-determination of behavior. *Psychological Inquiry, 11*(4), 227–268.

Dixon, M. A., Warner, S. M., & Bruening, J. E. (2008). More than just letting them play: Parental influence on women's lifetime sport involvement. *Sociology of Sport Journal, 25*(4), 538–559.

Dozier, S. G., Schroeder, K., Lee, J., Fulkerson, J. A., & Kubik, M. Y. (2020). The association between parents and children meeting physical activity guidelines. *Journal of Pediatric Nursing, 52*, 70–75.

Eccles, J. S. (1993). *School and family effects on the ontogeny of children's interests, self-perceptions, and activity choices.* Nebraska Symposium on Motivation, 1992: Developmental Perspectives on Motivation.

Eccles, J. S., Adler, T., Futterman, T., Goff, R., Kaczala, S., Meece, C., & Midgley, J. (1983). Expectations, values, and academic behaviors. *Achievement and Achievement Motivation*, 283–331.

Eccles, J. S., & Harold, R. D. (1991). Gender differences in sport involvement: Applying the Eccles' expectancy-value model. *Journal of Applied Sport Psychology, 3*(1), 7–35.

Eccles, J. S., & Wigfield, A. (2020). From expectancy-value theory to situated expectancy-value theory: A developmental, social cognitive, and sociocultural perspective on motivation. *Contemporary Educational Psychology*, 101859.

Eckelt, M., Hutmacher, D., Steffgen, G., & Bund, A. (2019). *Differences in physical activity among children with physically active and inactive parents*. Healthy & Active Children Lifespan Motor Development Science & Application, Verona, Italy. http://158.64.76.181/handle/10993/40642

Fraser-Thomas, J., Côté, J., & Deakin, J. (2008). Understanding dropout and prolonged engagement in adolescent competitive sport. *Psychology of Sport and Exercise, 9*(5), 645–662.

Fredricks, J. A., & Eccles, J. S. (2004). Parental influences on youth involvement in sports. In M. R. Weiss (Ed.), *Developmental sport and exercise psychology: A lifespan perspective* (pp. 145–164). Fitness Information Technology.

Fredricks, J. A., & Eccles, J. S. (2005). Family socialization, gender, and sport motivation and involvement. *Journal of Sport & Exercise Psychology, 27*(1), 3.

Harwood, C. G., & Knight, C. J. (2015). Parenting in youth sport: A position paper on parenting expertise. *Psychology of Sport and Exercise, 16*(Part 1), 24–35. https://doi.org/10.1016/j.psychsport.2014.03.001

Harwood, C. G., Knight, C. J., Thrower, S. N., & Berrow, S. R. (2019). Advancing the study of parental involvement to optimise the psychosocial development and experiences of young athletes. *Psychology of Sport and Exercise, 42*, 66–73.

Hellstedt, J. (1987). The coach/parent/athlete relationship. *The Sport Psychologist, 1*, 151–160.

Hopwood, M., Farrow, D., MacMahon, C., & Baker, J. (2015). Sibling dynamics and sport expertise. *Scandinavian Journal of Medicine & Science in Sports, 25*(5), 724–733.

Huxley, D. J., O'Connor, D., & Bennie, A. (2018). Olympic and World Championship track and field athletes' experiences during the specialising and investment stages of development: A qualitative study with Australian male and female representatives. *Qualitative Research in Sport, Exercise and Health, 10*(2), 256–272.

Johansson, E., Mei, H., Xiu, L., Svensson, V., Xiong, Y., Marcus, C., Zhang, J., & Hagströmer, M. (2016). Physical activity in young children and their parents—An early STOPP Sweden–China comparison study. *Scientific Reports, 6*, 29595.

Keegan, R. J., Harwood, C. G., Spray, C. M., & Lavallee, D. E. (2009). A qualitative investigation exploring the motivational climate in early career sports participants: Coach, parent and peer influences on sport motivation. *Psychology of Sport and Exercise, 10*(3), 361–372. https://doi.org/10.1016/j.psychsport.2008.12.003

Knight, C. J. (2019). Revealing findings in youth sport parenting research. *Kinesiology Review, 8*(3), 252–259.

Knight, C. J., Berrow, S. R., & Harwood, C. G. (2017). Parenting in sport. *Current Opinion in Psychology, 16*, 93–97.

Knight, C. J., Boden, C. M., & Holt, N. L. (2010). Junior tennis players' preferences for parental behaviors. *Journal of Applied Sport Psychology, 22*(4), 377–391.

Knight, C. J., & Holt, N. L. (2014). Parenting in youth tennis: Understanding and enhancing children's experiences. *Psychology of Sport and Exercise, 15*(2), 155–164. https://doi.org/10.1016/j.psychsport.2013.10.010

Knight, C. J., Neely, K. C., & Holt, N. L. (2011). Parental behaviors in team sports: How do female athletes want parents to behave? *Journal of Applied Sport Psychology, 23*(1), 76–92.

Lundy, G. I., Allan, V., Cowburn, I., & Cote, J. (2019). Parental support, sibling influences and family dynamics across the development of Canadian interuniversity student-athletes. *Journal of Athlete Development and Experience, 1*(2), 4.

McMinn, A. M., van Sluijs, E. M., Nightingale, C. M., Griffin, S. J., Cook, D. G., Owen, C. G., Rudnicka, A. R., & Whincup, P. H. (2011). Family and home correlates of children's physical activity in a multi-ethnic population: The cross-sectional Child Heart and Health Study in England (CHASE). *International Journal of Behavioral Nutrition and Physical Activity, 8*(1), 11.

Milošević, V., & Vesković, A. (2013). Family as an agent for sport socialization of youth. *Serbian Journal of Sports Sciences, 7*(3).

Nelson, K., & Strachan, L. (2017). Friend, foe, or both? A retrospective exploration of sibling relationships in elite youth sport. *International Journal of Sports Science & Coaching, 12*(2), 207–218.

Nicholls, J. G. (1989). *The competitive ethos and democratic education.* Harvard University Press.

O'Rourke, D. J., Smith, R. E., Smoll, F. L., & Cumming, S. P. (2014). Relations of parent- and coach-initiated motivational climates to young athletes' self-esteem, performance anxiety, and autonomous motivation: Who is more influential? *Journal of Applied Sport Psychology, 26*(4), 395–408.

Osai, K. V., & Whiteman, S. D. (2017). Family relationships and youth sport: Influence of siblings and parents on youth's participation, interests, and skills. *Journal of Amateur Sport, 3*(3), 86–105.

Partridge, J. A., Brustrad, R. J., & Babkes Stellino, M. (2008). Social influence in sport. In T. S. Horn (Ed.), *Advances in sport psychology* (3rd ed.). Human Kinetics.

Quested, E., & Duda, J. L. (2011). Enhancing children's positive sport experiences and personal development. *Coaching Children in Sport,* 123–138.

Ruiz, M. C., Robazza, C., Tolvanen, A., Haapanen, S., & Duda, J. L. (2019). Coach-created motivational climate and athletes' adaptation to psychological stress: Temporal motivation-emotion interplay. *Frontiers in Psychology, 10,* 617. www.frontiersin.org/articles/10.3389/fpsyg.2019.00617/full

Ryan, R. M., & Deci, E. L. (2019). Brick by brick: The origins, development, and future of self-determination theory. *Advances in Motivation Science, 6,* 111–156.

Sánchez-Miguel, P. A., Leo, F. M., Sánchez-Oliva, D., Amado, D., & García-Calvo, T. (2013). The importance of parents' behavior in their children's enjoyment and amotivation in sports. *Journal of Human Kinetics, 36*(1), 169–177.

Shen, B., Centeio, E., Garn, A., Martin, J., Kulik, N., Somers, C., & McCaughtry, N. (2018). Parental social support, perceived competence and enjoyment in school physical activity. *Journal of Sport and Health Science, 7*(3), 346–352.

Simpkins, S. D., Fredricks, J. A., & Eccles, J. S. (2012). Charting the Eccles' expectancy-value model from mothers' beliefs in childhood to youths' activities in adolescence. *Developmental Psychology, 48*(4), 1019–1032. https://doi.org/10.1037/a0027468

Straub, G. (2019). Parental (over-) ambition in competitive youth sport. *German Journal of Exercise and Sport Research, 49*(1), 1–10.

Tucker, R., & Collins, M. (2012). What makes champions? A review of the relative contribution of genes and training to sporting success. *British Journal of Sports Medicine, 46*(8), 555–561.

Ullrich-French, S., & Smith, A. L. (2006). Perceptions of relationships with parents and peers in youth sport: Independent and combined prediction of motivational outcomes. *Psychology of Sport and Exercise, 7*(2), 193–214.

Vallerand, R. J., Blais, M. R., Brière, N. M., & Pelletier, L. G. (1989). Construction et validation de l'échelle de motivation en éducation (EME) [Construction and validation of the Motivation toward Education Scale]. *Canadian Journal of Behavioural Science/Revue canadienne des sciences du comportement, 21*(3), 323–349. https://doi.org/10.1037/h0079855

Wang, M.-T., Chow, A., & Amemiya, J. (2017). Who wants to play? Sport motivation trajectories, sport participation, and the development of depressive symptoms. *Journal of Youth and Adolescence, 46*(9), 1982–1998. https://link.springer.com/article/10.1007/s10964-017-0649-9

Weiss, M. R. (2019). Youth sport motivation and participation: Paradigms, perspectives, and practicalities. *Kinesiology Review, 8*(3), 162–170.

CHAPTER 10

How Does the School Setting Influence Athletic Development?

Nichola Kentzer

Since children and young people spend a significant proportion of their lives in educational settings, the influence of schools on a young person's athletic development should not be ignored. What is more, researchers who have studied the career span of elite athletes consider education settings to be an important aspect of their development (e.g., Wylleman & Lavallee, 2004), where children often encounter their first experience of organised sport (Lovell et al., 2019). This chapter examines the social influence of the school setting on athletic development, focusing largely on physical education (PE) and school sport for those aged 5 to 18 years, in 'primary' and 'secondary' education (Wylleman & Lavallee, 2004).

Before we begin our exploration of the topic, we need to define what we mean by PE and school sport since some have claimed that the use of the two terms in conjunction could be "potentially misleading and may cause some confusion" (Stidder & Hayes, 2011, p. xix). The Association for Physical Education (AfPE; 2015, p. 3) offers suitable definitions for the purpose of the chapter:

> **Physical Education** is the planned, progressive learning that takes place in school curriculum timetabled time and which is delivered to all pupils.
> **School Sport** is the structured learning that takes place beyond the curriculum (i.e. in the extended curriculum) within school settings; this is sometimes referred to as out-of-school-hours learning.

The discussion of the social influence of PE and school sport on athletic development is structured by this book's framework of athletic development (adapted from Gagné, 2015), introduced in Chapter 1, with components of the model highlighted in *italics* throughout the chapter.

THE SOCIAL INFLUENCE OF EDUCATIONAL SETTINGS ON ATHLETIC DEVELOPMENT

Our adapted framework demonstrates how educational settings could have an influence on a young person's athletic development. Gagné (2015) highlighted schools as an *environmental catalyst* that could affect the athletic development process in a positive or negative way, influenced by factors such as setting (e.g., urban/rural), finances, culture, and policy. The framework also considers the following areas that will be discussed in this chapter:

- *Individual relations* are significant to athletic development, such as the teachers and coaches that deliver PE and school sport. These "significant persons" (Gagné, 2015, p. 22) not only create the environment but act as role models and can provide opportunities for athletic development. A second key influence is that of peers in the school setting. A third key influence is family. Parents can be key influences within PE and school sport and will be discussed where appropriate; for further detail on this area see Chapter 9.
- PE and school sport have the capacity to influence *mental catalysts*, identified in the framework. For example, schools can contribute to the development of psychosocial attitudes, behaviours, and skills important for athletic development. Linked to this is the mental health and *wellbeing* of athletes, discussed in Chapter 11, a topic which has become a key area of interest for researchers and practitioners alike. Experiences at school, including PE and school sport, can provide opportunities for personal development to support wellbeing, especially during adolescence (Eccles & Roeser, 2011). Given that 50% of all mental health problems have been established by the age of 14 years (Mental Health Taskforce, 2016), PE and school sport can have a significant role to play.

The framework demonstrates that *environmental catalysts*, *mental catalysts*, and *wellbeing* provide input to all three aspects of the *development journey*. For example, a young person's progress along the development journey will involve sport related progressions, such as a move from junior to senior level, but will also include school-based 'key moments' (Toms et al., 2009) with the transition from primary to secondary school and pressure points from examinations. The development journey can impact on wellbeing (and vice versa) and progress can be accelerated or slowed by positive and negative experiences.

There are other factors that will impact on this journey including whether the young person participates and competes in sporting activities outside of the school setting, often influenced by family and their circumstances (Bailey et al., 2010). However, Bailey and Morley (2006, p. 211) argue that PE is of "unique importance . . . within any talent development scheme", and as such this chapter will consider the *opportunities* afforded by PE and school sport based on the type of school attended (i.e., socioeconomic status) and geographical location (e.g., access to facilities) on the athletic development journey. In addition, we will explore the role of the PE teacher in talent identification and development and their influence on such *opportunities*. Furthermore, we will consider how PE and school sport can influence the young person as they *progress* on their athletic development journey.

THE SCHOOL ENVIRONMENT: A CATALYST FOR ATHLETIC DEVELOPMENT

The *investment* of time and money on the development journey from a PE and school sport perspective is influenced by government policy (different in each country), school/district budgeting, facilities available, and the type of school attended. It is important to note that a family's socioeconomic status will affect participation in sport, particularly outside of school, until later adolescence (Bailey et al., 2010). Also of note, PE and school sport are typically available at little, or no, cost (Bedard et al., 2020), in addition to there often being no requirement for transportation (Guèvremont et al., 2014). Moreover, school-based sport can offer opportunities for all children for long-term athletic development, in addition to offering a wide range of sports in which more able individuals could be challenged to develop their talents (Lovell et al., 2019).

Considerations of the global circumstances of sport more broadly demonstrate how the investment of time and money can have a strong bearing on the PE and school sport provision in the educational setting in an individual country. Indeed, as highlighted by Güllich and Cobley (2017) "significant social-ecological factors affecting the 'talent pool' that talented athletes can be drawn from" (p. 84) include:

- A country's population;
- Size of the country;
- The popularity of a sport;
- Mass participation in competitive sport; and
- General local training environments.

A country's PE and school sport provision could be a useful adjunct to this list, given that in England, for example, the Department for Culture, Media and Sport (2001) states that school-based PE can play an important role in both the identification and subsequent development of future champions. Hardman (2011) presents a useful snapshot of the global PE provision where the majority of countries have a legal requirement in place for PE in schools and where this is not the case, PE is generally taught as a matter of general practice. Of concern, however, are the gaps that exist globally between policy and actual practice, with PE lessons more likely to be cancelled than other subject areas, and low priority of PE reported in Africa, Asia, and Central and Latin America (Hardman, 2011). Unsurprisingly, the quality of PE provision, including the facilities and equipment available, was directly correlated in Hardman's research to the economic status of a country. Bailey and Morley (2006) highlight that children who do not have access to necessary equipment and support even at a basic level of participation, "will struggle to become aware of whatever talents they might possess" (p. 223).

When the difference between state- or government-funded educational settings (non–fee paying) and those that are privately funded (fee paying) is examined, an evident divide is seen in the investment of monies for the provision of PE and school sport. For example, despite a significant cash injection from government into school sport provision in the United Kingdom over the last 20 years, Team GB's Olympians are still four times more likely to have come from a private education background, particularly in hockey and rowing (The Sutton Trust, 2016).

Schools With a Distinct Sporting Focus

There are institutions that have a key focus on sport participation and talent development, where students develop their academic profile alongside their athletic development journey. Such settings can be termed dual career development environments (DCDEs), where a dual career can be defined as "a career with foci on sport and studies or work" (Stambulova & Wylleman, 2015, p. 1). Morris et al. (2020) sought to identify and classify different types of DCDEs found in seven

TABLE 10.1 Dual career development environment (DCDE) types for school ages

DC Institution Type	DC Institution Definition	European Examples
Sport-friendly schools	• Regional educational institutions that permit elite sport or align themselves with elite sport to provide academic flexibility for athletes to train and compete in their own sporting environment • Secondary and higher/further education • The support provisions are non-standardised between institutions in the same country—each is able to decide the provision of support they give to each athlete for themselves; they can, however, include similar features (e.g., sports facilities and sport science provision) • Academic flexibility is provided, although it is unlikely any formal arrangements between the school and sporting federations are formed	United Kingdom—Millfield School and Hartpury College Talented Athlete Scholarship Scheme Accredited Schools and Colleges, including Loughborough College and Stoke-on-Trent College Sweden—Sandagymnasiet Finland—Hämeenlinnan Lyseon Lukio, Jyväskylän Normaalikoulu, Pihtiputaan Lukio
Elite sports schools/ colleges	• Purposefully developed for elite athletes who wish to combine their athletic and academic careers by providing a combination of sport and academic support (e.g., elite coaching and an adapted timetable for studies) • Secondary and higher education • The support provisions as sport-friendly schools • Formal communication with sport federations and the school will often receive funding from the body they link with	United Kingdom—Scottish Football Association Performance Schools Belgium—Stedelijk Lyceum Topsport Sweden—Gudlav Bilderskolan Denmark—Marseiliesborg School Finland—Kilpisen Koulu, Sotkamon Lukio, Jyväskylän Koulutuskuntayhtymä Gradia

Source: Adapted from Morris et al., 2020, pp. 7–8

European countries. The researchers identified eight types of DCDEs, of which three were classified as 'education led': elite sport schools/colleges, sport-friendly schools/colleges, and sport-friendly universities. The two that include school-aged provision are detailed in Table 10.1.

It could be argued that the young people attending these sport-focused institutions would have access to a superior environment for their athletic development, as discussed by Oakley in Chapter 1 in his consideration of *chance*. Indeed, Bailey and Morley (2006) argued that the opportunity to study at a school where teachers and coaches have specialist skills and have high expectations for their students can make a significant contribution to performance. For example, in 2020, Millfield School in England boasted five age group international rugby union players as well as several young Olympians from a range of different sports (Gallagher, 2020), with access to a variety of support mechanisms (see Morris et al., 2020).

While these specialised environments offer a focus for the student-athletes on their athletic development journey, we must understand their influence on the development of psychosocial attitudes, behaviours and skills (*mental catalysts*), and *wellbeing*. For example, Stambulova et al. (2020) argued that dual career athletes usually recognise that it is not possible to fully invest, and continuously so, in both sport and education, highlighting the need for supporting the development of coping skills and dual career competencies (Stambulova & Wylleman, 2019; Henriksen et al., 2020). Indeed, while pursuing an academic career alongside their sporting focus can help maintain perspective for athletes (Aquilina, 2013) and support a more successful transition out of sport (Torregrosa et al., 2015), an inability to cope with the demands of such an environment can impact mental health and lead to increased stress, burnout and, ultimately, dropping out of the sport entirely (Stambulova et al., 2020).

Student-Athletes and Their Identities

In addition to the potential conflict between school and sport pressures, student-athletes could be more likely to form a stronger athletic identity than students attending more traditional educational settings. Indeed, often student-athletes are in late adolescence, a period that is recognised as a key time for establishing a sense of personal identity (Erikson, 1959). These identities are created through social interactions, and the nature of these social interactions student-athletes can experience are influenced by the worlds they inhabit (Eccles & Roeser, 2011)—for example, the DCDE. Research has identified a fluidity to the levels of athletic identity reported by student-athletes, with higher levels at the beginning and end of the academic year, but with inter- and intra- individual differences in between (Stambulova et al., 2015).

Optimal development of identity requires exploring a variety of activities and interacting with people from different backgrounds which provides opportunities for young people to "make informed decisions about their personal values, interests and skills" and "develop coping strategies and confidence in their abilities to be successful in adult life" (Brewer & Pepitas, 2017, p. 118). When based in a performance-focused environment, peers and teachers/coaches having the same focus could mean the student-athlete is at a greater risk of athletic identity foreclosure—"a state in which individuals are strongly committed to the athlete role without having engaged in exploratory behaviour" (Brewer & Pepitas, 2017, p. 120)—than with other leisure pursuits such as music and art. Through their exploration of the research literature, the authors concluded that athletic identity foreclosure had four key features (Table 10.2).

Sorkkila et al. (2018) examined the development of school and sport burnout in student-athletes using burnout profiles and exploring the demands placed on the elite junior athletes and their available resources (e.g., level of motivation and social support). Those student-athletes identified as at risk of burnout reported experiencing school-related stress and described having more demands than resources, with the researchers contending that it is possible "that school burnout generalises to the sport context" (p. 127). Perhaps compounding this further, concerns from parents over the ability of their children to manage sport and school pressures has been highlighted (Harwood et al., 2010), which can become amplified as children commit further to their sports and progress through the education system (Harwood & Knight, 2009).

TABLE 10.2 Features of athletic identity foreclosure
• Prominent during late adolescence; • Affected by changes in the athletes' status regarding sport participation; • Relates to a range of academic, social, cognitive/motivational, and emotional/affective factors; and • Associated with potential consequences in the domains of substance use, career development, burnout, and adjustment to sport transition.
Source: Brewer & Pepitas, 2017, pp. 120–121

Developing an Appropriate Skill Set

For student-athletes, the sport domain may be more prominent than school (Ryba et al., 2016). Perhaps unsurprisingly, therefore, one of Henriksen et al.'s (2014) features of a successful athletic talent development environment was where "school, family members, friends and others acknowledge and accept the athletes dedication to sport" (p. 145), along with an integrated approach with coordination and communication between family, sport, school, and other factors. Thus, suggesting that synergy surrounding the student-athlete, in addition to them developing an appropriate mental skill set, would allow them to concentrate on, and balance, both sporting and academic performance.

While we previously argued that the DCDEs may place greater pressure on the student-athlete, they may in fact offer support in a way that traditional school settings might not. For example, in an attempt to provide instruction and guidance for student-athletes to support their athletic development, Kiens and Larsen (2020) implemented a mental skills training programme in an elite sport school in Estonia. This is explained in the spotlight.

Spotlight On: Developing Student-Athletes' Mental Skills

To address some of the concerns in the literature regarding the experience of student-athletes, Kiens and Larsen (2020) implemented a mental skills training programme at an elite sport school in Estonia where Kiens was an established sport psychology practitioner (SPP). The student-athletes at this school, aged 15 to 19 years, lived on site and had access to a range of support staff. Entry to the school was on acceptance from the Estonian Olympic Committee in conjunction with sport federations.

The programme was developed as "a normal part of their development instead of adding an extra thing on top" (p. 3). The programme for 39 student-athletes consisted of 16 small group sessions, held twice a week over the academic year. Each session had a clear structure with a focus on reflective practice, psychoeducation, and goal setting.

> Overall, the programme was seen to be effective in developing basic mental skills (e.g., self-awareness), concentration skills, the management of emotions, improved self-control, and a more developed sense of self in the student-athletes.
>
> Reflecting on the programme, the SPP was faced with sessions being cancelled and had to adjust to the needs of the student-athletes (in terms of being flexible with timings). The reflections highlighted the importance of collaborating with other staff members to integrate efforts and the value of peer support in the process.
>
> Although this research examines one cohort of student-athletes, the study provides an insight into the practicalities of implementing a support programme for student-athletes.

This section has largely focused on student-athletes in elite school sport environments. However, the concepts and *mental catalysts* of athletic development discussed could also impact on pupils in state-funded schools who pursue their sporting focus and, therefore, the development of their mental skills could be beneficial. The students at the elite school featured in Kiens and Larsen's (2020) research had access to a sport psychologist, but would there be an appropriately trained staff member to offer training of this nature in more traditional, state-funded school settings? For a programme of this nature to be integrated into a PE and school sport curriculum, it is more likely that it would be delivered by a PE teacher. Before we examine the role of the PE teacher in supporting athletic development in more depth, we look now to the curricula and discuss how it, and the opportunity for talent identification and development in PE and school sport, could influence the athletic development journey.

PE AND SCHOOL SPORT: DEVELOPING A TALENT POOL

While many countries claim to commit to a "broad and balanced" (Hardman, 2011, p. 19) PE curriculum, there is evidence of a focus on performance sport with a significant proportion of schools globally focusing on games, track and field athletics, and gymnastics, and there have been issues raised of relevance and quality of the curriculum. Further, divided approaches to delivering PE within education systems could be evident as a result of a lack of empirical-based evidence for best practices in PE (Giblin et al., 2014). Consequently, how PE is experienced by pupils can influence their engagement and motivation to pursue sport outside of curriculum time (Ommundsen & Kvalø, 2007), thus missing *opportunities* to *progress* along any potential athletic development journey.

Where different approaches to teaching PE exist globally, and indeed within countries, an important question is, 'Are we all starting from the same place'? The International Position Statement on Physical Education (International Council of Sport Science and Physical Education, ICSSPE, 2010) states that:

> Physical education develops physical competence so that all children can move efficiently, effectively and safely and understand what they are doing. The outcome, physical literacy, is an essential basis for their full development and achievement.

It contributes to children's confidence and self-esteem; enhances social development by preparing children to cope with competition, winning and losing; and cooperation and collaboration.

In this statement there is a focus on the physical, mental, and social components of athletic development, including an outcome of physical literacy, confidence, and self-esteem, with consideration of working with others. Of interest in this description is the use of the term physical literacy (PL) as the outcome of PE. The concept has been claimed as a "core element of early learning" (Department for Education, 2019, p. 8), and a "foundation pillar of long-term athletic development" (Long Term Athletic Development, 2020). However, when investigating PL in relation to athletic development, multiple definitions and differing uses of the term in the literature are encountered (Edwards et al., 2017; Bailey et al., 2019), which "has led some to question the concept's current capacity to act as the basis of a coherent programme" (Bailey, 2020, p. 1). For the purpose of our discussion, we will consider that PL is concerned with the broad areas of physical, psycho-social (affect), and cognitive and integrated (holistic) development as identified by Bailey et al. (under review) and correlates with *mental catalysts* and *wellbeing* that can influence the athletic development journey.

A second noteworthy feature of the ICSSPE definition is the use of competition, particularly as the definition posits that PE helps to prepare children to 'cope' with competition. PE takes place in a more public environment than typical classroom-based subjects (Spray et al., 2013), and this, in addition to its competitive element, may lead to increased pupil concerns over ability and performance (Yli-Piipari et al., 2009). Indeed, carefully managed competition can be a valuable educational experience for pupils, but "should not be at the expense of their holistic development" (Stidder and Hayes, 2013, p. 2), and caution is needed to ensure that it does not foster bullying (Jiménez-Barbero et al., 2020). Moreover, although competition may be viewed as meaningful for many youth sport participants (e.g., Gledhill and Harwood, 2014), Beni et al.'s (2017) findings suggest this is not the case for students in PE. It is, therefore, important for schools to consider the role competition plays in athletic development.

Using a Model of Talent Development in PE

In an attempt to "address the imbalance" from an almost sole focus on out of school clubs as a talent development mechanism when preparing for adult elite sport, Bailey and Morley (2006, p. 211) proposed a model of talent development in PE (Figure 10.1). The model was designed by the authors drawing on a number of sources and exemplars, largely from sport and education, including the work of Gagné, hence a number of similar features to the book's framework of athletic development, including 'abilities' and 'environmental characteristics'. In the PE context, the identification and development of talent can be influenced by the school, and those within it—for example, the teachers. The authors argue that talent development, "an integral feature" (Bailey & Morley, 2006, p. 224) of PE programmes, is part of differentiated practice, functioning to meet the individual needs of the pupils to achieve the 'outcomes' in the model (right-hand side of Figure 10.1). This would include the more able pupils aiming towards 'elite sport performance' and, equally important, the programme encouraging outcomes of enjoyment and lifelong participation.

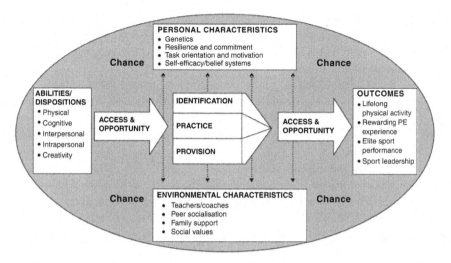

FIGURE 10.1 A model of talent development in physical education

Source: Bailey & Morley, 2006, p. 212

The model is applied to the following case study where we examine the experiences of one teacher supporting an emerging talent (**bold** is used within the narrative to highlight where the features of the model are applied).

CASE STUDY 10.1

Identifying Talent in PE and School Sport

Ashley was known at his school—a non–fee paying comprehensive (secondary) school in a rural area of northern England—for his poor behaviour. He was also known as a talented sprinter, with the **ability** to run faster than anyone in his year group, indeed faster than anyone in the older year groups. This level of speed was indicated early in his PE classes by the results of baseline fitness tests.

While speed can be used advantageously in many team sports (e.g., rugby), Ashley did not demonstrate some of the **personal characteristics** required to make him an effective part of a squad, particularly regarding **commitment**, **task-orientation**, and communication with others.

Despite his talent being identified in PE lessons at the age of 11, the **opportunity** for this to be nurtured did not arise until Ashley was 15 years old, when contact was made by his PE teacher with a local female athlete who represented her country as part of the 4x100m relay squad. This led to Ashley being invited to meet with her coach at a local athletics track, due to the lack of appropriate facilities (**access**) at the school. However, the PE teacher—in his own time and with his own transport—had to take Ashley himself, due to his mother being unable to do so.

Where the PE and school sport programme at the school did not have the scope to provide the **practice** and **provision** to support Ashley's talent, the coach at the track agreed that the student had potential. He attended specific training sessions twice a week and was entered into national age group events, both indoor and outdoor, and enjoyed a good level of success.

The relationship and trust that had developed between the PE teacher and Ashley was key to the success of this situation. Ashley, having largely poor relationships with the other teachers in the school, was afforded in PE a "stimulating, challenging and revealing environment" (Bailey & Morley, 2006, p. 217), whereby his abilities were able to be nurtured. Where the researchers discussed that often the **provision** stage of the process is "less problematic" (p. 218) for schools, in this case study, due to the rural location of the school and a focus on athletics not being supported by the school's own facilities, it was down to the teacher to source the **practice** and **provision** from outside the school. Arguably, without the intervention of PE and the school environment, Ashley's talent would not have been identified nor nurtured, supporting Bailey and Morley's (2006) belief that PE can play a critical role in talent identification.

This case study highlighted the role of the PE teacher in the identification and development of a student's talent and how they were able to support the young person's athletic development journey. As Bailey and Morley's (2006) model indicates, the outcome of the process also includes enjoyment and lifelong participation, both shaped by the PE environment, including the influence of PE teacher. Indeed, Domville et al. (2019) identified teacher behaviour as one of three key factors that influence a child's perceived PE enjoyment, in addition to peer behaviour and individual preferences. We will now explore two of these factors—the role of the PE teacher and relations with peers—in more detail.

INDIVIDUAL RELATIONS

Influential individuals, in the PE and school sport context, are the teachers/coaches and the young person's peer group. The teachers and coaches in schools are often in the best position to stimulate pupils' early interest and enthusiasm for play, physical activity, PE, and school sport (Office for Standards in Education, Children's Services and Skills, OfSTED, 2013), and can influence a young person's athletic development journey as evidenced in Case Study 10.1. The next two subsections examine who delivers PE and school sport and how this might influence the sporting experiences of those who participate. The final subsection considers an approach to PE and school sport delivery that allows for a positive experience for those on their athletic development journey.

Primary Physical Education

At primary level, PE delivery in most countries is led by general classroom teachers (who teach all subjects; 71%) and/or specialist PE teachers (67%), in comparison to secondary level where predominantly specialist PE teachers (98%) are used (Hardman, 2011). Globally, it is at primary level, however, where concerns over the inadequacies of teaching personnel for PE classes have consistently been raised (e.g., Jones & Green, 2017). Such concerns highlight that generalist teachers can lack the knowledge and skills associated with PE curriculum development (Jess et al., 2016), in addition to an increasing tendency to use external organisations to deliver both PE and school-based sport (Griggs, 2016).

Jones and Green (2017) identified the primary PE workforce in their study in England to include: in 69% of the schools examined, the delivery of PE involved a generalist plus one model; where the additional other was either a sports coach (44% of schools) or a specialist PE teacher (25%). This use of coaches, or outsourcing to external providers (EPs), is also on the rise in New Zealand where Dyson et al. (2016) sought the views of teachers in over 130 schools on this practice. While teachers valued the expertise of the EPs, and the range of sports they offer to the pupils, there were criticisms about the pedagogical approaches used and the EPs' knowledge of the curriculum. Where the use of coaches might provide links to sports clubs, and enhance the engagement with sport along the young person's athletic development journey, Jones and Green (2017) argue that this outsourcing of primary PE provision is creating "a pale imitation" (p. 759) of the more focused secondary provision. A further consequence of the outsourcing of primary PE provision to coaches was highlighted by Randall and Griggs (2020) who, in their examination of over 1,000 pre-service primary school teachers in England, found that almost 50% (48.9%) of the respondents reported no opportunity to teach PE on placement.

Secondary Physical Education

At secondary school level, Camire et al. (2017) reported that, from surveying almost 4,000 high school teacher-coaches in Canada, the majority (60%) were not trained PE teachers, in comparison with global data from Hardman (2011) where 98% of secondary provision was led by a PE specialist teacher. It is important to note that in North America, high school sport refers to school-sponsored sports that take place outside regular classes where students compete in organised leagues, and so is heavily performance focused. Of interest, however, those participants in Camire et al.'s (2017) research that were teacher trained, and were coaching high school sport, reported having more benefits from holding both positions, including maintaining a productive class atmosphere and higher levels of coaching efficacy than their non–teacher trained counterparts.

A Focus on Mastery for Effective Athletic Development

Regardless of who delivers the PE and school sport provision—teacher or coach—it is their approach and the relationships that are built with the students that are key for successful athletic development. Erikson's (1950) developmental stages of childhood highlight the importance of the primary years where the central task is for children, as they grow, to develop a sense of competence and mastery. Positive reinforcement from both teacher and peers is influential during this time as it can help develop confidence and competence (Erikson, 1950). It is important then, given our previous discussion of the inclusion of competition as part of the PE curriculum, that teachers can still emphasise the mastery elements of effort and participation (Pangrazi, 2001) and promote an overall mastery-involving climate (Morgan et al., 2005), where the teacher values and praises an individual's effort and improvements. Furthermore, PE teachers can plan how competition is presented with pupils preferring that an emphasis is placed on the challenges within the process of competing rather than on the outcome (i.e., winning and losing; Beni et al., 2017).

One mechanism through which a PE teacher, or coach, can create a mastery climate is to adopt the TARGET framework in their teaching practice (Ames, 1992), drawn from Self-Determination Theory (Deci & Ryan, 1985; Ryan & Deci, 2000) and Achievement Goal Theory (Nicholls, 1989)—for details on the underlying theory, see Chapter 8. The acronym TARGET refers to Task, Authority, Recognition, Grouping, Evaluation, and Time, and Morgan (2019) proposed this as a pedagogical framework for PE teachers to use to enhance students' physical literacy in the PE curriculum (Table 10.3), where both the teacher and peer group can have an influence.

TABLE 10.3 The TARGET structure manipulated to enhance physical literacy

TARGET Structure	Mastery Climate	How the Structure Can Be Manipulated to Enhance Physical Literacy
Task	A variety and range of tasks set that are differentiated* to the students' individual needs * where differing student needs are catered for by offering a variety of teaching techniques and lesson adaptations	Share lesson learning outcomes with the students Teach students to set goals (SMART) Use differentiation Use a range and variety of tasks
Authority	Students are involved in decision making and are given leadership roles	Encourage decision making in students Provide choice to support autonomy Create opportunities for leadership Adopt student-centred delivery styles
Recognition	Individualised recognition of improvement and effort Developing nurturing relationships with learners	Recognise students for their individual learning, and value them equally Encourage students to track their own progress and avoid comparison with others Educate the students to understand they are at different stages of personal development Develop effective relationships by getting to know the students
Grouping	Mixed-ability and co-operative groups	Vary grouping and regroup regularly (within and between lessons) Encourage cooperative groups by implementing the cooperative learning model (Dyson & Casey, 2012)

TARGET Structure	Mastery Climate	How the Structure Can Be Manipulated to Enhance Physical Literacy
Evaluation	Self-evaluation Individual feedback by the teacher based on improvement and effort	Base rewards on improvement, progress towards own/team goal, participation, and effort Use formative assessment strategies Track and plan for student progress collaboratively on their individual learning journey
Time	Flexible time for task completion	Allow flexible learning time Include extension tasks, and allow additional practice/learning time where required Encourage students to be as physically active for as long as possible during lessons while also allowing for learning opportunities

Source: Adapted from Morgan, 2019, pp. 10–14

Morgan (2019) emphasised treating each student as an individual and setting goals accordingly but also encouraging appropriate and carefully managed cooperation between peers. Indeed, where students have a strong relationship with both teachers and peers, they are likely to have the most positive PE experiences (Cox & Ullrich-French, 2010), and can have enhanced motivation (Shen et al., 2012). Furthermore, Warburton (2017) highlighted that peers, alongside teachers and parents, can be influential in the perceptions of students in terms of mastery or performance climates in PE, with Agans et al. (2018) highlighting that high school athletes who perceived mastery-orientated peer climates demonstrated the most positive character.

Two dimensions of peer climate in youth sport (Ntoumanis & Vazou, 2005) can be discussed in the PE and school sport context. As Morgan (2019) outlines, PE teachers are advised to avoid ego-involving climates where there is an emphasis of competition among classmates, where peers can engage in negative behaviour such as being unsupportive and criticising each other (Ntoumanis & Vazou, 2005). The emphasis, therefore, should be on a mastery (task-involving) climate where autonomy, cooperative group learning, and personal improvement and effort are championed. In this climate, peers can offer encouragement to each other to improve and learn to value and accept one another (Ntoumanis & Vazou, 2005). With positive peer relationships, an individual may encourage a peer to join a team, allowing them to feel valued (Bedard et al., 2020) and, arguably, more likely to pursue opportunities on their athletic development journey.

CLOSING THOUGHTS

It is argued that PE and school-based sport afford opportunities for young people on their sporting journey and provide an integral contribution to childhood experiences of athletic development. Not only are these movement and sporting experiences some of the first encountered by these young people, but PE and school-based sport offers a structured environment in which personal skills, such as communication, can be developed, and a wide range of sports can be experimented with. Furthermore, the relationships experienced in the school environment can influence not only immediate emotional responses (e.g., enjoyment of sessions) but also future sport participation both in school-based sport and more broadly in out-of-school sport. Teachers can play an important role in talent identification and development through creating optimal mastery environments involving positive peer interaction, ultimately allowing effective progress on the athletic development journey.

REFERENCES

Agans, J. P., Su, S., & Ettekal, A. V. (2018). Peer motivational climate and character development: Testing a practitioner-developed youth sport model. *Journal of Adolescence, 62*, 108–115.

Ames, C. (1992). Achievement goals, motivational climate, and motivational processes. In G. C. Roberts (Ed.), *Motivation in sport and exercise* (pp. 161–176). Human Kinetics.

Aquilina, D. (2013). A study of the relationship between elite athletes' educational development and sporting performance. *The International Journal of the History of Sport, 30*(4), 374–392.

Association for Physical Education (AfPE). (2015). Health position paper. *Association for Physical Education.* www.afpe.org.uk/physical-education/wp-content/uploads/afPE_Health_Position_Paper_Web_Version.pdf

Bailey, R. P. (2020). Defining physical literacy: Making sense of a promiscuous concept. *Sport in Society*, 1–18. https://doi.org/10.1080/17430437.2020.1777104

Bailey, R. P., Collins, D., Ford, P., MacNamara, Á., Toms, M., & Pearce, G. (2010). Participant development in sport: An academic review. *Sports Coach UK, 4*, 1–134.

Bailey, R. P., Glibo, I, & Koenen, K. (2019). Some Questions about physical literacy. *International Journal of Physical Education, 56*(4), 2–6.

Bailey, R. P., Glibo, I., & Koenen, K. (under review). What is physical literacy? A review and analysis of definitions. *Research Papers in Education.*

Bailey, R. P., & Morley, D. (2006). Towards a model of talent development in physical education. *Sport Education and Society, 11*, 211–230. https://doi.org/10.1080/13573320600813366

Bedard, C., Hanna, S., & Cairney, J. (2020). A longitudinal study of sport participation and perceived social competence in youth. *Journal of Adolescent Health, 66*(3), 352–359. https://doi.org/10.1016/j.jadohealth.2019.09.017

Beni, S., Fletcher, T., & Ní Chróinín, D. (2017). Meaningful experiences in physical education and youth sport: A review of the literature. *Quest, 69*(3), 291–312. https://doi.org/10.1080/00336297.2016.1224192

Brewer, B. W., & Pepitas, A. J. (2017). Athletic identity foreclosure. *Current Opinion in Psychology, 16*, 118–122.

Camire, M., Rocchi, M., & Kendellen, K. (2017). A comparative analysis of physical education and non-physical education teachers who coach high school sports teams. *International Journal of Sports Science & Coaching, 12*(5), 557–564.

Cox, A. E., & Ullrich-French, S. (2010). The motivational relevance of peer and teacher relationship profiles in physical education. *Psychology of Sport and Exercise, 11*, 337–344. http://doi.org/10.1016/j.psychsport.2010.04.001

Deci, E. L., & Ryan, R. M. (1985). *Intrinsic motivation and self-determination in human behavior.* Freeman.

Department for Culture, Media and Sport. (2001). *A sporting future for all. The Government's plan for sport.* Department for Culture, Media and Sport.

Department for Education. (2019). *School sport and activity action plan.* Department for Education.

Domville, M., Watson, P. M., Richardson, D., & Graves, L. E. F. (2019). Children's perceptions of factors that influence PE enjoyment: A qualitative investigation. *Physical Education and Sport Pedagogy, 24*(3), 207–219.

Dyson, B., & Casey, A. (2012). *Cooperative learning in physical education: A research based approach.* Routledge.

Dyson, B., Gordon, B., Cowan, J., & McKenzie, A. (2016). External providers and their impact on primary physical education in Aotearoa/New Zealand. *Asia-Pacific Journal of Health, Sport and Physical Education, 7*(1), 3–19.

Eccles, J. S., & Roeser, R. W. (2011). Schools as developmental contexts during adolescence. *Journal of Research on Adolescence, 21*(1), 225–241. https://doi.org/10.1111/j.1532-7795.2010.00725.x

Edwards, L. C., Bryant, A. S., Keegan, R. J., Morgan, K., & Jones, A. M. (2017). Definitions, foundations and associations of physical literacy: A systematic review. *Sports Medicine, 47*(1), 113–126.

Erikson, E. H. (1950). *Childhood and society.* Norton.

Erikson, E. H. (1959). Identity and the life cycle: Selected papers. *Psychological Issues, 1*, 1–71.

Gagné, F. (2015). From genes to talent: The DMGT/CMTD perspective. De los genes al talento: la perspectiva DMGT/CMTD. *Revista de Educación, 368*, 12–37.

Gallagher, B. (2020, June 14). Gareth's team start Millfield's dynasty. *The Rugby Player, 113.*

Giblin, S., Collins, D., MacNamara, A., & Kiely, J. (2014). "Deliberate preparation" as an evidence-based focus for primary physical education. *Quest, 66*(4), 385–395.

Gledhill, A., & Harwood, C. (2014). Developmental experiences of elite female youth soccer players. *International Journal of Sport and Exercise Psychology, 12*(2), 150–165.

Griggs, G. (2016). Spending the primary physical education and sport premium: A West Midlands case study. *Education 3–13, 44*(5), 547–555. http://doi.org/10.1080/03004279.2016.1169485

Guèvremont, A., Findlay, L., & Kohen, D. (2014). Organized extracurricular activities: Are in-school and out-of-school activities associated with different outcomes for Canadian youth?. *Journal of School Health, 84*(5), 317–325.

Güllich, A., & Cobley, S. (2017). On the efficacy of talent identification and talent development programmes. In J. Baker, S. Cobley, J. Schorer, & N. Wattie (Eds.). *Routledge handbook of talent identification and development in sport* (pp. 80–98). Routledge.

Hardman, K. (2011). Global issues in the situation of physical education in schools. In K. Hardman & K. Green (Eds.), *Contemporary issues in physical education: International perspectives* (pp. 11–32). Meyer & Meyer Verlag.

Harwood, C., Drew, A., & Knight, C. J. (2010). Parental stressors in professional youth football academies: A qualitative investigation of specialising stage parents. *Qualitative Research in Sport and Exercise, 2*(1), 39–55. https://doi.org/10.1080/19398440903510152

Harwood, C., & Knight, C. (2009). Stress in youth sport: A developmental investigation of tennis parents. *Psychology of Sport and Exercise, 10*(4), 447–456. https://doi.org/10.1016/j.psychsport.2009.01.005

Henriksen, K., Larsen, C. H., & Christensen, M. K. (2014). Looking at success from its opposite pole: The case of a talent development golf environment in Denmark. *International Journal of Sport and Exercise Psychology*, *12*(2), 134–149. https://doi.org/10.1080/16121 97X.2013.853473

Henriksen, K., Storm, L. K., Kuettel, A., Linnér, L., & Stambulova, N. (2020). A holistic ecological approach to sport and study: The case of an athlete friendly university in Denmark. *Psychology of Sport and Exercise*, *47*, 101637.

International Council of Sport Science and Physical Education. (2010). *International Position Statement on Physical Education*. www.icsspe.org/sites/default/files/International%20Position%20 Statement%20on%20Physical%20Education.pdf

Jess, M., Carse, N., & Keay, J. (2016). The primary physical education curriculum process: More complex than you might think! *Education 3–13*, *44*(5), 502–512. http://doi.org/10.1080/03 004279.2016.1169482

Jiménez-Barbero, J. A., Jiménez-Loaisa, A., González-Cutre, D., Beltrán-Carrillo, V. J., Llor-Zaragoza, L., & Ruiz-Hernández, J. A. (2020). Physical education and school bullying: A systematic review. *Physical Education and Sport Pedagogy*, *25*(1), 79–100.

Jones, L., & Green, K. (2017). Who teaches primary physical education? Change and transformation through the eyes of subject leaders. *Sport, Education and Society*, *22*(6), 759–771.

Kiens, K., & Larsen, C. H. (2020). Provision of a mental skills intervention program in an elite sport school for student-athletes. *Journal of Sport Psychology in Action*, 1–15. https://doi.org/10 .1080/21520704.2020.1765925

Long Term Athletic Development. (2020). Physical literacy. *Alpine Canada Association*. https://ltad. alpinecanada.org/athletes/athleticism-developing

Lovell, T. W. J., Fransen, J., Bocking, C. J, & Coutts, A. (2019). Factors affecting sports involvement in a school-based youth cohort: Implications for long-term development. Journal of Sport Sciences, *37*(22), 2522–2529. https://doi.org/10.1080/02640414.2019.1647032

Mental Health Taskforce. (2016). *The five year forward for mental health*. London: National Health Service. www.england.nhs.uk/wp-content/uploads/2016/02/Mental-Health-Taskforce-FYFV-final.pdf

Morgan, K. (2019). Applying the TARGET pedagogical principles in physical education to enhance students' physical literacy. *Journal of Physical Education, Recreation & Dance*, *90*(1), 9–14.

Morgan, K., Sproule, J., Weigand, D., & Carpenter, P. (2005). A computer-based observational assessment of the teaching behaviours that influence motivational climate in physical education. *Physical Education & Sport Pedagogy*, *10*(1), 83–105.

Morris, R., Cartigny, E., Ryba, T. V., Wylleman, P., Henriksen, K., Torregrossa, M., Lindahl, K., & Erpič, S. C. (2020). A taxonomy of dual career development environments in European countries. *European Sport Management Quarterly*, 1–18. https://doi.org/10.1080/16184742.20 20.1725778

Nicholls, J. G. (1989). *The competitive ethos and democratic education*. Harvard University Press.

Ntoumanis, N., & Vazou, S. (2005). Peer motivational climate in youth sport: Measurement development and validation. *Journal of Sport and Exercise Psychology*, *27*(4), 432–455.

Office for Standards in Education. (2013). *Beyond 2012—outstanding physical education for all. Physical education in schools 2008–12*. www.gov.uk/government/publications/beyond-2012-outstanding-physical-education-for-all

Ommundsen, Y., & Kvalø, S. E. (2007). Autonomy-mastery supportive or controlling: Differential teacher behaviours and pupils' outcomes of physical education. *Scandinavian Journal of Educational Research, 51*(5), 385–413.

Pangrazi, R. P. (2001). *Dynamic physical education for elementary school children.* Allyn and Bacon.

Randall, V., & Griggs, G. (2020). Physical education from the sidelines: Pre-service teachers opportunities to teach in English primary schools. *Education 3–13,* 1–14.

Ryan, R. M., & Deci, E. L. (2000). Self-determination theory and the facilitation of intrinsic motivation, social development, and well-being. *American Psychologist, 55*(1), 68–78. https:// doi.org/10.1037/0003-066X.55.1.68

Ryba, T. V., Aunola, K., Kalaja, S., Selanne, H., Ronkainen, N. J., & Nurmi, J. E. (2016). A new perspective on adolescent athletes' transition into upper secondary school: A longitudinal mixed methods study protocol. *Cogent Psychology, 3*(1), 1142412. https://doi.org/10.1080/2 3311908.2016.1142412

Shen, B., McCaughtry, N., Martin, J. J., Fahlman, M., & Garn, A. C. (2012). Urban high-school girls' sense of relatedness and their engagement in physical education. *Journal of Teaching in Physical Education, 31*(3), 231–245.

Sorkkila, M., Ryba, T. V., Selanne, H., & Aunola, K. (2018). Development of school and sport burnout in adolescent student-athletes: A longitudinal mixed-methods study. *Journal of Research on Adolescence, 30*(1), 115–133.

Spray, C. M., Warburton, V. E., & Stebbings, J. (2013). Change in physical self-perceptions across the transition to secondary school: Relationships with perceived teacher-emphasised achievement goals in physical education. *Psychology of Sport and Exercise, 14*(5), 662–669.

Stambulova, N. B., Engström, C., Franck, A., Linnér, L., & Lindahl, K. (2015). Searching for an optimal balance: Dual career experiences of Swedish adolescent athletes. *Psychology of Sport and Exercise, 21,* 4–14. https://doi.org/10.1016/j.psychsport.

Stambulova, N. B., Ryba, T. V., & Henriksen, K. (2020). Career development and transitions of athletes: The international society of sport psychology position stand revisited. *International Journal of Sport and Exercise Psychology,* 1–27.

Stambulova, N. B., & Wylleman, P. (2015). Dual career development and transitions (editorial). *Psychology of Sport and Exercise, 21,* 1–3.

Stambulova, N. B., & Wylleman, P. (2019). Psychology of athletes' dual careers: A state-of-the-art critical review of the European discourse. *Psychology of Sport and Exercise, 42,* 74–88.

Stidder, G., & Hayes, S. (Eds.). (2011). *The really useful physical education book: Learning across the 7–17 age range.* Routledge.

Stidder, G., & Hayes, S. (Eds.). (2013). *Equity and inclusion in physical education and sport.* Routledge.

The Sutton Trust (2016, October 22). Educational backgrounds of Olympic medallists. *The Sutton Trust.* www.suttontrust.com/our-research/education-backgrounds-of-olympic-medallists/

Toms, M., Bridge, M., & Bailey, R. (2009). *A developmental perspective of sports participation in the UK: Implications for coaching,* 7th International Council for Coach Education Conference, Vancouver, Canada.

Torregrosa, M., Ramis, Y., Pallarés, S., Azócar, F., & Selva, C. (2015). Olympic athletes back to retirement: A qualitative longitudinal study. *Psychology of Sport and Exercise, 21,* 50–56. https:// doi.org/10.1016/j.psychsport.2015.03.003.

Warburton, V. E. (2017). Peer and teacher influences on the motivational climate in physical education: A longitudinal perspective on achievement goal adoption. *Contemporary Educational Psychology, 51,* 303–314.

Wylleman, P., & Lavallee, D. (2004). A developmental perspective on transitions faced by athletes. In M. Weiss (Ed.), *Developmental sport and exercise psychology: A lifespan perspective* (pp. 507–527). Fitness Information Technology.

Yli-Piipari, S., Watt, A., Jaakkola, T., Liukkonen, J., & Nurmi, J. E. (2009). Relationships between physical education students' motivational profiles, enjoyment, state anxiety, and self-reported physical activity. *Journal of Sports Science & Medicine, 8*(3), 327.

SECTION III

Mental Health and Wellbeing on the Athlete's Journey

Caroline Heaney

Mental health and wellbeing is a highly contemporary topic in sport and an essential consideration as the athlete progresses on their journey through sport. In recent times awareness of mental health, wellbeing, and related topics has grown as athletes have spoken out about the challenges they have faced. Many athletes have shared their experiences of mental health disorders (e.g., depression), whilst others have spoken about toxic sports environments and cultures that have challenged their mental health and welfare. For example, following the release of the documentary *Athlete A* in 2020, several gymnasts from around the world have spoken out about the culture of abuse in their sport prompting independent reviews in some countries such as the UK (Kavanagh et al., 2020).

Whilst sport can provide a nurturing environment that can positively enhance mental health and allow the athlete to thrive, it can also provide an environment that threatens mental health. There has been much debate around whether the 'winning at all costs' approach traditionally adopted in many high-performance sport environments has benefited (e.g. medal success, development of skills such as resilience and mental toughness) or damaged athletes by compromising their welfare and negatively impacting on their wellbeing and mental health. It has been implied, by some media outlets, that athlete welfare and athlete success are at odds, a notion contested by British Olympic medallist Cath Bishop in the following quote.

> Katherine Grainger, my Olympic crew-mate and close friend, has been clear in her position as chair of UK Sport that it's not a choice between high performance and wellbeing, you can have both. I believe that we must have both, and wellbeing must come first as the foundation on which high performance is built. As I've said, I don't think that needs to harm performance, quite the opposite. Wellbeing, self-esteem and respect enable an athlete to tap into deeper sources of motivation than purely medals—yes, there are other reasons to do elite sport—and to have a longer and more fulfilling career.
>
> (Bishop, 2020)

This quote suggests that athletes can be successful in elite sport without compromising their mental health and wellbeing, and that environments which positively influence mental health can allow athletes to thrive and fulfil their full sporting potential. The research explored in this section of this book strongly supports this perspective.

There are a multitude of factors that can potentially threaten the mental health of an athlete. These include more obvious and predictable factors, such as anxieties related to the pressure of competition, as well as less predictable events, such as the unprecedented global COVID-19 pandemic of 2020. The latter event led to the postponement of many sporting events, including the Olympic and Paralympic Games, and required athletes to adapt their training schedules as many training facilities were forced to temporarily close. In the face of such adversity athletes need to be resilient in order to protect their mental health and potentially grow from their experiences.

This section of the book aims to explore mental health and wellbeing in sport and the closely related and interlinked topics of resilience, thriving, and athlete welfare. In Chapter 11, *Understanding Mental Health and Wellbeing in Sport*, Caroline Heaney sets the scene by introducing mental health in athletes and coaches. The chapter examines the prevalence of mental health difficulties, with a focus on the eleven mental health conditions identified in the International Olympic Committee (IOC) consensus statement on mental health in elite athletes (Reardon et al., 2019), and explores the reasons why athletic populations may be at risk of experiencing mental health difficulties. The chapter concludes by considering the treatment and prevention of mental health conditions, highlighting the importance of mental health literacy and creating environments, systems, and processes that promote positive wellbeing alongside performance enhancement. This is further explored in the subsequent chapters where the need for sporting organisations to prevent mental health difficulties by creating an environment in which athletes can thrive (see Chapter 13), feel safe (see Chapter 14), and be resilient to the stresses placed on them (see Chapter 12) are discussed.

In order to protect their mental health on their journey through sport athletes need to be able to cope with the potential stressors they will be exposed to. In Chapter 12, *Developing Resilience on the Athlete's Journey*, Karen Howells explores the relatively new concept of psychological resilience in sport. Resilience is considered to be an important quality for athletes to possess in order to cope with the challenges and setbacks that are part of sport. The chapter critically examines psychological resilience, exploring what it is, its application in sport, and how it can be developed. In considering how resilience can be developed, the ethics of deliberately inducing adversity in order to facilitate the development of resilience are discussed, including the potential for negative impacts on athlete welfare, thriving, and mental health.

Competitive sport can create a high-pressure environment. In order to promote positive mental health and wellbeing it is important that athletes and support staff are able to thrive under this pressure rather than just survive. In Chapter 13, *Thriving in Athletic Development Environments*, Daniel J. Brown explores the novel area of thriving and its application in sport, considering what thriving is and what characterises it, including links with mental toughness and adversity (see Chapter 12). The chapter concludes by reflecting on how thriving can be predicted and promoted in sports environments in order to facilitate optimal performance, welfare (see Chapter 14), and wellbeing.

With several high-profile athlete welfare and abuse cases in the media in recent years in this final chapter of the section Chapter 14, *Athlete Welfare for Optimal Athletic Development*, Daniel J. A. Rhind examines the important topic of safeguarding and welfare in sports environments in the context of athletic development. The chapter considers what athlete welfare is, why it is important to athletic development, and potential threats to athlete welfare. It revisits the debate discussed earlier about welfare versus winning, drawing on the duty of care organisations and individuals (e.g., coaches) have to protect athletes, and discusses the strategies that can be put in place to promote athlete welfare in sporting environments.

Collectively, the chapters in this section of the book demonstrate how mental health, resilience, thriving, and athlete welfare are interrelated and impact on the wellbeing of the athlete on their journey through sport.

REFERENCES

Bishop, C. (2020). Greedy Britain's focus on medals creates a culture of fear when winning is the end that justifies any means. *Mail Online.* www.dailymail.co.uk/sport/article-8537087/CATH-BISHOP-Greedy-Britains-focus-medals-creates-culture-fear.html

Kavanagh, E., Adams, A., & Adams, A. (2020). Winning at all costs—How abuse in sport has become normalised. *The Conversation.* Retrieved July 9, 2020, from https://theconversation.com/winning-at-all-costs-how-abuse-in-sport-has-become-normalised-142739

Reardon, C. L., Hainline, B., Aron, C. M., Baron, D., Baum, A. L., Bindra, A., . . . & Engebretsen, L. (2019). Mental health in elite athletes: International Olympic Committee consensus statement (2019). *British Journal of Sports Medicine, 53*(11), 667–699. https://doi.org/10.1136/bjsports-2019-100715

CHAPTER 11

Understanding Mental Health and Wellbeing in Sport

Caroline Heaney

According to the World Health Organization (2018) mental health can be defined as "a state of wellbeing in which an individual realises his or her own abilities, can cope with the normal stresses of life, can work productively and is able to make a contribution to his or her community". This definition acknowledges that mental health is more than the absence of mental disorders (Galderisi et al., 2015) and shows that sport can potentially create situations that challenge mental health where, for example, the athlete is unable to cope with the stresses of training and competition. Athletes, like all members of society, can be affected by mental health difficulties. Mental health is perhaps best conceptualised as a continuum ranging from negative (ill health) to positive (good health/mental wealth; Kuettel & Larsen, 2019), where both clinically diagnosed mental health disorders and subclinical symptoms can have an impact on an individual's quality of life. Indeed, research has explored both clinical and subclinical symptoms in athletes and, consequently, throughout this chapter the term *mental health difficulties* is used to describe both clinically diagnosed mental health conditions and subclinical symptoms. The chapter explores the mental health of athletes by examining the prevalence of mental health difficulties in athletes, the mental health difficulties that can affect athletes, why athletes might be vulnerable to these, how they can be prevented or treated, and how positive mental health and wellbeing can be promoted in sporting environments. This will be further explored in Chapters 12 to 14 which investigate resilience, thriving, and athlete welfare which are all closely allied to mental health.

Traditionally sport and exercise psychology research exploring mental health has predominantly focused on physical activity as a treatment modality in the prevention and treatment of mental health difficulties. However, in recent years, interest has been sparked in the role of sport as a potential causative factor in the development of mental health difficulties and how sporting environments can be shaped to impact positively on mental health. This interest has been fuelled by an ever-increasing number of high-profile athletes openly discussing their mental health challenges. This chapter is focused on the mental health of athletes, rather than on the role of exercise in treating mental health in non-athletic populations. The rising interest in the mental health of athletes is evidenced by a recent explosion in research in this area (Poucher et al., 2019) and the large number of position, consensus, and expert statements that have been published on the topic in recent years. Nine examples of these, published between 2018 and 2020, are shown in Table 11.1. The volume of these statements indicates the growing recognition of the importance of mental health in athletes amongst researchers and sporting bodies and the need to raise awareness regarding mental health issues within the world of sport.

TABLE 11.1 Position statements on mental health in sport

International Organisations:

International Olympic Committee (IOC) consensus statement: Mental health in elite athletes (Reardon et al., 2019)

FEPSAC position statement: Mental health disorders in elite athletes and models of service provision (Moesch et al., 2018)

International Society of Sport Psychology (ISSP) position stand: Athletes' mental health, performance, and development (Schinke et al., 2018)

Sample Statements From National Organisations:

British Association of Sport and Exercise Sciences (BASES) expert statement: Mental health literacy in elite sport (Gorczynski et al., 2019)

American Medical Society for Sports Medicine (AMSSM) position statement: Mental health issues and psychological factors in athletes: detection, management, effect on performance, and prevention (Chang et al., 2020)

Canadian Centre for Mental Health and Sport (CCMHS) position statement: Principles of mental health in competitive and high-performance sport (Van Slingerland et al., 2019)

Other:

International consensus statement on the psychosocial and policy-related approaches to mental health awareness programmes in sport (Breslin et al., 2019)

Athlete mental health in the Olympic/Paralympic quadrennium: a multi-societal consensus statement (Henriksen et al., 2020)

Consensus statement on improving the mental health of high performance athletes (Henriksen et al., 2019)

The recognition that athletes can experience mental health difficulties challenges the commonly held perception that athletes, particularly those competing at elite level, are unbreakable superior beings both physically and mentally (Hainline & Reardon, 2019). As will be explored later in this chapter, this perception can create a culture that exacerbates the development of mental health difficulties, as can be seen with the stigma attached to seeking help (Bauman, 2016). There are signs that this culture is changing and the world of sport is evolving and becoming more aware and accepting of mental health difficulties. This chapter seeks to provide an overview of our current knowledge on the topic of mental health in sport. Whilst it will focus predominantly on athlete mental health, it will also consider the mental health of support staff such as coaches. We will begin this journey by exploring what mental health difficulties athletes can be affected by and their prevalence.

THE PREVALENCE OF MENTAL HEALTH DIFFICULTIES IN SPORT

There has been much debate over whether athletes are more vulnerable or less vulnerable to developing mental health difficulties than the general population (Moesch et al., 2018). Hainline and Reardon (2019) suggest that although elite athletes generally experience several mental health difficulties at the same rate as the general population, there are some that are more common in sport (e.g., eating disorders, substance abuse). In this section we will explore some of the data examining the prevalence of mental health disorders, but before doing so it is important to acknowledge some of the challenges in collecting such data which may affect its credibility. Firstly, despite recent advances in understanding there is still a stigma attached to mental ill health, particularly in sporting environments, which can lead to the underreporting of mental health difficulties (Bauman, 2016). This is not exclusive to sporting domains; it has been suggested that mental health difficulties and disorders are underdiagnosed in the population as a whole (Hainline & Reardon, 2019). However, sport represents a unique environment in which a culture of mental toughness is often promoted which may be in conflict with disclosing mental health concerns (Rao & Hong, 2020). Secondly, there are differences in the reporting of clinical and subclinical symptoms, with some studies only reporting data where the clinical threshold of a mental health disorder has been reached whilst others, recognising the impact of subclinical symptoms, reporting symptoms below the criteria for formal diagnosis (Moesch et al., 2018). Finally, Reardon et al. (2019) suggest that data comparing the prevalence with the general population is limited due to most athlete studies lacking reference groups from the general population, different measures of mental health difficulties being used in different studies (e.g., self-report vs medical diagnosis), and failure to consider cultural differences in the meaning of mental health difficulties.

In their systematic review and meta-analysis of research exploring both current and former elite athletes from a range of sports, Gouttebarge et al. (2019) found that the prevalence of mental health difficulties ranged from 19% to 34% in current athletes, and 16% to 26% in former athletes. They suggested that this was slightly higher than the general population, although they acknowledged the difficulties in making comparisons. In their systematic review, Rice et al. (2016) concluded that elite athletes experience a similar prevalence of mental health difficulties, such as anxiety and depression, to the general population and that they are vulnerable to a wide range of mental health difficulties. In their review of the literature examining elite athletes, Poucher et al. (2019) concluded that mental health difficulties generally appeared to be more prevalent in female athletes, although this could be due to female athletes being more willing to disclose difficulties.

There may also be further differences in prevalence between able-bodied and disabled athletes, and elite and lower level athletes. Swartz et al. (2019) identified a lack of research exploring the mental health of disabled athletes and a need for more research exploring the prevalence of mental health difficulties in this group who may experience additional stressors beyond those that able-bodied athletes encounter. Similarly, Vella and Swann (2020) have critiqued the lack of research exploring lower level athletes. Whilst much of the research focuses on elite athletes, it is important to recognise that lower level athletes are not immune to developing mental health difficulties and those supporting athletes of any level need to be aware of mental health struggles.

Like the general population, athletes can be affected by a broad range of mental health difficulties. The IOC consensus statement on mental health in elite athletes (Reardon et al., 2019, p. 671) identified eleven groups of mental health disorders that can be experienced by athletes:

1. Sleep disorders and concerns
2. Major depressive disorder and depression symptoms
3. Suicide
4. Anxiety and related disorders

5. Post-traumatic stress disorder and other trauma-related disorders

6. Eating disorders

7. Attention deficit hyperactivity disorder (ADHD)

8. Bipolar and psychotic disorders

9. Sport-related concussion

10. Substance use and substance use disorders

11. Gambling disorder and other behavioural addictions

The prevalence of each of these in athletic populations is briefly explored here. It is important to note that this is not an exhaustive list and that often these disorders can occur alongside each other rather than in isolation.

Sleep Disorders and Concerns

Sleep is considered to be a key determinant of athlete wellbeing, performance, and health (Kroshus et al., 2019), yet insufficient sleep (less than 7 hours per night) and sleep disturbances appear to be common amongst athletes (Reardon et al., 2019). For example, in their study of 317 Olympic athletes preparing to compete at the 2016 games, Drew et al. (2018) found that the prevalence of poor sleep quality was high with 49% of athletes reaching the threshold for clinical diagnosis. Athletes commonly report sleep difficulties such as trouble sleeping the night before competition or maintaining sleep patterns whilst travelling (Reardon et al., 2019). Poor sleep can be indicative of a mental health disorder or can exacerbate existing mental health difficulties and so is an important consideration in the mental health of an athlete (Asplund & Chang, 2020). Athletes who suffer from poor sleep quality are much more likely to suffer from conditions such as anxiety and depression than those with good sleep quality (Asplund & Chang, 2020).

Depression

The term depression can cover a range of disorders that are generally characterised by a reduction in functioning and symptoms such as low mood, sadness, decreased energy, and feelings of worthlessness (Doherty et al., 2016). Depressive disorders are one of the most common mental health disorders experienced by athletes and rates of depression are thought to be equal to or higher than the general population, and on the rise amongst both groups (Wolanin, 2020). In their study of 465 collegiate athletes, Wolanin et al. (2016) found a 23.7% rate of clinical symptoms of depression and a 6.3% rate of moderate depression symptoms. Similarly, Beable et al. (2017) reported a 21% rate of depressive symptoms in elite athletes. In their meta-analysis of depressive symptoms in high-performance athletes Gorczynski et al. (2017) found that both male and female athletes were no more likely than non-athletes to report mild or severe depressive symptoms but found that male athletes were 52% less likely to report depressive symptoms than female athletes. However, they critiqued some of the existing literature for an overreliance on self-report measures and called for more research exploring clinically diagnosed depression in athletes. Wolanin (2020) suggests that rates of depression may be higher in individual sport athletes compared to team sport athletes and identified that factors such as injury, retirement, and poor performance can lead to depressive symptoms.

Suicide

Suicidal thoughts can be a symptom of depression and other mental health disorders (Doherty et al., 2016) and, consequently, athletes with depression are potentially at risk of suicide. According to Rao (2020) 20% of the general population have a mental health disorder that places them at risk of suicide, which is an alarming figure. Comparable data on athlete populations is not available, but sadly, the world of sport has seen high profile instances of suicide such as the tragic deaths of 18-year-old British snowboarder Ellie Soutter in 2018 and former World Judo Champion Craig Fallon in 2019. Male athletes appear to be at greater risk of suicide than their female counterparts, which matches the general population where young males are most at risk (Rao, 2020). This may be due to a greater willingness amongst female athletes to seek support for mental health difficulties such as depression (Gorczynski et al., 2017). In their study of collegiate athletes, Rao et al. (2015) found that the annual suicide rate for male athletes was 1.35/100,000 compared to 0.37/100,000 in female athletes.

Anxiety

Anxiety disorders are different from performance anxiety which is a common occurrence in competitive sport (Reardon et al., 2019). Anxiety disorders include generalised anxiety disorder (GAD), social anxiety, obsessive-compulsive disorder, and panic disorder (Reardon et al., 2019). GAD which is characterised by excessive anxiety and worry has been reported to have a prevalence of between 6 and 14.6% in athletes, with female athletes and injured athletes being at greatest risk (Reardon et al., 2019). There is less research on the other disorders but the prevalence for these from self-reported data is: social anxiety (14.7%), obsessive-compulsive disorder (5.2%), and panic disorder (4.5%; Reardon et al., 2019). In their systematic review and meta-analysis of anxiety in elite athletes, Rice et al. (2019) concluded that athletes and non-athletes experience a similar prevalence of anxiety disorders, and that athletes who are dissatisfied, female, younger, injured, or have experienced a recent adverse life event are more prone to anxiety. Anxiety can have a negative impact on cognitive and overall functioning in the general population and can lead to negative performance in athletes (Reardon et al., 2019). It is important to note that anxiety does not always occur in isolation and may occur alongside other mental health disorders such as depression (Reardon et al., 2019).

Trauma

According to Reardon et al. (2019) trauma-related disorders such as post-traumatic stress disorder (PTSD) are relatively common in elite sport. PTSD can be defined as at least a month of negative mental health symptoms following exposure to a trauma (Reardon et al., 2019). Symptoms that last for less than a month are instead categorised as acute stress disorder (Reardon et al., 2019). In their review of the literature, Aron et al. (2019) concluded that elite athletes may have higher rates of PTSD (13–25%) and other trauma-related disorders than the general population.

Athletes can encounter traumatic events both inside and outside of the sporting domain that can lead to trauma-related disorders. Examples of traumatic events in the sporting domain include sports injury and abusive relationships/environments (Aron et al., 2019). Equally, athletes can be affected by traumatic events outside of sport such as adverse childhood experiences (e.g., domestic violence, child abuse, neglect).

Eating Disorders

Both eating disorders (anorexia nervosa, bulimia nervosa, and binge eating disorder) and disordered eating (subclinical symptoms that do not meet the criteria for diagnosis but are still of concern) are common in athletes (Reardon et al., 2019) and are thought to be more prevalent in athletes compared to non-athletes (Joy et al., 2016). These conditions can have a significant negative impact on the mental and physical health of the athlete and are reported to have a prevalence of 0 to 19% in male athletes and 6 to 45% in female athletes (Bratland-Sanda & Sundgot-Borgen, 2013). Whilst female athletes are more vulnerable to eating disorders, male athletes are still affected and are at more risk than males from the general population (Souter et al., 2018). Additionally, athletes from endurance (e.g., distance running), aesthetic (e.g., gymnastics), and weight-controlled sports (e.g., combat sports) appear to be at greater risk (Bratland-Sanda & Sundgot-Borgen, 2013).

ADHD

ADHD is a brain development disorder characterised by persistent inattention and hyperactivity-impulsivity causing dysfunction in various settings (Han et al., 2019). ADHD in athletes has received limited research interest in comparison to other mental health disorders (Moesch et al., 2018). Its inclusion in the IOC position statement may surprise some since it is deemed to have both positive and negative impacts on sports performance (Han et al., 2019). In their narrative review of the literature Han et al. (2019) reported the prevalence of ADHD to be around 7 to 8% in elite and college athletes and suggested that ADHD may be more common in athletes than the general population. This may be because those with ADHD are naturally drawn to sport (Han et al., 2019). In their systematic review Poysophon and Rao (2018) found a prevalence rate of 4.2 to 8.1% in young athletes which they concluded was similar to the general population. Although predominantly considered a childhood condition it has been suggested that around 30% of those diagnosed in childhood continue to meet the diagnostic criteria in adulthood (Han et al., 2019).

Bipolar and Psychotic Disorders

Bipolar disorders are characterised by episodes of extreme changes in mood (e.g., mania or depressed mood) and associated functional impairment (Currie, Gorczynski et al., 2019). Psychotic disorders (e.g., schizophrenia) are characterised by symptoms such as delusions and hallucinations (Reardon et al., 2019). Whilst much is known about bipolar and psychotic disorders in the general population, little is known about their prevalence and impact in athletes; however, there are anecdotal reports of athletes having such conditions and as the peak age of onset crosses over the peak age of performance in most sports these conditions are a consideration (Currie,

Gorczynski et al., 2019). These conditions are likely to have a significant impact on sports performance as the conditions are often chronic and the symptoms enduring, although some athletes have had successful sports careers despite this (Reardon et al., 2019). Bipolar and psychotic disorders can be categorised as primary or secondary, with secondary often induced through substance abuse (Currie, Gorczynski et al., 2019). Currie, Gorczynski et al. (2019) report that the prevalence of bipolar disorder in the general population is 0.4 to 0.6% and 0.5% for psychotic disorders.

Concussion

Sport-related concussion can lead to changes in mood, emotions, and behaviour and those affected can develop anxiety, depression, and other mental health difficulties (Reardon et al., 2019). Such symptoms appear to be more prevalent when an athlete has had multiple concussions (Reardon et al., 2019). In their systematic review exploring concussion and mental health, Rice et al. (2018) concluded that depression symptoms were the most commonly reported mental health outcome of concussion. Although reported less frequently, the other outcomes identified in the studies reviewed were anxiety, impulsivity, aggression, and apathy (Rice et al., 2018). Some studies have shown that ADHD can increase the risk of concussion and impact recovery (Ströhle, 2019).

Substance Use

In their review of substance use in elite athletes, McDuff et al. (2019) reported that a range of substances were used by elite athletes, both recreational and ergogenic. They identified alcohol, cannabis, tobacco, prescribed opioids, and stimulants as the substances most frequently used by elite athletes but noted that the prevalence of their use was lower than in non-athletes (McDuff et al., 2019). However, they also found that the rates of alcohol, oral tobacco, non-prescription opioids, and anabolic-androgenic steroid use were higher in athletes compared to non-athletes, despite the fact that some of these substances are banned by the World Anti-Doping Agency (WADA; McDuff et al., 2019). Various risk factors have been identified that place athletes at greater risk of substance abuse. These include a culture of substance abuse in a sport, male gender, and injury (Reardon et al., 2019).

Behavioural Addictions

Athletes are recognised to commonly have risk factors for addictive behaviours such as sensation seeking tendencies and young age (Grall-Bronnec et al., 2016). Behavioural addictions that can affect athletes include those to gaming and social media; however, it is gambling addiction that has received the most research attention (Reardon et al., 2019). In their study of European professional athletes, Grall-Bronnec et al. (2016) reported the prevalence of either past or present problem gambling as 8.2% compared to 0.15 to 6.6% in the general population. Similarly, in their narrative review Derevensky et al. (2019) concluded that rates of gambling disorders are higher amongst elite athletes than non-athletes. Gambling addictions can be associated with several negative mental health outcomes such as anxiety, depression, irritability, and substance abuse (Derevensky et al., 2019).

So far, this section has focused on the prevalence of mental health difficulties in athletes, but other people involved in sport, such as coaches, also experience difficulties as explored in the spotlight box that follows.

Spotlight On: Coach Mental Health

Whilst most of the research exploring mental health in sport focuses on athletes, it is important to be aware that all those involved in sport are potentially vulnerable to mental health difficulties. Here we look at mental health in sports coaches, using the case study of Lance.

Lance is a high-performance coach in an Olympic sport. He has successfully worked in this environment for several years, but in recent months has been finding it increasingly difficult to cope with the demands being placed on him and constantly feels under pressure. This has led to feelings of anxiety, depression, and exhaustion, which are having a negative impact on his motivation and enjoyment of coaching. He describes his job as '24-7' and therefore finds it hard to switch off his mind and relax.

Lance's experiences are not unique. Coaches work in environments where they are exposed to a large amount of pressure and stress (Fletcher & Scott, 2010). The demands of coaching in high-performance sport make it difficult to achieve an appropriate work-life balance (Carson et al., 2018), and this is negatively impacting Lance's mental health and wellbeing. Lance is not alone in feeling this way. In a study of 103 UK coaches 49.5% indicated that they were experiencing symptoms of a mental health disorder (Gorczynski et al., 2020).

Most of the research exploring the mental health of coaches has focused on burnout and, after talking to the medical team, this is what the doctor has suggested Lance might be suffering from. In their study of 25 full-time and 45 part-time coaches exploring stress and burnout, Altfeld et al. (2015) concluded that full-time coaches such as Lance experience higher levels of emotional stress and have insufficient recovery time during the competitive season, highlighting the importance of recovery and self-care in protecting mental health. Stress and burnout scores were particularly high towards the end of the season. The prevention and treatment options discussed later in this chapter should also be considered for coaches and other support staff.

WHY ARE ATHLETES VULNERABLE?

The previous section suggests that athletes are at least as vulnerable as the general population when it comes to experiencing mental health difficulties, with some research showing that they are more vulnerable. So why is that the case when exercise is known to have a positive impact on mental health? One explanation is that the peak age of athletic performance in most sports tends to coincide with the peak age for risk of developing mental health difficulties (Rao & Hong, 2020). Additionally, Moesch et al. (2018) suggest that elite sport environments and the stressors experienced by athletes can trigger mental health difficulties.

Research has shown that there are multiple factors in sport that could potentially increase an athlete's risk of developing mental health difficulties. Some of these are summarised in Figure 11.1. Arnold and Fletcher (2012) identified 640 distinct organisational stressors that can be experienced by sports performers. These stressors were split into four categories: leadership and personnel; cultural and team; logistical and environmental; and performance and personal. Gouttebarge et al. (2019) suggest that in addition to generic adverse life events, elite athletes can be

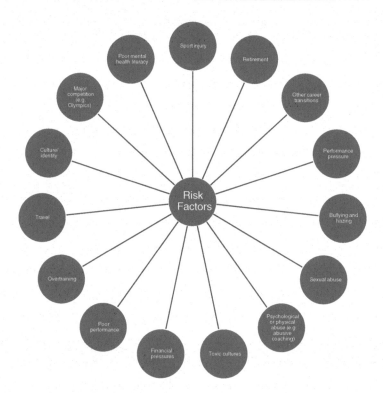

FIGURE 11.1 Sample mental health risk factors

Sources: Gouttebarge et al., 2019; Henriksen et al., 2020; Howells & Lucassen, 2018; Jeckell et al., 2020; Kuettel & Larsen, 2019; Moesch et al., 2018; Poucher et al., 2019; Putukian, 2020; Rao, 2020; Reardon et al., 2019; Rice et al., 2019; Rice et al., 2016; Sarac et al., 2018; Schinke et al., 2018; Souter et al., 2018; Van Slingerland et al., 2019

exposed to a wealth of sport-specific stressors. Some of these stressors (e.g., pushing oneself to the extreme) are created by the culture of sport (Hainline & Reardon, 2019). Key stressors appear to include those linked to career transitions such as sport injury and retirement from sport (Gouttebarge et al., 2019). Sport injury can lead to several mental health symptoms such as depression and anxiety (Putukian, 2020). Additionally, the existence of mental health symptoms can increase the risk of injury (Reardon et al., 2019). Retirement from sport is associated with an increased risk of developing mental health difficulties, particularly for those experiencing an unplanned retirement (e.g., career-ending injury) or with a strong athletic identity (Reardon et al., 2019). Disabled athletes are likely to be affected by additional stressors such as chronic pain and logistical difficulties (Reardon et al., 2019). Schinke et al. (2018) suggest that culture, identity, and mental health are inextricably linked, and that where sporting environments are not accepting of an athlete's diversity (e.g., disability, gender, ethnicity, sexual orientation, nationality) mental health can be negatively impacted. Awareness of the factors that may make athletes vulnerable to developing mental health difficulties is important to help facilitate the prevention of such difficulties.

Case Study 11.1 shows a case study of an athlete who has reflected on how sport added to her mental health difficulties. A sport injury, lack of support, and a culture of not wanting to show weakness all appear to have contributed to her symptoms.

CASE STUDY 11.1

Priscilla

Over the last few months, I've been feeling really down—I've been experiencing feelings of depression and anxiety. I guess it really started when I first got injured. I got what I thought was a minor hamstring injury and whilst I was a bit angry and frustrated about it, I was determined to get back—and I did. But it turns out that I came back too soon, pushed too hard, and made it much worse. I now have a significant muscle tear and am going to miss the first part of the season. I'm now starting to question whether I will recover and whether I will re-injure my hamstring again. That fear is playing on my mind and making me really anxious. My sport is everything to me and the thought of not having it in my life is really depressing. I feel sad every day and I don't know what to do with myself. I feel like I've got no one to talk to about how I feel. I pretend to my teammates that everything is okay, because I don't want to show weakness, but inside it's not. I haven't spoken to my coach for weeks—it's like I'm no use to him at the moment. I feel worthless.

—Priscilla

PREVENTING AND TREATING MENTAL HEALTH DIFFICULTIES

It is important that sports organisations and coaching environments put in place structures and strategies that both (a) help prevent mental health difficulties occurring in the first place, and (b) support the athlete appropriately when they do occur. Whilst this section is predominantly written with the athlete in mind it also applies to support staff who are vulnerable to mental health difficulties as well.

Prevention of Mental Health Difficulties

One of the main ways to prevent mental health difficulties is to create an environment which promotes and supports mental wellbeing and helps individuals to cope with the stressors they face (Hainline & Reardon, 2019). This requires a cultural shift towards an environment where mental health is openly discussed and there is no stigma attached to mental health or seeking help (Schinke et al., 2018). Mental health literacy is considered key to achieving this. Mental health literacy can be defined as awareness of mental health disorders and symptoms, and knowledge of when and where to seek help (Rao & Hong, 2020). Castaldelli-Maia et al. (2019) found that stigma and poor mental health literacy were the most significant barriers to athletes seeking support for mental health difficulties. Seeking such support early can help prevent a more serious mental health disorder. It has been suggested that both athletes and coaches have limited understanding of mental health (Biggin et al., 2017). However, coaches are considered to be well positioned to act as gatekeepers in facilitating athletes accessing mental health support (Brown et al., 2017). Therefore, education interventions aimed at increasing the mental health literacy of athletes, coaches, and other staff are advocated (Breslin et al., 2017). In their systematic review of such interventions, Breslin et al. (2017) found that they can be effective in increasing mental health awareness, reducing stigma, enhancing help-seeking intentions, improving wellbeing, and increasing self-efficacy to provide help; however, they critiqued the quality of the studies reviewed and called for further research.

It has been suggested that in order for mental health literacy training to be effective it needs to be ongoing (starting at an early training age), specific to the needs of the organisation, and focus on the mental health of all involved (e.g., athletes, coaches, support staff, family), and not just the athlete (Gorczynski et al., 2019). Such training should be considered as an investment as mental health is an important resource throughout the individual's career and beyond (Henriksen et al., 2019). In their international consensus statement, Breslin et al. (2019) make several recommendations for the design of rigorous evidence-based mental health awareness programmes in sport. For example, they suggest that any programme should be underpinned by appropriate theories and models (e.g., Theory of Planned Behaviour, Self-Determination Theory, Integrated Behaviour Change Model) and led by appropriately qualified individuals with an understanding of the culture of sport.

Changing the environment to be more aware, accepting, and supportive of mental health difficulties goes beyond the coach and athlete. It requires all stakeholders, such as support staff, governing bodies, sport associations, clubs, and the media to acknowledge their role to make systemic changes (Breslin et al., 2019). The aim is to create an environment in which athletes can thrive (see Chapter 13), feel safe (see Chapter 14), and be resilient to the stresses placed on them (see Chapter 12). Henriksen et al. (2019) suggest that sporting environments can either "nourish" or "malnourish" the athlete (p. 5). Environments that negatively impact on mental health, such as those with a culture of bullying or abuse, can be considered to malnourish the athlete and those around them (Henriksen et al., 2019). In recent years there have been several high-profile examples of environments that have been deemed as malnourishing such as British cycling and USA gymnastics, where cultural changes have been recommended.

Improving mental health literacy and creating environments that promote wellbeing will encourage all stakeholders to better recognise and respond to mental health difficulties. Screening also has a role in identifying those at risk, although many tools still need to be validated for sporting populations and should only be administered by an appropriately qualified person (Trojian, 2020). The Baron Depression Screener for Athletes (Baron et al., 2013) is an example of a self-report screening tool and is advocated in the IOC consensus statement. An athlete scoring highly on the tool should be assessed by a mental health professional (Reardon et al., 2019).

When an individual identifies signs of mental health difficulties—for example in an athlete they coach—they need to elicit an appropriate response. In a mental health literate environment, there may be a structure and system in place to help facilitate a response. Responses essentially fall into two categories—self-help/self-care advice or referral. Self-care advice might be administered where symptoms are very mild and could, for example, involve giving an athlete experiencing mild sleep issues advice on good sleep hygiene (Reardon et al., 2019). Depending on the nature of the symptoms and the country of residence referral could be to a range of professionals including the sport psychologist, psychotherapist, clinical psychologist, or medical doctor (e.g., general practitioner, psychiatrist, or sports medicine physician; Moesch et al., 2018). For those making decisions about whether referral is necessary or not, it is important to consider that symptoms can manifest in a different way in athletes compared to the general population. For example, in their study Doherty et al. (2016) found that athletes with depression outwardly masked their symptoms (e.g., performing at a high level, interacting with teammates) creating a mismatch with the internal stress they were experiencing.

Treatment of Mental Health Difficulties

Once an athlete has been referred to a mental health professional there are a multitude of treatment options available depending on the nature and extent of their symptoms. It is beyond the scope of this chapter to provide a comprehensive analysis of the various treatment options available for a diverse range of mental health difficulties, but treatments can be broadly split into pharmacological interventions and talking therapies (Reardon et al., 2019). When prescribing medication for a mental health disorder in an athlete, additional consideration has to be given to the potential impact of that medication on the athlete's performance and whether the athlete is permitted to use that medication by WADA (Chang et al., 2020). Talking therapies used can include psychotherapy and counselling (Ströhle, 2019). In their review of the literature, Stillman et al. (2019) concluded that psychotherapy can be effectively used to treat a range of mental health difficulties in elite athletes and suggested that an athlete's treatment should be managed by a multidisciplinary team with a thorough understanding of their specific needs. This multidisciplinary team should work with the athlete to decide if it is appropriate for an athlete to continue training and competing during treatment, whether that be pharmacological, talking therapy, or combination (pharmacological and talking therapy) based (Moesch et al., 2018).

Response to a mental health emergency is an important consideration for those involved in sport who may need to make a quick decision about how to react to such an event. A mental health emergency can be defined as a situation where an "individual presents with an acute disturbance in mental state associated with either an underlying mental health or other medical disorder" (Currie, McDuff et al., 2019, p. 772). Such disturbances could manifest as agitation, aggression, or violence, and place the individual or those around them at immediate risk of harm, thus requiring immediate intervention (Currie, McDuff et al., 2019). An athlete who attempts to take their own life whilst at a training camp is an example of a mental health emergency. Organisations should have mental health emergency plans in place to guide responses, which should cover protocols for responding to events such as suicidal thoughts, sexual assault, paranoia, extreme agitation, delirium, intoxication, or drug overdose (Currie, McDuff et al., 2019). An appropriate response to an emergency is one that avoids physical/emotional harm; uses a person-centred approach; establishes safety; and encourages hope, recovery, and resilience (Currie, McDuff et al., 2019). When travelling with athletes it is also recommended that staff are familiar with local emergency services and legislation (Reardon et al., 2019).

CLOSING THOUGHTS

The aim of this chapter was to help you to recognise the importance of mental health in sport and the need to understand the uniqueness of the sporting environment and its potential impact on mental health. Mental health is a complex area and those involved in sport (e.g., coaches and support staff) are not expected to have a detailed understanding of the area that extends beyond their professional boundaries but should have a basic understanding that includes awareness of warning signs, sources of support, referral networks, and mental health emergency plans. Such mental health literacy will allow individuals to perform in environments that nourish their mental health as well as their sports performance. Mental health is best viewed as a continuum that extends from negative (ill health) to positive (good health). At the negative end are clinically diagnosed mental health disorders, which everyone recognises as problematic, but extending further along the continuum, before we reach good health, we also have negative mental health symptoms at a subclinical level. Whilst these symptoms are subclinical, as we have seen in this chapter, they can still have a significant impact on wellbeing and sports performance. It is perhaps in this zone that we can have the most impact by developing systems and environments that catch and support those individuals before their symptoms escalate to a clinical level.

REFERENCES

Altfeld, S., Mallett, S. J., & Kellmann, M. (2015). Coaches' burnout, stress, and recovery over a season: A longitudinal study. *International Sport Coaching Journal, 2*(2), 137–151. https://doi.org/10.1123/iscj.2014-0113

Arnold, R., & Fletcher, D. (2012). A research synthesis and taxonomic classification of the organizational stressors encountered by sport performers. *Journal of Sport and Exercise Psychology, 34*(3), 397–429. https://doi.org/10.1123/jsep.34.3.397

Aron, C. M., Harvey, S., Hainline, B., Hitchcock, M. E., & Reardon, C. L. (2019). Post-traumatic stress disorder (PTSD) and other trauma-related mental disorders in elite athletes: A narrative review. *British Journal of Sports Medicine, 53*(12), 779–784. https://doi.org/10.1136/bjsports-2019-100695

Asplund, C., & Chang, C. J. (2020). The role of sleep in psychological well-being in athletes. In E. Hong & A. L. Rao (Eds.), *Mental health in the athlete* (pp. 277–290). Springer.

Baron, D. A., Baron, S. H., Tompkins, J., & Polat, A. (2013). Assessing and treating depression in athletes. In D. A. Baron, C. L. Reardon, & S. H. Baron (Eds.), *Clinical sports psychiatry* (pp. 65–78). Wiley. https://doi.org/10.1002/9781118404904.ch7

Bauman, N. J. (2016). The stigma of mental health in athletes: Are mental toughness and mental health seen as contradictory in elite sport? *British Journal of Sports Medicine, 50*(3), 135–136. http://libezproxy.open.ac.uk/login?url=https://search.ebscohost.com/login.aspx?direct=true&db=s3h&AN=112867033&site=ehost-live&scope=site

Beable, S., Fulcher, M., Lee, A. C., & Hamilton, B. (2017). SHARPSports mental Health Awareness Research Project: Prevalence and risk factors of depressive symptoms and life stress in elite athletes. *Journal of Science and Medicine in Sport, 20*(12), 1047–1052. https://doi.org/10.1016/j.jsams.2017.04.018

Biggin, I. J. R., Burns, J. H., & Uphill, M. (2017). An investigation of athletes' and coaches' perceptions of mental ill-health in elite athletes. *Journal of Clinical Sport Psychology, 11*(2), 126–147. https://doi.org/10.1123/jcsp.2016-0017

Bratland-Sanda, S., & Sundgot-Borgen, J. (2013). Eating disorders in athletes: Overview of prevalence, risk factors and recommendations for prevention and treatment. *European Journal of Sport Science, 13*(5), 499–508. https://doi.org/10.1080/17461391.2012.740504

Breslin, G., Shannon, S., Haughey, T., Donnelly, P., & Leavey, G. (2017). A systematic review of interventions to increase awareness of mental health and well-being in athletes, coaches and officials. *Systematic Reviews, 6*(1), 177. https://doi.org/10.1186/s13643-017-0568-6

Breslin, G., Smith, A., Donohue, B., Donnelly, P., Shannon, S., Haughey, T. J., . . . & Leavey, G. (2019). International consensus statement on the psychosocial and policy-related approaches to mental health awareness programmes in sport. *BMJ Open Sport & Exercise Medicine*, *6*(1), e000585. https://doi.org/10.1136/bmjsem-2019-000585

Brown, M., Deane, F. P., Vella, S. A., & Liddle, S. K. (2017). Parents views of the role of sports coaches as mental health gatekeepers for adolescent males. *International Journal of Mental Health Promotion*, *19*(5), 239–251. https://doi.org/10.1080/14623730.2017.1348305

Carson, F., Walsh, J., Main, L. C., & Kremer, P. (2018). High performance coaches' mental health and wellbeing: Applying the areas of work life model. *International Sport Coaching Journal*, *5*(3), 293–300. http://libezproxy.open.ac.uk/login?url=https://search.ebscohost.com/login.asp x?direct=true&db=s3h&AN=132369747&site=ehost-live&scope=site

Castaldelli-Maia, J. M., Gallinaro, J. G. d. M. e., Falcão, R. S., Gouttebarge, V., Hitchcock, M. E., Hainline, B., Reardon, C. L., & Stull, T. (2019). Mental health symptoms and disorders in elite athletes: A systematic review on cultural influencers and barriers to athletes seeking treatment. *British Journal of Sports Medicine*, *53*(11), 707–721. https://doi.org/10.1136/bjsports-2019-100710

Chang, C., Putukian, M., Aerni, G., Diamond, A., Hong, G., Ingram, Y., Reardon, C. L., & Wolanin, A. (2020). Mental health issues and psychological factors in athletes: Detection, management, effect on performance and prevention: American Medical Society for Sports Medicine position statement—executive summary. *British Journal of Sports Medicine*, *54*(4), 216–220. https://doi.org/10.1136/bjsports-2019-101583

Currie, A., Gorczynski, P., Rice, S. M., Purcell, R., McAllister-Williams, R. H., Hitchcock, M. E., Hainline, B., & Reardon, C. L. (2019). Bipolar and psychotic disorders in elite athletes: A narrative review. *British Journal of Sports Medicine*, *53*(12), 746–753. https://doi.org/10.1136/bjsports-2019-100685

Currie, A., McDuff, D., Johnston, A., Hopley, P., Hitchcock, M. E., Reardon, C. L., & Hainline, B. (2019). Management of mental health emergencies in elite athletes: A narrative review. *British Journal of Sports Medicine*, *53*(12), 772–778. https://doi.org/10.1136/bjsports-2019-100691

Derevensky, J. L., McDuff, D., Reardon, C. L., Hainline, B., Hitchcock, M. E., & Richard, J. (2019). Problem gambling and associated mental health concerns in elite athletes: A narrative review. *British Journal of Sports Medicine*, *53*(12), 761–766. https://doi.org/10.1136/bjsports-2019-100668

Doherty, S., Hannigan, B., & Campbell, M. J. (2016). The experience of depression during the careers of elite male athletes [Original Research]. *Frontiers in Psychology*, *7*(1069). https://doi.org/10.3389/fpsyg.2016.01069

Drew, M., Vlahovich, N., Hughes, D., Appaneal, R., Burke, L. M., Lundy, B., . . . & Waddington, G. (2018). Prevalence of illness, poor mental health and sleep quality and low energy availability prior to the 2016 Summer Olympic Games. *British Journal of Sports Medicine*, *52*(1), 47–53. https://doi.org/10.1136/bjsports-2017-098208

Fletcher, D., & Scott, M. (2010). Psychological stress in sports coaches: A review of concepts, research, and practice. *Journal of Sports Sciences*, *28*(2), 127–137. https://doi.org/10.1080/02640410903406208

Galderisi, S., Heinz, A., Kastrup, M., Beezhold, J., & Sartorius, N. (2015). Toward a new definition of mental health. *World Psychiatry: Official Journal of the World Psychiatric Association (WPA)*, *14*(2), 231–233. https://doi.org/10.1002/wps.20231

Gorczynski, P., Coyle, M., & Gibson, K. (2017). Depressive symptoms in high-performance athletes and non-athletes: A comparative meta-analysis. *British Journal of Sports Medicine*, *51*(18), 1348–1354. https://doi.org/10.1136/bjsports-2016-096455

Gorczynski, P., Gibson, K., Clarke, N., Mensah, T., & Summers, R. (2020). Examining mental health literacy, help-seeking behaviours, distress, and wellbeing in UK coaches. *European Physical Education Review, 26*(3), 713–726. https://doi.org/10.1177/1356336X19887772

Gorczynski, P., Gibson, K., Thelwell, R., Papathomas, A., Harwood, C., & Kinnafick, F. (2019). The BASES expert statement on mental health literacy in elite sport. *Sport & Exercise Scientist, 59*, 6–7. http://libezproxy.open.ac.uk/login?url=https://search.ebscohost.com/login.aspx?direct=true&db=s3h&AN=135074674&site=ehost-live&scope=site

Gouttebarge, V., Castaldelli-Maia, J. M., Gorczynski, P., Hainline, B., Hitchcock, M. E., Kerkhoffs, G. M., Rice, S. M., & Reardon, C. L. (2019). Occurrence of mental health symptoms and disorders in current and former elite athletes: A systematic review and meta-analysis. *British Journal of Sports Medicine, 53*(11), 700–706. https://doi.org/10.1136/bjsports-2019-100671

Grall-Bronnec, M., Caillon, J., Humeau, E., Perrot, B., Remaud, M., Guilleux, A., Rocher, B., Sauvaget, A., & Bouju, G. (2016). Gambling among European professional athletes. Prevalence and associated factors. *Journal of Addictive Diseases, 35*(4), 278–290. https://doi.org/10.1080/10550887.2016.1177807

Hainline, B., & Reardon, C. L. (2019). Breaking a taboo: Why the International Olympic Committee convened experts to develop a consensus statement on mental health in elite athletes. *British Journal of Sports Medicine, 53*(11), 665–666. https://doi.org/10.1136/bjsports-2019-100681

Han, D. H., McDuff, D., Thompson, D., Hitchcock, M. E., Reardon, C. L., & Hainline, B. (2019). Attention-deficit/hyperactivity disorder in elite athletes: A narrative review. *British Journal of Sports Medicine, 53*(12), 741–745. https://doi.org/10.1136/bjsports-2019-100713

Henriksen, K., Schinke, R., McCann, S., Durand-Bush, N., Moesch, K., Parham, W. D., . . . & Hunziker, J. (2020). Athlete mental health in the Olympic/Paralympic quadrennium: A multi-societal consensus statement. *International Journal of Sport and Exercise Psychology, 18*(3), 391–408. https://doi.org/10.1080/1612197X.2020.1746379

Henriksen, K., Schinke, R., Moesch, K., McCann, S., Parham, William, D., Larsen, C. H., & Terry, P. (2019). Consensus statement on improving the mental health of high performance athletes. *International Journal of Sport and Exercise Psychology*, (6), 1–8. https://doi.org/10.1080/1612197X.2019.1570473

Howells, K., & Lucassen, M. (2018). 'Post-Olympic blues'—The diminution of celebrity in Olympic athletes. *Psychology of Sport and Exercise, 37*, 67–78. https://doi.org/10.1016/j.psychsport.2018.04.008

Jeckell, A. S., Copenhaver, E. A., & Diamond, A. B. (2020). Hazing and bullying in athletic culture. In E. Hong & A. L. Rao (Eds.), *Mental health in the athlete* (pp. 165–179). Springer.

Joy, E., Kussman, A., & Nattiv, A. (2016). 2016 update on eating disorders in athletes: A comprehensive narrative review with a focus on clinical assessment and management. *British Journal of Sports Medicine, 50*(3), 154–162. https://doi.org/10.1136/bjsports-2015-095735

Kroshus, E., Wagner, J., Wyrick, D., Athey, A., Bell, L., Benjamin, H. J., . . . & Hainline, B. (2019). Wake up call for collegiate athlete sleep: Narrative review and consensus recommendations from the NCAA interassociation task force on sleep and wellness. *British Journal of Sports Medicine, 53*(12), 731–736. https://doi.org/10.1136/bjsports-2019-100590

Kuettel, A., & Larsen, C. H. (2019). Risk and protective factors for mental health in elite athletes: A scoping review. *International Review of Sport and Exercise Psychology*, 1–35. https://doi.org/10.1080/1750984X.2019.1689574

McDuff, D., Stull, T., Castaldelli-Maia, J. M., Hitchcock, M. E., Hainline, B., & Reardon, C. L. (2019). Recreational and ergogenic substance use and substance use disorders in elite athletes: A narrative review. *British Journal of Sports Medicine, 53*(12), 754–760. https://doi. org/10.1136/bjsports-2019-100669

Moesch, K., Kenttä, G., Kleinert, J., Quignon-Fleuret, C., Cecil, S., & Bertollo, M. (2018). FEP-SAC position statement: Mental health disorders in elite athletes and models of service provision. *Psychology of Sport and Exercise, 38*, 61–71. https://doi.org/10.1016/j.psychsport.2018. 05.013

Poucher, Z. A., Tamminen, K. A., Kerr, G., & Cairney, J. (2019). A commentary on mental health research in elite sport. *Journal of Applied Sport Psychology*, 1–23. https://doi.org/10.1080/104 13200.2019.1668496

Poysophon, P., & Rao, A. L. (2018). Neurocognitive deficits associated with ADHD in athletes: A systematic review. *Sports Health, 10*(4), 317–326. https://doi.org/10.1177/1941738117751387

Putukian, M. (2020). The psychological response to injury and illness. In E. Hong & A. L. Rao (Eds.), *Mental health in the athlete* (pp. 95–101). Springer.

Rao, A. L. (2020). Athletic suicide. In E. Hong & A. L. Rao (Eds.), *Mental health in the athlete* (pp. 39–56). Springer.

Rao, A. L., Asif, I. M., Drezner, J. A., Toresdahl, B. G., & Harmon, K. G. (2015). Suicide in National Collegiate Athletic Association (NCAA) Athletes: A 9-year analysis of the NCAA resolutions database. *Sports Health, 7*(5), 452–457. https://doi.org/10.1177/1941738115587675

Rao, A. L., & Hong, E. (2020). Overcoming the stigma of mental health in sport. In E. Hong & A. Rao (Eds.), *Mental health in the athlete* (pp. 1–10). Springer.

Reardon, C. L., Hainline, B., Aron, C. M., Baron, D., Baum, A. L., Bindra, A., . . . & Engebretsen, L. (2019). Mental health in elite athletes: International Olympic Committee consensus statement (2019). *British Journal of Sports Medicine, 53*(11), 667–699. https://doi.org/10.1136/ bjsports-2019-100715

Rice, S. M., Gwyther, K., Santesteban-Echarri, O., Baron, D., Gorczynski, P., Gouttebarge, V., Reardon, C. L., Hitchcock, M. E., Hainline, B., & Purcell, R. (2019). Determinants of anxiety in elite athletes: A systematic review and meta-analysis. *British Journal of Sports Medicine, 53*(11), 722–730. https://doi.org/10.1136/bjsports-2019-100620

Rice, S. M., Parker, A. G., Rosenbaum, S., Bailey, A., Mawren, D., & Purcell, R. (2018). Sport-related concussion and mental health outcomes in elite athletes: A systematic review. *Sports Medicine, 48*(2), 447–465. https://doi.org/10.1007/s40279-017-0810-3

Rice, S. M., Purcell, R., De Silva, S., Mawren, D., McGorry, P. D., & Parker, A. G. (2016). The mental health of elite athletes: A narrative systematic review. *Sports Medicine, 46*(9), 1333–1353. https://doi.org/10.1007/s40279-016-0492-2

Sarac, N., Sarac, B., Pedroza, A., & Borchers, J. (2018). Epidemiology of mental health conditions in incoming division I collegiate athletes. *The Physician and Sportsmedicine, 46*(2), 242–248. https://doi.org/10.1080/00913847.2018.1427412

Schinke, R. J., Stambulova, N. B., Si, G., & Moore, Z. (2018). International society of sport psychology position stand: Athletes' mental health, performance, and development. *International Journal of Sport and Exercise Psychology, 16*(6), 622–639. https://doi.org/10.1080/16121 97X.2017.1295557

Souter, G., Lewis, R., & Serrant, L. (2018). Men, mental health and elite sport: A narrative review. *Sports Medicine—Open, 4*(1), 57. https://doi.org/10.1186/s40798-018-0175-7

Stillman, M. A., Glick, I. D., McDuff, D., Reardon, C. L., Hitchcock, M. E., Fitch, V. M., & Hainline, B. (2019). Psychotherapy for mental health symptoms and disorders in elite athletes: A narrative review. *British Journal of Sports Medicine, 53*(12), 767–771. https://doi.org/10.1136/bjsports-2019-100654

Ströhle, A. (2019). Sports psychiatry: Mental health and mental disorders in athletes and exercise treatment of mental disorders. *European Archives of Psychiatry and Clinical Neuroscience, 269*(5), 485–498. https://doi.org/10.1007/s00406-018-0891-5

Swartz, L., Hunt, X., Bantjes, J., Hainline, B., & Reardon, C. L. (2019). Mental health symptoms and disorders in Paralympic athletes: A narrative review. *British Journal of Sports Medicine, 53*(12), 737–740. https://doi.org/10.1136/bjsports-2019-100731

Trojian, T. H. (2020). Screening for mental health conditions in athletes. In E. Hong & A. L. Rao (Eds.), *Mental health in the athlete* (pp. 11–24). Springer.

Van Slingerland, K. J., Durand-Bush, N., Bradley, L., Goldfield, G., Archambault, R., Smith, D., . . . & Kenttä, G. (2019). Canadian Centre for Mental Health and Sport (CCMHS) position statement: Principles of mental health in competitive and high-performance sport. *Clinical Journal of Sport Medicine, 29*(3), 173–180. https://journals.lww.com/cjsportsmed/Fulltext/2019/05000/Canadian_Centre_for_Mental_Health_and_Sport.1.aspx

Vella, S. A., & Swann, C. (2020). Time for mental healthcare guidelines for recreational sports: A call to action. *British Journal of Sports Medicine.* https://doi.org/10.1136/bjsports-2019-101591

Wolanin, A. T. (2020). Depression in athletes: Incidence, prevalence, and comparisons with the nonathletic population. In E. Hong & A. Rao (Eds.), *Mental health in the athlete* (pp. 25–37). Springer.

Wolanin, A. T., Hong, E., Marks, D., Panchoo, K., & Gross, M. (2016). Prevalence of clinically elevated depressive symptoms in college athletes and differences by gender and sport. *British Journal of Sports Medicine, 50*(3), 167–171. https://doi.org/10.1136/bjsports-2015-095756

World Health Organization. (2018, March 30). *Mental health: Strengthening our response.* www.who.int/news-room/fact-sheets/detail/mental-health-strengthening-our-response

CHAPTER 12

Developing Resilience on the Athlete's Journey

Karen Howells

The postponement of the 2020 Tokyo Olympic and Paralympic Games as a result of the global COVID-19 pandemic threw national governing bodies, performance directors, coaches, and athletes into a situation that had not been experienced in the modern Olympic Games. It was an adversity that challenged the toughest of athletes, shattered their dreams and expectations, and catapulted them into a period of uncertainty. At the time of writing this chapter, we cannot envisage the full emotional, performance-related, and financial consequences of the global pandemic and what it has meant for domestic and international sport at all levels. What we can surmise is that the experiences and decisions made in light of the pandemic will have been perceived as a negative event or an adversity by many of the athletes who had been training for the 2020 Olympic/Paralympic Games for a significant proportion of their lives, and for those at the start of their athletic journey. Furthermore, we know that the research tells us that there are some of those athletes who will have bounced back from such an adversity and who will have come back psychologically and physically stronger than they were before (cf. Fletcher & Sarkar, 2012). This bounceback capability is conceptualised in the academic literature and in the public understanding as *resilience*. An athlete's resilience, that is the extent to which they can use their personal qualities to withstand pressure (Fletcher & Sarkar, 2016), will perhaps be key to determining whether the situation in which they find themselves in is facilitative or detrimental to their ongoing journey through sport.

An athlete's journey, whether it is focused on the outcome of Olympic success or on the process of an intrinsically motivated desire to engage in sport (at any level), will be characterised by highs and lows (Howells & Fletcher, 2016). The lows may involve stressors, adversities, traumas, or failures (Galli & Gonzalez, 2015). These experiences which are all perceived to be negative in nature may be analogous with those experienced by the wider population such as bereavement (e.g., Simpson & Elberty, 2018), interpersonal difficulties (e.g., Lamont et al., 2019), poor mental health (e.g., Newman et al., 2016), or the social isolation and lack of control encountered in a global pandemic. The experiences may also involve adversities that are specific to the athlete experience such as performance slumps (e.g., C.J. Brown et al., 2020), sport injury (e.g., Cavallerio et al., 2016), post-Olympic blues (e.g., Howells & Lucassen, 2018), or organisational stressors (e.g., Arnold et al., 2017). Although it is acknowledged that there are some differences in the terminology used to describe these experiences that are perceived as negative (see Howells et al., 2017), this chapter will refer to them as adversities, except where authors of studies cited use one of the alternative terms (e.g., stressors; Fletcher & Sarkar, 2012).

Irrespective of whether the adversities are specific to sport or those shared with the wider population, they can play a fundamental role in the process of resilience and in the development of a similar, but distinct, concept of adversarial growth (for a distinction between resilience and growth see D.J. Brown et al., 2020). Understanding resilience is vital for anyone, such as coaches, parents, practitioners, or sport science staff, who is involved in an athlete's journey as it may be fundamental in facilitating ongoing success and positive mental wellbeing. Resilience, in a sporting context, is two-dimensional; it relates to an individual's capability to handle the pressure of the routine stressors of training and competition and is indicative of an individual's psychological characteristics that are required to overcome potentially more extreme stressors (e.g., long-term illness; Gould et al., 2002). To facilitate a more in-depth understanding of resilience, this chapter will explain what resilience comprises and then, informed by the wider academic literature, identify a number of ways that coaches and practitioners can develop resilience during athletes' journeys. Specifically, it will address the use of mental fortitude training (e.g., Fletcher & Sarkar, 2016), planned disruptions (e.g., Kegelaers et al., 2019), and rational-emotive behaviour therapy (e.g., Wood et al., 2017).

WHAT IS RESILIENCE?

There are multiple definitions of resilience which have informed research and practice over the years (for an in-depth discussion of the definitions of resilience, see Fletcher & Sarkar, 2013; Sisto et al., 2019). The abundance of definitions has meant that there is a lack of consensus about what resilience is and, consequently, this has been problematic for researchers interested in conducting research into resilience. Fletcher and Sarkar (2013) explained that, in the absence of a consensus about how resilience is defined, it can be conceptualised as a trait, a process, or an outcome and this can lead to a tendency to misuse the term (e.g., conceptualising resilience as a fixed trait, as in 'a resilient individual'). However, where there is consensus most definitions are consistent in noting the fundamental components of adversity and positive adaptation, where adversity is the main antecedent and positive adaptation is the main consequence (Fletcher & Sarkar, 2013).

In relation to sport performers, Fletcher and Sarkar (2012) coined a definition of resilience that encompasses both the qualities of resilience and its benefits; they defined it as "the role of mental processes and behaviour in promoting personal assets and protecting an individual from the potential negative effect of stressors" (p. 675). This definition of psychological resilience (thereby distinguishing it from other forms of resilience such as physical or molecular resilience) has been broadly accepted by the sport and performance psychology community and is useful to inform applied practice. In later research, Fletcher and Sarkar (2016) distinguished between *robust resilience* and *rebound resilience*. Robust resilience, they argued, refers to resilience providing protection to the individual which is identifiable in the maintenance of wellbeing and performance levels whilst under pressure. Rebound resilience refers to the bounceback characteristics reflected in the minimal impact that adversity has on an individual's wellbeing or performance. What is interesting and important for those involved in sport to appreciate relating to both concepts is they are not purely focused on the performance outcomes of athletes. Instead, both types of resilience adopt a more holistic view of the athlete incorporating the athlete's wellbeing.

Although resilience research and its application in the sporting context has grown almost exponentially in the last decade, resilience is still a relatively new concept in sport psychology. The first systematic approach to consider resilience in sport was by Galli and Vealey (2008) who used Richardson et al.'s (1990) resiliency model as a guiding theoretical framework to explore college and professional athletes' perceptions and experiences of resilience. Based on the findings of their qualitative study with ten high level athletes, the authors rejected the notion of resilience as a trait. Rather, they conceptualised resilience as a process that involves both environmental (e.g., social support) and internal (e.g., competitiveness, confidence, being positive) processes that require cognitive appraisals and coping strategies to "mediate the relationship between personal and environmental resources and psychological outcomes of adversity" (p. 328).

Later, in a grounded theory examination of psychological resilience in Olympic champions, Fletcher and Sarkar (2012) progressed the literature on resilience in sport by moving away from Galli and Vealey's (2008) linear stage framework which they argued was biased towards coping focused processes. Fletcher and Sarkar (2012) interviewed twelve Olympic champions (eight men and four women) from a range of sports regarding their experiences of withstanding pressure during their sporting careers. Their analytical process involved a variant of grounded theory (cf. Strauss & Corbin, 1998), a research method that is concerned with the generation of theory which is *grounded* in data that has been systematically collected and analysed (see Chapter 5 for a more detailed overview of grounded theory). In contrast to the deductive scientific method, it is inductive in nature. Specifically, in Fletcher and Sarkar's (2012) research, the analysis of the data from one interview often informed the direction and content of the next.

The researchers identified numerous psychological factors that protect the world's best athletes from the potential negative effect of stressors. They posited that central to their theory of resilience is the positive evaluation and meta-cognition (i.e., evaluation of own thoughts) of the stressors experienced by the individual. They referred to the positive evaluation as a challenge appraisal which occurs when the stressor (or adversity) is relevant to the individual's goals and the individual perceives that their resources are sufficient to cope with the demands placed upon them. In addition to these positive evaluations, Fletcher and Sarkar (2012) highlighted that in their study, elite athletes were able to withstand the demands of their experiences through meta-cognition. In addition to positive evaluation and meta-cognition, they argued that an integral aspect of withstanding pressure are the psychological characteristics that individuals high in resilience possess. They refer to five psychological factors, namely: positive personality, motivation, confidence, focus, and perceived social support. The relationship between challenge appraisal, meta-cognition, and individual characteristics (e.g., positive personality, confidence, focus) can be seen in Figure 12.1.

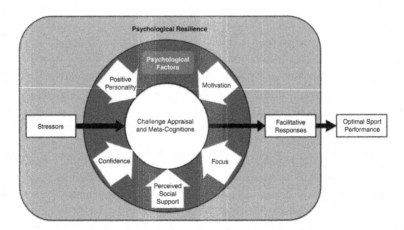

FIGURE 12.1 A grounded theory of psychological resilience and optimal sport performance

Source: Fletcher & Sarkar, 2012, p. 672

PREPARATION TO BUILD RESILIENCE

Resilience as a positive and desirable virtue has become internalised and normalised in the public's understanding and, increasingly, practitioners and coaches have searched for ways of promoting resilience in athletes. Over the last decade there has been a burgeoning of resilience programmes developed in a multitude of contexts, such as the military (e.g., Meredith et al., 2011) and the workplace (e.g., King et al., 2016), and for a number of different purposes, such as to develop sustained performance in sport (e.g., Fletcher & Sarkar, 2016) or to manage childhood adversity (e.g., Fritz et al., 2018). However, before jumping on the proverbial bandwagon and embarking on the development of a resilience programme, coaches and practitioners should ask themselves two pertinent questions: (1) Should we aspire to facilitate resilience? and (2) What is the motivation for building resilience?

Should We Aspire to Facilitate Resilience?

The first question may, at first sight, appear redundant; the development of resilience is intuitively both positive and protective, and may therefore be an attractive proposition for practitioners who aspire to improve some aspect of athletes' lives. However, there are several issues that should be addressed before embarking on an intervention. The first issue relates to the requirement of adversity to facilitate and build resilience (D.J. Brown et al., 2020), and the second relates to the relationship that resilience has with (adversarial or posttraumatic) growth (D.J. Brown et al., 2020). In respect of the former, Howells and Wadey (2020) identified that national governing bodies, performance directors, sport science practitioners, and coaches might be enticed by the transformational qualities of the positive outcomes following experiences of adversity in sport. This is supported by research by Sarkar and Hilton (2020) who identified that elite coaches often create a challenging but supportive environment to facilitate athletes' personal and athletic progression. However, Howells and Wadey (2020) cautioned against an intrinsic belief that introducing, reinforcing, and/or perpetuating current harsh practices (cf. Cavallerio et al., 2016) into training and competition will facilitate enhanced sporting performance and thus promote certain key performance indicators (e.g., heightened podium potentials, improved positioning in medal tables).

Indeed, Kegelaers et al. (2019) warned that increasing pressure on athletes "without sufficient support in place may lead to an unrelenting environment, characterised by unhealthy outcomes such as conflicts, unhealthy competition, blaming, and little attention for mental well-being" (n.p.). In respect of the second issue regarding the relationship with growth, in addressing the similarities and differences between thriving (see Chapter 13), resilience, and growth, D.J. Brown et al. (2020) identified that resilience may prevent growth occurring at an individual (as opposed to a team) level. Growth occurs when an individual's assumptive world (that is, their beliefs, values, and identity) is shattered by an adversity (cf. Janoff-Bulman, 1992) that is accompanied by significant ongoing distress. Following a period of cognitive processing (e.g., reflective pondering) and disclosure, facilitated by enhanced social support, a higher level of functioning, including superior performance, may ensue (cf. Howells et al., 2017); this higher level of functioning is conceptualised as *growth*. Resilience, as a consequence of its protective qualities, may impede this process as it has the potential to impact the individual's perception of an adversity as not being sufficiently negative to involve a shattering of assumptions. Rather, the robust individual is protected from the impact of the adversity and therefore growth, with its increased level of functioning and potentially superior performance (Howells et al., 2017), does not occur. Accordingly, before embarking on an intervention to facilitate resilience, one should question whether it is ethical to introduce adversities in the form of challenges and whether resilience is preferable to growth in a particular context.

What Is the Motivation for Building Resilience?

This second question relates to addressing a number of key issues in respect of the rationale and motivation for the aspiration to build resilience. Before embarking on a systematic (or otherwise) approach to developing resilience, a number of key issues should be addressed. Firstly, Fletcher and Sarkar (2016) emphasise that resilience training is not a panacea for all mental health or performance problems and that any programme should be part of a larger holistic programme of psychosocial support to develop well-adjusted performers. Secondly, coaches and practitioners need to be cognisant of why they are proposing such an intervention. For example, we may reflect on whether the goal of an intervention is to enhance or deliver optimal performance or whether it is to create a shield that protects the athlete from the negative impact that adversities can have on their emotional and psychological wellbeing. Reflection on this question is an important stage in the development of an effective and timely intervention. To elaborate, Fletcher and Sarkar (2016) discuss an evidence-based approach to developing psychological resilience specifically to facilitate sustained success, and therefore the timing of an intervention is critical.

Thirdly, the decision to implement a resilience intervention or programme should be made whilst being cognisant of the dynamic psychosocial and political nuances in an organisation, for example, the extent to which an organisation is open to sport psychology support. As Bell et al. (2020) report "Overall perceptions of sport psychology [are] varied, with multiple factors impacting upon them including the use and understanding of sport psychology, as well as coaches' perceptions" (n.p.). Finally, for sport psychology practitioners, it is important that one's professional philosophies are acknowledged as this will impact of whether a resilience intervention is considered appropriate and if so, what content it will include. For example, Gonzalez et al. (2016) reported upon a number of case studies involving intervention strategies where they reported their philosophical approach as being eclectic (i.e., drawing on multiple schools of thought) and involved them using a psychological skills training (PST) model to develop resilience in athletes. Alternatively, consultants identifying with a cognitive-behavioural philosophical approach would assume that an individual's beliefs and thoughts influence their behaviour. A consultant working within this paradigm may utilise rational emotive behaviour therapy (REBT) which proposes that an "individual's beliefs (rational versus irrational beliefs) are associated with emotions and action tendencies that are divergent in their functionality (functional versus dysfunctional) towards goal achievement" (Wood et al., 2017, p. 265). To illustrate, irrational beliefs can lead to dysfunctional cognitive, emotional, and behavioural responses that can be detrimental to an individual achieving their goals. In contrast, rational beliefs can facilitate positive functional cognitive, emotional, and behavioural responses that can help an individual to reach their goals.

BUILDING RESILIENCE

In considering the development of resilience interventions in athletes, Fletcher and Sarkar (2012) argued that the intervention development should be grounded in systematic resilience programmes and conceptual and theoretical advances. Later they specified that programmes should take both robust and rebound resilience into account (Fletcher & Sarkar, 2016). In this latter paper, they acknowledged that it is arguably easier to research and write about resilience than to incorporate it into practice to bring about positive change. However, the research in the area has grown substantially and there is now a burgeoning body of evidence to inform practitioners on how to create rigorous and systematic intervention programmes. This section will address three different intervention strategies that may be useful in developing resilience in athletes through their sporting journeys, namely mental fortitude training, planned disruptions, and rational-emotive behaviour therapy (REBT). Nevertheless, irrespective of the approach used any resilience training should be transparent about explaining what resilience is and what it is not (Fletcher & Sarkar, 2016).

Mental Fortitude Training

Fletcher and Sarkar (2016) developed the principles for an evidenced-based "mental fortitude training" (p. 136) programme for performers who wished to develop resilience, that is to withstand and thrive on pressure, to facilitate sustained success. Concentrating on the dual-dimensional aspect of resilience (i.e., robust and rebound), they argued that training should be proactive to encourage and develop robust resilience (i.e., the protective quality) and reactive (i.e., the rebound quality). Accordingly, they argued performers should be targeted before, during, and after adverse experiences and that any intervention will need to identify timing and type of resilience being developed. Their reflections on the development of the programme, which was partially informed by the authors' own sport psychology practice in the elite sport environment, resulted in a number of recommendations for practitioners in this area.

The programme focused on three specific areas to enhance performers' ability to withstand pressure: (1) personal qualities, (2) facilitative environment, and (3) challenge mindset. In the first instance they endorsed the importance of training programmes focusing on an individual's personal qualities which can protect them from negative consequences. They proposed gradually increasing the pressure on an individual(s) through challenges and the manipulation of the environment. They suggested that this could be achieved in two ways: firstly, by increasing the demand of the stressors, through their type (e.g., competitive), property (e.g., novelty), or dimension (e.g., frequency). Secondly, by increasing the significance of the appraisals, through their relevance (e.g., beliefs), importance (e.g., goals), and consequences (e.g., punishment). In developing the intervention, they suggest that the aim of a training programme should be to optimise an individual's qualities with the acknowledgement that any individual will have their own breaking point where they succumb to extreme hardship and/or adversity. They distinguished between personality characteristics that can be resistant to change (e.g., being a perfectionist, being competitive), psychological skills (e.g., goal setting, attentional control) and desirable outcome (e.g., enhancing confidence, emotional regulation). This distinction is important as, for example, personality characteristics (e.g., believing in oneself) are less amenable to change than psychological skills (e.g., goal setting). At any given time these qualities, which vary in relevance and importance dependent on the context, may be tested by adversities and supported by social and environmental resources. To illustrate this latter point, Sarkar and Hilton (2020) posited that elite coaches have a role to play in developing resilience in athletes through developing a strong coach-athlete relationship (see Chapter 6) and creating a facilitative environment (see Figure 12.2). The relevance and importance of qualities varies across contexts and will depend on the preferred outcomes of any intervention programme.

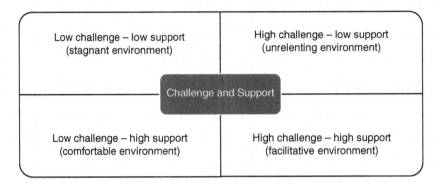

FIGURE 12.2 A visual representation of Fletcher and Sarkar's (2016) four challenge and support environments

Fletcher and Sarkar (2016) illustrate that withstanding training-related stressors is likely to require a different focus from those who need to withstand competition stressors.

Fletcher and Sarkar (2016) acknowledged that resilience is essentially a cognitive-affective (loosely defined as thinking and feeling) construct but that it is positively or negatively impacted upon by environmental factors. They suggest that an environment that fosters the development of resilience is facilitative, but with a focus on the protective elements of resilience, they endorsed the importance of challenge and support in that environment. The nature of that challenge varies; one example is covered in the next section where planned disruptions are discussed. To inform an understanding of the relationship between challenge and support and how they impact on the athletic environment, Fletcher and Sarkar drew upon Sanford's (1967) theory of challenge and support which allowed them to differentiate between four quadrants, each representing a different environment (see Figure 12.2). Resilience, they argued, is developed in a high-challenge, high-support and, therefore, facilitative environment.

Planned Disruptions

Planned disruptions involve the exposure of athletes to structured and deliberate training activities comprising increased and/or changing demands under controlled circumstances (Kegelaers et al., 2020) and can be used to facilitate the development of athletes' resilience (e.g., Fletcher & Sarkar, 2016; Galli & Gonzalez, 2015). Planned disruptions can take many forms, such as manipulating the physical and mental demands on the athlete including disrupting sleep or adding consequences to certain behaviours. In a qualitative study that explored coaches of elite athletes' use of planned disruptions, Kegelaers et al. (2020) identified nine types of planned disruptions namely, location, competition simulation, punishments and rewards, physical strain, stronger competition, distractions, unfairness, restrictions, and outside the box (i.e., non-sport-specific activities). When these planned disruptions are combined with formal reflection to create athlete awareness of their responses under pressure then they can be used to promote resilient qualities in athletes. An example of this in practice can be seen in the experiences of Richard Parks, a former Wales international rugby player who retired from professional rugby following a career ending injury and who, following a period of depression and agoraphobia, turned to adventure physical activity and became an extreme environment athlete (see Case Study 12.1).

CASE STUDY 12.1

Richard Parks—Pushing the Bounds of Human Endurance

Richard Parks is a former Wales international rugby player and extreme environment athlete who takes part in expeditions that push the boundaries of human endurance. His successes involve completing the 737 challenge where he was the first person ever to climb the highest mountain on each of the world's seven continents and stand on all three poles (the North Pole, the South Pole, and the summit of Everest) within seven months.

In a BBC Learning production, Richard talked about the use of planned disruptions to prepare for his extreme adventure expedition. He referred to this as 'deprivation training' and used the example of reducing his body to clinical hypothermia through submersion in an ice bath to learn how to control emotions, cognition, and anxieties. This specific deprivation training, he believes, allowed him to manage a fall into a crevasse in Alaska and successfully facilitate a rescue.

Source: www.bbc.co.uk/programmes/p02xc4pk

In a study that utilised a mixed methods quasi-experimental design, Kegelaers et al. (2019) evaluated the effectiveness of a pressure training intervention for elite level female basketball players with a specific focus on planned disruptions. They measured resilience using the unidimensional 10-item Connor-Davidson resilience scale (CD-RISC-10; Campbell-Sills & Stein, 2007) and through qualitative interviews. Their findings were inconclusive. Thematic analysis of their interview data indicated that their intervention was effective in developing certain resilient qualities and they interpreted that it may have a positive impact on a team's ability to deal with competitive stressors. However, improvements in these psychosocial processes were not necessarily reflected by the answers on the CD-RISC-10. Although the authors hypothesised why this inconsistency occurred, they suggested that the intervention may have been more successful in having an impact on collective (e.g., team), rather than individual, processes. This is an important observation as the design of any intervention should be specific about whether the development of resilience is targeted at an individual or collective level. Furthermore, they noted that the CD-RISC-10 is not specific to sport and therefore given the wording, which is specific to general life stressors, may not necessarily reflect sport-specific competitive stressors. This study illustrates the importance of ensuring a theoretically informed design and appropriate measurement of resilience in any intervention programme.

Rational-Emotive Behaviour Therapy

REBT is a form of cognitive-behavioural therapy that is becoming increasingly popular in sport psychology. Practitioners who use REBT start with the assumption that many of the problems that an individual may experience in the sporting environment can be attributed to irrational thinking. REBT practitioners employ an ABC (DE) framework where A is the antecedent (adversity), B is the belief (irrational and/or rational), C is the consequence, D involves disputation and E a new effective rational belief. Importantly, REBT does not dispute the perception of the adversity (A); it assumes that the adversity is true and accepts that it is negative for the individual involved (even if others may not perceive the event or experience to be negative in nature). Rather, it is the beliefs (B) about the adversity that are disputed (D) and should be replaced with new effective beliefs (E). From an REBT perspective:

> Resilience comprises a set of flexible cognitive, behavioural and emotional responses to acute or chronic adversities that can be unusual or commonplace. These responses can be learned and are within the grasp of everyone. While many factors affect the development of resilience, the most important one is the belief that the person holds about the adversity. Therefore, belief is the heart of resilience.
>
> (Dryden, 2011, p. 134)

In a study involving five elite athletes who were low in resilient qualities as measured by the CD-RISC-10 (Campbell-Sills & Stein, 2007), an REBT intervention was shown to reduce irrational beliefs and enhance resilient qualities in athletes (Deen et al., 2017).

Wood et al. (2017) suggest that the nature of elite sport may perpetuate an athlete's irrational beliefs; specifically, the transition to elite sport may involve a shift into a period fixated on success, failure, and perceived self-worth. When faced with setbacks (adversity) athletes may become susceptible to more irrational beliefs which, in turn, result in unhealthy emotions and maladaptive behaviours. By addressing an individual's propensity to irrational beliefs and adopting strategies that allow a disruption to create new effective beliefs, the individual will become resilient to (as in protected against) further adversity. In Wood et al.'s (2017) intervention, a young cricketer developed a new formed rational philosophy that allowed him to "weather" (p. 274) further setbacks. Locating this within Fletcher and Sarkar's (2016) dual conceptualisation of resilience (i.e., robust and rebound), REBT may address both aspects. Through addressing the irrationals beliefs (B), the potential for rebound is enhanced, and through development of disruption strategies, robust resilience may be developed.

Irrespective of the type of intervention that a practitioner deems appropriate, sport psychologists have to be flexible and respond to a multitude of different factors in developing an effective intervention. The ability to deal with the unexpected is as important to the practitioner as it is to the athlete. This chapter opened with the impact that the COVID-19 pandemic in 2020 had on athletes. Practitioners also have to respond to unforeseen events and this applies to the interventions that are developed to facilitate athlete resilience. In the spotlight box, an example of how sport psychologists responded to developing resilience in a socially distanced world is presented.

Spotlight On: Developing Resilience in a Socially Distanced World

Practitioners often have to overcome challenges themselves to deliver effective interventions to athletes. Because of socially distanced COVID-19 2020, sport psychologists had to come up with innovative ways of developing resilience using socially distanced online platforms. One such example came from Swim England and sport psychologists Hannah Stoyel and Helen Davis who, informed by academic empirical evidence, encouraged swimmers to develop a personal highlight reel to develop resilience. They encouraged swimmers to:

1. Write down some of the things in your life that you are proud of. Add pictures and stories where possible.
2. Circle the highlights that involved a challenge that you had to overcome.
3. Then list what skills, actions, and personal characteristics you used to overcome these challenges. Think about which of these you can build on to use again in the future.

Source: www.swimming.org/sport/resilience-personal-highlight-reel/

CLOSING THOUGHTS

This chapter has provided an empirically informed explanation of what resilience is, a discussion around whether it should be developed, and described three intervention strategies that could be developed to facilitate resilience in athletes. The chapter has predominantly focused on the individual (or interpersonal) experience, however, for coaches and practitioners working in team sports, understanding resilience at a team or dyad level is also important. For readers interested in team resilience, research by Morgan et al. (2013) would be a good starting point. As alluded to in the chapter, attempts to develop resilience should be informed by reflecting on the motivations that have informed the desire to facilitate resilience. Perhaps, closing on Fletcher and Sarkar's (2016) warning to practitioners is salient here. They warned:

> Resilience is not about choosing to place one's (or others') health, wellbeing, or even life at risk. Confusion occurs when, paradoxically, weakness is misconstrued as strength. Examples include being under stress and denying it, [and] being so single-minded and focused on performance that everything else is ignored. . . . Scholars, practitioners, and others working with performers should distinguish between resilience and weakness to minimize misunderstanding.
>
> (Fletcher & Sarkar, 2016, p. 150)

REFERENCES

Arnold, R., Wagstaff, C. R., Steadman, L., & Pratt, Y. (2017). The organisational stressors encountered by athletes with a disability. *Journal of Sports Sciences, 35,* 1187–1196. https://doi.org/10.1080/02640414.2016.1214285

Bell, A. F., Knight, C. J., Lovett, V. E., & Shearer, C. (2020). Understanding elite youth athletes' knowledge and perceptions of sport psychology. *Journal of Applied Sport Psychology,* 1–23. https://doi.org/10.1080/10413200.2020.1719556

Brown, C. J., Butt, J., & Sarkar, M. (2020). Overcoming performance slumps: Psychological resilience in expert cricket batsmen. *Journal of Applied Sport Psychology*, *32*, 277–296. https://doi.org/10.1080/10413200.2018.1545709

Brown, D. J., Sarkar, M., & Howells, K. (2020). Growth, resilience, and thriving: A jangle fallacy? In R. Wadey, M. Day, & K. Howells (Eds.). *Growth following adversity: A mechanism to positive change in sport* (pp. 59–72). Routledge.

Campbell-Sills, L., & Stein, M. B. (2007). Psychometric analysis and refinement of the Connor—Davidson resilience scale (CD-RISC): Validation of a 10-item measure of resilience. *Journal of Traumatic Stress: Official Publication of the International Society for Traumatic Stress Studies*, *20*(6), 1019–1028. https://doi.org/10.1002/jts.20271

Cavallerio, F., Wadey, R., & Wagstaff, C. R. (2016). Understanding overuse injuries in rhythmic gymnastics: A 12-month ethnographic study. *Psychology of Sport and Exercise*, *25*, 100–109. https://doi.org/10.1016/j.psychsport.2016.05.002

Deen, S., Turner, M. J., & Wong, R. S. (2017). The effects of REBT, and the use of credos, on irrational beliefs and resilience qualities in athletes. *The Sport Psychologist*, *31*(3), 249–263. https://doi.org/10.1123/tsp.2016-0057

Dryden, W. (2011). *Understanding psychological health: The REBT perspective*. Taylor & Francis.

Fletcher, D., & Sarkar, M. (2012). A grounded theory of psychological resilience in Olympic champions. *Psychology of Sport and Exercise*, *13*, 669–678. https://doi.org/10.1016/j.psychsport.2012.04.007

Fletcher, D., & Sarkar, M. (2013). Psychological resilience: A review and critique of definitions, concepts, and theory. *European Psychologist*, *18*(1), 12–23. https://doi.org/10.1027/1016-9040/a000124

Fletcher, D., & Sarkar, M. (2016). Mental fortitude training: An evidence-based approach to developing psychological resilience for sustained success. *Journal of Sport Psychology in Action*, *7*, 135–157. http://doi.org10.1080/21520704.2016.1255496

Fritz, J., de Graaff, A. M., Caisley, H., Van Harmelen, A. L., & Wilkinson, P. O. (2018). A systematic review of amenable resilience factors that moderate and/or mediate the relationship between childhood adversity and mental health in young people. *Frontiers in Psychiatry*, *9*, 230. https://doi.org/10.3389/fpsyt.2018.00230

Galli, N., & Gonzalez, S. P. (2015). Psychological resilience in sport: A review of the literature and implications for research and practice. *International Journal of Sport and Exercise Psychology*, *13*, 243–257. http://doi.org/10.1080/1612197X.2014.946947

Galli, N., & Vealey, R. S. (2008). "Bouncing back" from adversity: Athletes' experiences of resilience. *The Sport Psychologist*, *22*, 316–335. https://doi.org/10.1123/tsp.22.3.316

Gonzalez, S. P., Detling, N., & Galli, N. A. (2016). Case studies of developing resilience in elite sport: Applying theory to guide interventions. *Journal of Sport Psychology in Action*, *7*, 158–169. https://doi.org/10.1080/21520704.2016.1236050

Gould, D., Dieffenbach, K., & Moffett, A. (2002). Psychological characteristics and their development in Olympic champions. *Journal of Applied Sport Psychology*, *14*(3), 172–204. https://doi.org/10.1080/10413200290103482

Howells, K., & Fletcher, D. (2016). Adversarial growth in Olympic swimmers: Constructive reality or illusory self-deception? *Journal of Sport & Exercise Psychology*, *38*, 173–186. http://doi.org/10.1123/jsep.2015-0189

Howells, K., & Lucassen, M. (2018). Post-Olympic blues—The diminution of celebrity in Olympic athletes. *Psychology of Sport and Exercise, 37*, 67–78. http://doi.org/10.1016/j.psychsport.2018.04.008

Howells, K., Sarkar, M., & Fletcher, D. (2017). Can athletes benefit from difficulty? A systematic review of growth following adversity in competitive sport. *Progress in Brain Research*, 117–159. https://doi.org/10.1016/bs.pbr.2017.06.002

Howells, K., & Wadey, R. (2020). Nurturing growth in the aftermath of adversity: A narrative review of evidence-based practice. In R. Wadey, M. Day, & K. Howells (Eds.). *Growth following adversity: A mechanism to positive change in sport* (pp. 219–234). Routledge.

Janoff-Bulman, R. (1992). *Shattered assumptions: Towards a new psychology of trauma.* The Free Press.

Kegelaers, J., Wylleman, P., Bunigh, A., & Oudejans, R. R. (2019). A mixed methods evaluation of a pressure training intervention to develop resilience in female basketball players. *Journal of Applied Sport Psychology*. https://doi.org/10.1080/10413200.2019.1630864

Kegelaers, J., Wylleman, P., & Oudejans, R. R. (2020). A coach perspective on the use of planned disruptions in high-performance sports. *Sport, Exercise, and Performance Psychology, 9*, 29–44. https://doi.org/10.1037/spy0000167

King, D. D., Newman, A., & Luthans, F. (2016). Not if, but when we need resilience in the workplace. *Journal of Organizational Behavior, 37*, 782–786. https://doi.org/10.1002/job.2063

Lamont, M., Kennelly, M., & Moyle, B. (2019). Perspectives of endurance athletes' spouses: A paradox of serious leisure. *Leisure Sciences, 41*, 477–498. https://doi.org/10.1080/01490400.2017.1384943

Meredith, L. S., Sherbourne, C. D., Gaillot, S. J., Hansell, L., Ritschard, H. V., Parker, A. M., & Wrenn, G. (2011). Promoting psychological resilience in the US military. *Rand Health Quarterly, 1.* www.ncbi.nlm.nih.gov/pmc/articles/PMC4945176/

Morgan, P. B., Fletcher, D., & Sarkar, M. (2013). Defining and characterizing team resilience in elite sport. *Psychology of Sport and Exercise, 14*(4), 549–559. https://doi.org/10.1016/j.psychsport.2013.01.004

Newman, H. J., Howells, K. L., & Fletcher, D. (2016). The dark side of top level sport: An autobiographic study of depressive experiences in elite sport performers. *Frontiers in Psychology, 7*, 868. https://doi.org/10.3389/fpsyg.2016.00868

Richardson, G. E., Neiger, B. L., Jensen, S., & Kumpfer, K. L. (1990). The resiliency model. *Health Education, 21*(6), 33–39. https://doi.org/10.1080/00970050.1990.10614589

Sanford, N. (1967). *Where colleges fail: A study of student as person.* Jossey-Bass.

Sarkar, M., & Hilton, N. K. (2020). Psychological resilience in Olympic medal–winning coaches: A longitudinal qualitative study. *International Sport Coaching Journal, 7(2)*, 209–219. https://doi.org/10.1123/iscj.2019-0075

Simpson, D., & Elberty, L. P. (2018). A phenomenological study: Experiencing the unexpected death of a teammate. *Journal of Clinical Sport Psychology, 12*, 97–113. https://doi.org/10.1123/jcsp.2017-0026

Sisto, A., Vicinanza, F., Campanozzi, L. L., Ricci, G., Tartaglini, D., & Tambone, V. (2019). Towards a transversal definition of psychological resilience: A literature review. *Medicina, 55*(11), 745.

Strauss, A., & Corbin, J. (1998). *Basics of qualitative research: Grounded theory procedures and techniques* (2nd ed.). Sage.

Wood, A. G., Barker, J. B., & Turner, M. J. (2017). Rational emotive behaviour therapy to help young athletes build resilience and deal with adversity. In C. J. Knight, C. G. Harwood, & D. Gould (Eds.). *Sport psychology for young athletes* (pp. 265–276). Routledge.

CHAPTER 13

Thriving in Athletic Development Environments

Daniel J. Brown

Within the media and in advertising we often see statements like 'don't survive, thrive', and 'together we thrive'. But what do these statements mean? What does it mean to *thrive on pressure*? What would it look like, feel like, sound like even? What do we mean when we describe a player as *thriving* as opposed to merely *surviving*? What is different in their response and why may this have occurred? Was it something about the player, the environment they operate in, or the combination of the player and environment? How about *together we thrive*; does this mean we thrive as a team rather than as individuals? Does it mean we depend on our teammates to thrive or just that our personal chance of thriving is in some way enhanced by the presence of others? These are some of the questions that we are seeking to better understand in research but, first, let's set the scene for why *thriving* is in vogue.

Humans are regularly exposed to challenging situations that require them to respond adaptively to experience positive outcomes. Sport is no exception, with competition creating high-pressure environments requiring athletes to manage stressors effectively to elicit high-level performance. Understanding how people can experience these positive outcomes and be more productive and fulfilled within their lives has historically been a key mission for psychologists; yet, this message was lost and neglected for many decades following World War II with resources instead diverted towards psychopathology and rehabilitation (Seligman & Csikszentmihalyi, 2000).

In 1998, Martin Seligman used his American Psychological Association presidential address to re-ignite this mission through the advent of a positive psychology movement (Seligman, 1999). Defined as "the scientific study of optimal human functioning" (Linley et al., 2006, p. 8), positive psychology seeks to go beyond restorative and pathological understanding and instead elicit new knowledge on the promotion of valued subjective experiences and thriving in individuals, families, and communities. Since Seligman's speech, knowledge on positive psychology and thriving has grown rapidly with researchers studying it across the human lifespan (e.g., infants, adolescents, older adults; Brown, Arnold, Fletcher et al., 2017).

This chapter will outline how a similar pattern of growth has occurred in sport-based thriving research. It will first discuss the conceptualisation of thriving and offer a definition for it. Second, literature on thriving in sport will be reviewed to describe how thriving has been characterised in athletes and coaches, and to highlight mechanisms through which thriving can be predicted and promoted. Lastly, future research directions will be offered to identify areas where thriving research can progress further.

WHAT IS THRIVING?

Examples of the various interest in human thriving can be observed through the growing bodies of literature on positive youth development (e.g., Bowers et al., 2014), thriving at work (e.g., Kleine et al., 2019), and adaptive outcomes following adversity (see, for a discussion, Brown, Sarkar et al., 2020). Within this work scholars have based their conceptualisations of thriving within the context that they are working and have consequently ascribed the word to capture differing experiences (see Box 13.1). For positive youth development researchers, thriving represents either a healthy, positive developmental process whereby a young person moves towards an idealised adult state (Lerner et al., 2003, 2010) or it represents the exhibition of a collection of positive 'vital signs' or markers (e.g., positive emotionality, purpose, prosocial orientation; Benson & Scales, 2009). In contrast, Spreitzer et al. (2005) considered thriving at work to be "a psychological state in which individuals experience both a sense of vitality and a sense of learning" (p. 538). A third approach has seen the term 'thriving' used to describe "a higher level of functioning in some life domain following a stressful encounter" (Park, 1998, p. 269). Although these conceptual examples illustrate how thriving may be understood in specific situations, they do not allow us to describe what it means to thrive holistically as a human being. Thus, following their review of literature on thriving, Brown, Arnold, Fletcher et al. (2017) suggested that human thriving can be broadly defined as "the joint experience of development and success" (p. 168).

Moving beyond its broad definition, thriving can be considered as a manifestation of an individual's functioning (Brown, Sarkar et al., 2020). Specifically, thriving is believed to describe an experience when an individual is functioning to his or her fullest extent (Ryan & Deci, 2017) and holistically across various dimensions (e.g., feeling happy, sense of accomplishment; Brown, Arnold, Fletcher et al., 2017; Su et al., 2014). Importantly, individuals need to exhibit full functioning across all dimensions to thrive, rather than experiencing high levels on some dimensions but not others (Brown, Arnold, Fletcher et al., 2017).

Box 13.1 The Semantics of Thriving

Semantically, *thriving* can either be considered as an adjective or as the present participle of the verb *to thrive*. When used as an adjective, *thriving* describes something characterised by success or prosperity (e.g., a thriving business). Comparatively, when used in verb form, *thriving* represents being fortunate or successful, and growing and developing vigorously (e.g., she is thriving). When used in the context *thriving on/off*, it can describe doing well in a particular kind of situation (e.g., thriving on pressure).

WHAT CHARACTERISES THRIVING IN SPORT?

Mirroring literature on human thriving across the lifespan, those studying thriving within sport have adopted various interpretations of what it means to thrive as a sport performer. These interpretations can be broadly categorised into associations with mental toughness, thriving as a response to adversity, applications of a positive youth development lens, thriving as full and holistic functioning, and applications of a thriving at work perspective.

Associations With Mental Toughness

Some of the earliest academic mentions of thriving in sport appear in the conceptual work on mental toughness by Jones et al. (2002) and Bull et al. (2005). Within their study, Jones et al. (2002) identified *thriving on the pressure of competition* as one of 12 distinct mental toughness attributes, which reflected the athletes' ability to "raise their game" (p. 212) when the occasion required it. Similarly, Bull et al. (2005) described how mentally tough elite cricketers were able to *thrive on competition* as reflected by their clear attitude, positive intent, and ability to rise to the occasion. This usage of thriving was subsequently incorporated into a scale of mental toughness, where it represented a mental toughness factor labelled *thrive through challenge* (Gucciardi et al., 2009).

Since this early work, the suggested association between mental toughness and thriving has been repeated; however, the nature of this association has varied. To elaborate, some researchers have maintained the argument that thriving, along with striving and surviving, characterises mental toughness (Mahoney et al., 2014), whereas others have considered mental toughness as an indicator of thriving within certain contexts (e.g., youth sport; Gucciardi & Jones, 2012). Most recently, however, the conjoined characterisation of thriving and mental toughness has been replaced with thriving representing a distinct outcome from mental toughness (Gucciardi et al., 2017). The association between thriving and challenging situations has also been discussed within the context of adversity.

Thriving as a Response to Adversity

Thriving has been used in the context of athlete adversity and trauma to describe an elevation in functioning as a result of an adverse experience such as injury (e.g., Wadey & Hanton, 2014). This perspective stemmed from early work by O'Leary and Ickovics (1995) and Carver (1998) who described the occurrence of positive outcomes (e.g., resilience/recovery, thriving) following life crises. Three sport-based studies exist that have considered thriving within the context of such hardship and challenge (e.g., geographic relocation, retirement from sport).

In a pair of studies, Harris et al. (2012a, 2012b) constructed a *thriving transition cycle* from the accounts of elite Australian football players relocating as part of their contract with their football club. The cycle comprised four stages that players experienced during their transition: Preparation, Encounter, Adjustment, and Stabilisation. Across the four stages 16 qualities were described that enabled some performers to thrive during the transition (i.e., display positive outcomes), where others experienced less positive (i.e., survived), or negative (i.e., languished) outcomes. Examples of these qualities included *readiness for challenge* in the Preparation stage, *sense making* when in the Encounter stage, *role development* during the Adjustment stage, and *relationship building* in the Stabilisation stage. In the third study, van Rens and Filho (2020) documented the experiences of elite gymnasts on their retirement from sport and transition to becoming professional circus artists. The athletes were described as moving through a three-phase career transition of realising-adapting-thriving. The latter thriving phase was characterised by experiences of freedom, personal development, and social connectedness.

Although thriving can be experienced following crises and significant challenge, it has been acknowledged that thriving is not dependent on trauma (Carver, 1998) and the occurrence of elevated functioning following adversity is now more appropriately described as growth (Brown, Sarkar et al., 2020). Instead, thriving can occur following both life adversity and life opportunity (Feeney & Collins, 2015), and this latter, positive context aligns with the positive youth development lens adopted by some scholars to understand thriving in sport.

Applications of a Positive Youth Development Lens

Two studies have drawn from the positive youth development (PYD) literature when considering thriving in youth sport populations (Gucciardi & Jones, 2012; Jones & Lavellee, 2009). Within the earliest of these studies, Jones and Lavellee (2009) built from the belief that behaviours developed during adolescence provide the foundation for thriving in adulthood (Lerner et al., 2006) to identify the interpersonal and personal life skill needs of British adolescent athletes. In total, four interpersonal life skills (i.e., social skills, respect, leadership, and family interaction skills) and six personal life skills (i.e., self-organisation skills, discipline, self-reliance, goal-setting, managing performance outcomes, and motivation) were described.

In the second study, Gucciardi and Jones (2012) drew on the developmental asset framework (Benson, 1997, 2002) to assess the relationship between mental toughness and variables associated with thriving. More specifically, they separated a sample of 226 cricketers into three groups labelled as high, moderate, and low for mental toughness and examined whether significant differences existed between the groups on the possession of 40 developmental assets considered to be 'building blocks' for human development (e.g., family support, resistance skills, self-esteem). Gucciardi and Jones (2012) found that the high mental toughness cluster generally reported significantly higher levels of the developmental assets than the moderate and low mental toughness groups.

In addition to these empirical studies, Kerr et al. (2017) interpreted thriving via a PYD lens in their chapter on promoting an athlete-centred approach to enhancing thriving for both athletes and coaches. This approach tapped into the PYD belief that thriving involves the mutual enhancement of an individual and their environment, thereby capturing the bi-directional influences of an athlete and a coach on each other's experience of thriving. Moreover, they considered thriving to be a developmental construct along an upwards trajectory whereby individuals pursue optimal development across all life domains. This latter notion of thriving involving multiple domains or areas also relates to the perspective of thriving as full and holistic functioning.

Thriving as Full and Holistic Functioning

This interpretation of thriving in sport has seen athletes' and coaches' experiences of thriving viewed through the lens of functioning. For example, Sarkar and Fletcher (2014) defined thriving as "a sustained high level of functioning and performance" (p. 47) in their paper on resilience and thriving in high achievers. Furthermore, Brown, Arnold, Standage et al. (2017) measured functioning using subjective scales of performance and wellbeing, and identified thriving performers as those who report highest levels across subjective performance (via performance satisfaction), eudaimonic wellbeing (via subjective vitality), and hedonic wellbeing (via positive affect) dimensions. Qualitative support has also been provided for thriving being characterised by both high-level performance and dimensions of wellbeing via interview data collected with athletes, coaches, and sport psychology practitioners operating in elite sport (Brown et al., 2018).

Beyond the study of thriving in athletes, it is also becoming increasingly important to better understand the experiences of others involved in sport (e.g., coaches, performance directors, science, and medicine staff). In their study with Canadian development and high-performance sport coaches, McNeill et al. (2018) asked coaches to complete measures for illbeing and wellbeing to allow the researchers to investigate coaches' profiles of psychological functioning. Cluster analyses favoured the creation of three profiles (or clusters), which the authors labelled as *thriving*, *depleted*, and *at-risk*. The largest cluster was the thriving profile with coaches scoring highest on personal accomplishment, emotional wellbeing, social wellbeing, and psychological wellbeing and lowest on emotional exhaustion and depersonalisation dimensions. Thus, as with the work on athletes, coaches were perceived to be thriving if they scored fully and holistically for functioning.

Applications of a Thriving At-Work Perspective

The last interpretation of thriving adopted by sport-based scholars has been Spreitzer et al.'s (2005) definition of thriving at work. This context-specific definition forwards vitality and learning as two dimensions of thriving (Spreitzer et al., 2005) and has resulted in the development of the Thriving at Work Scale (Porath et al., 2012). Gucciardi et al. (2015) and Gucciardi et al. (2017) used an adaptation of this multidimensional scale to examine the relationships between self-reported mental toughness, vitality, and learning in adolescent netballers. In the first of these studies, Gucciardi et al. (2015) showed that netballers who held an incremental theory for mental toughness (i.e., that mental toughness was changeable) reported significantly higher levels of vitality and learning than those who held an ambivalent theory (i.e., mixed feelings about whether mental toughness was fixed or changeable). The second of the studies examined whether mental toughness moderated the effect of controlling coach behaviours on vitality and learning. Gucciardi et al. (2017) found levels of mental toughness to be positively related to both dimensions of thriving, and that mental toughness buffered the detrimental effects of controlling coach behaviours on learning, but not vitality.

Understanding what it means to thrive and deciding on how you intend to operationalise it has important implications for its promotion in sports contexts. The spotlight box discusses the relevance of these issues for coaches and performance directors attempting to instigate a positive change in their environments to facilitate thriving.

Spotlight On: Initiating Thriving in British Athletics

> [M]y overriding ambition has always been about creating an environment where our athletes and staff thrive and deliver continued success both individually and collectively.
>
> Sara Symington, British Athletics Performance Director (Scott, 2020)

This quote from Sara Symington came shortly after she was appointed as the new performance director for British Athletics. Her appointment followed a turbulent time for British Athletics after a series of controversies and resignations, and the subsequent publication of an independent review of the organisation's decision-making processes and areas requiring reform. Within her new role, Symington was tasked with achieving success in major games and championships and developing a long-term plan for the sport. To achieve these objectives, Symington highlights her ambition to provide an environment where athletes and staff thrive.

To create an environment for thriving, Symington, along with any other coaches and performance directors in similar positions, first needs to establish what her athletes' and staff's experiences of thriving represents. For example, will she deem her environment to be suitable when her staff exhibit learning and vitality as stipulated by Spreitzer et al. (2005) in their definition of thriving at work? Alternatively, will she determine the environment's adequacy when her athletes and staff are fully functioning as per Brown, Arnold, Fletcher et al. (2017)? If the latter approach, how will functioning be determined? If via indices of subjective performance and wellbeing, will these scales be tailored to the different roles occupied by athletes and staff alike (e.g., performance as an athlete vs. performance as a coach)? Defining and clarifying these measures will provide a clear boundary for what is desired and offer a mechanism for determining when it has been achieved.

Irrespective of the approach taken by Symington to characterise thriving, effectively operationalising the desired 'thriving' outcome will also be critical for ensuring that she can monitor and evaluate the effectiveness of any changes that she makes to the environment. Not only will this enable her to see what strategies are working, but it will also help identify approaches that require amending or are, perhaps, impeding progress.

Thus, possessing a clear idea of what it means to thrive and how to record its occurrence will enable Symington to identify the best strategies for promoting thriving and, in turn, support her ambition of enabling her athletes and staff to thrive.

HOW CAN WE PREDICT AND PROMOTE THRIVING IN SPORT?

Although various interpretations of thriving exist, researchers and practitioners have begun to identify a variety of ways in which thriving can be predicted and promoted in athletes (for a review, Brown et al., 2021). These approaches can be broadly categorised in personal enablers, contextual enablers, and process variables.

Personal Enablers

Personal enablers represent the intrapersonal factors (e.g., attitudes, behaviours, cognitions) that help an individual to thrive (Brown, Arnold, Fletcher et al., 2017). Characteristics previously mentioned in relation to thriving in sport include, but are not limited to, narcissism (Roberts et al., 2013), resilient qualities (e.g., Brown, Arnold, Standage et al., 2017), mental toughness (e.g., Gucciardi et al., 2017), use of psychological skills and self-regulatory processes (e.g., McNeill et al., 2018),

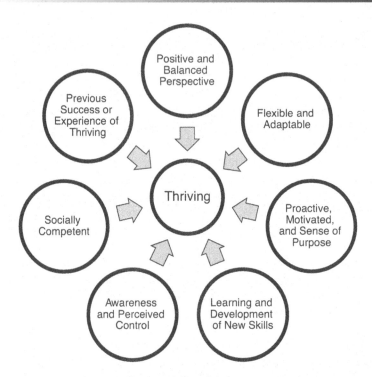

FIGURE 13.1 A summary of the personal enablers of thriving

and the development of life skills (e.g., Jones & Lavellee, 2009). Although some of these personal enablers are more enduring and trait-like (e.g., narcissism), others can be considered malleable and trainable (e.g., psychological skills). Figure 13.1 displays some of these personal enablers.

Possessing a *positive and balanced perspective* captures the importance of performers being confident, optimistic, and trusting of the circumstances in which they find themselves. For example, athletes interviewed in Brown et al. (2018) suggested that if you were happy and enjoying what you were doing, then you were more likely to do well. Being *flexible and adaptable* reflects how thriving can be promoted by being able to manage and respond appropriately to challenge and potentially negative performance outcomes. For participants in Sarkar and Fletcher's (2014) study, examples of this enabler included creative problem solving and proficiency when learning new work practices. Performers who are *proactive, motivated, and have a sense of purpose* are those who are purposeful and goal-driven in their action, forward-focused, and disciplined. Reflecting this enabler, McNeill et al. (2018) found that coaches in a thriving profile had significantly higher levels of self-regulation capacity (e.g., use of goal-setting) than those in the at-risk and depleted profiles. In addition, coaches interviewed in Brown et al. (2018) emphasised the need for athletes to be intrinsically motivated to be able to make the best use of available support and to, ultimately, thrive.

Learning and development of new skills reflects a capacity and willingness to learn from experiences. During significant change and upheaval, performers who thrive have shown an ability to develop an understanding and mastery of their new environment and, in so doing, are able to move on from old habits and make a clean separation from their old setting (Harris et al., 2012b). Establishing mastery also enables individuals to have an *awareness and perceived control* of the situation they are in, by having an understanding of the demands and significant factors present, and by having a sense of self-assuredness and self-reliance. Recognising that individuals rarely act in isolation, those who are *socially competent* are able to identify support systems and feel connected with others, which is thought to enable thriving. Indeed, participants in Jones and Lavellee (2009) argued that social skills, with a particular focus on communication, were the most important skills for British adolescent athletes to learn to thrive in later life. Lastly, *previous success or experience of thriving* has been suggested to positively support future experiences of thriving by fostering a sense of self-belief and confidence (e.g., Brown et al., 2018).

Contextual Enablers

Contextual enablers are the interpersonal interactions and environmental features that support an individual to thrive. Although work within this area has been limited to date, initial qualitative research on the promotion of thriving has highlighted the importance of establishing and maintaining high-quality (i.e., trusting) relationships with teammates, coaching staff, support staff, and family (e.g., Brown et al., 2018). In addition, exposure to appropriate levels of challenge and operating within supportive training environments were shown to assist thriving (e.g., McHenry et al., 2020). A summary of some of these contextual enablers are displayed in Figure 13.2.

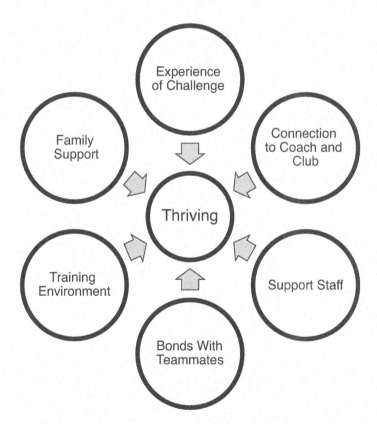

FIGURE 13.2 A summary of the contextual enablers of thriving

The *experience of challenge* captures the need for performers to operate in environments that are honest (e.g., instil appropriate performance standards) and hold athletes accountable (e.g., to behaviours that support progress; McHenry et al., 2020). Critical to this experience, is the *connection to coach and club* felt by performers. To elaborate, it has been suggested that coaches need to hold effective relationships with each player (playing and non-playing members of the training squad), facilitate enjoyment, and provide players with agency to enable thriving (Brown & Arnold, 2019). A connection to coach and club could also foster player development on- and off-pitch, for both now and the future. This may include clubs working with sponsors in professional sport to develop players' skills for life after retirement (e.g., accounting, business; Brown & Arnold, 2019) or by supporting players to give back to their sport through acquiring coaching and officiating qualifications (Kerr et al., 2017).

Along with their coaches, performers also hold relationships with other key *support staff* such as physiotherapists, strength and conditioning coaches, and psychologists. For athletes operating at the highest level of sport the physical and emotional support offered by these individuals has been suggested to complement and enhance that provided by the coaches to, ultimately, enable the athletes to thrive (Brown et al., 2018).

The presence of and *bonds with teammates* support thriving through the perceived benefits from having training partners (Brown et al., 2018) and the enabling effect of possessing collective goals with others, receiving senior player guidance, and experiencing equality in the training squad (Brown & Arnold, 2019). For example, professional rugby union players interviewed in Brown and Arnold (2019) spoke of the importance of removing a sense of hierarchy in the playing squad to allow new and younger squad members to integrate effectively with existing team members and to come together to thrive.

With numerous individuals actively supporting (or undermining) thriving in sport, it is important that they come together harmoniously to create a *training environment* which is integrated, inclusive, and trusting. Moreover, this environment should foster opportunities for interaction between groups to establish a collective culture. Brown and Arnold (2019) identified a variety of approaches that could be used for these interactions ranging from overt activities such as training trips away from the main base and team bonding socials, to more subtle and informal 'touchpoints' such as meeting for coffee after training and asking players to move around in team meetings and to sit in different seats.

In addition to the individuals who performers interact with in their sporting environment, continued *family support* via emotional, logistical, and financial means was considered important for thriving. Indeed, players interviewed by Brown and Arnold (2019) spoke of the importance of their partners in enabling them to thrive in their sport by acting as a source of pressure relief and of how clubs could further enable player thriving by encouraging greater inclusivity of players' families.

Process Variables

In addition to the personal and contextual enablers that have been suggested to facilitate thriving in sport, two process variables have been proposed as key mechanisms in the thriving experience: basic psychological needs and stress appraisals (Brown, Arnold, Fletcher et al., 2017).

According to self-determination theory, humans are thought to be affected by the satisfaction of the basic psychological needs of autonomy, competence, and relatedness (Ryan & Deci, 2017). Autonomy describes the need for volitional, congruent, and integrated functioning; competence captures the need to feel mastery; and relatedness is the need to feel socially connected and cared for. Ryan and Deci (2017) argue that satisfaction of these needs is a "necessary condition for human thriving" (p. 242) and that the needs are the essential psychological factors for predicting indicators reflective of functioning.

To test the role of basic psychological need satisfaction on thriving in sport, Brown and colleagues have conducted two studies looking at the relationship cross-sectionally (Brown, Arnold, Standage et al., 2017) and prospectively (Brown, Arnold et al., 2020). Within the first of these studies, Brown, Arnold, Standage et al. (2017) surveyed 535 sport performers and identified a thriving profile with high levels of subjective performance, subjective vitality, and positive affect. Importantly, basic psychological need satisfaction was a significant, positive predictor of the performers' membership in the thriving profile when compared to three other profiles: an 'above average' profile which had subjective performance, subjective vitality, and positive affect scores marginally above the mean; a 'below average' profile which had scores across all three scales marginally below the mean; and a 'low functioning' profile which had scores well below the mean. In the second study, elite hockey players reported their daily levels of need satisfaction in the week before an important match. Brown, Arnold et al. (2020) showed that levels of need satisfaction remained stable over the week and that pre-match levels of autonomy, competence, and relatedness satisfaction positively predicted in-match thriving. Taken collectively, these findings position basic psychological need satisfaction as a reliable and highly important predictor of thriving in sport.

Stress appraisals describe the judgements or evaluations that humans make when faced with a situation that has relevance for personal wellbeing (Lazarus & Folkman, 1984). These appraisals can be classified as challenge, benefit, harm/loss, and threat. Most relevant to thriving are the challenge appraisals that occur when the personal significance of the stressor is in proportion to the available coping resources, resulting in the belief that gain or growth may occur (Didymus & Jones, 2021). Perceiving a situation as a challenge is, therefore, likely to encourage engagement and create opportunities for positive change (Carver, 1998). In addition to considering basic psychological need satisfaction in their aforementioned studies, Brown, Arnold, Standage et al. (2017) and Brown, Arnold et al. (2020) also looked at the role that challenge appraisals played in predicting thriving in sport. Within the former study, higher levels of challenge appraisal significantly predicted membership to the thriving profile when compared to the low-functioning profile. In the latter study, challenge appraisals were shown to increase as the match approached, with pre-match levels of challenge appraisals positively predicting in-match thriving. Encouraging athletes to interpret upcoming events or ongoing demands as a challenge—as opposed to a threat—therefore appears to offer coaches and practitioners an additional mechanism through which to support thriving.

With literature on thriving in sport starting to build, researchers are establishing a foundation upon which players, coaches, practitioners, and management can draw to foster thriving in their environments. The following applied case study (Case Study 13.2) provides a hypothetical example of how this may occur.

CASE STUDY 13.2

Thriving in Tennis

Fred is a coach at a tennis club and oversees the club's performance in a national league. Many of the players have received individual accolades and won championships as junior performers, while the senior team has successfully reached international competitions in the past. The club, as a whole, are performing well, but the qualification for an international competition is approaching and Fred wants to ensure that the players have the best opportunity to thrive in their matches. Fred approaches a sport psychologist to better understand what he can do to promote thriving and, if necessary, what he can do to remove any barriers.

The psychologist begins by speaking to each of the players to capture their ongoing experiences of the environment and to collect their opinions of what they believe they will need to thrive. She then speaks to Fred to better understand the environment he is trying to create, the processes that he is already implementing, and the resources (i.e., time, budget) that are available. Based on her discussions, the psychologist identified two key areas for improvement and formulated a set of feasible suggestions for how Fred could promote future in-match thriving:

Key Areas for Improvement

- Although some of the players had competed for the club league team for many years, other, newer members of the team were more used to training and competing individually. As a result, conflict occasionally arose when the players spent extended periods of time together on away trips, which undermined cohesion within the group and compromised thriving.
- Some of the younger players expressed concern about their ability to cope with the pressures of the upcoming qualification matches and the impact that this may have on their performances.

Suggestions

- To create a greater sense of unity within the team and to aid the integration of new team members, the psychologist suggested that Fred create more opportunities for interaction between players via team-bonding exercises. Examples could include a team quiz, an 'away day', or a mutual disclosure exercise. She suggested to Fred that fostering better connections between players would enhance their sense of relatedness to one another, while also fostering the players' perception of social support when they were evaluating their ability to cope with a match.
- In addition to creating an enhanced network of social support to assist coping, the psychologist recommended that Fred made use of planned (e.g., last-minute changes to logistics) and incidental (e.g., injuries) disruptions to foster learning and the development of coping skills (as discussed in Chapter 12). These skills would offer players a greater suite of resources to draw on if needed during competition, meaning they were more flexible, adaptable, and would perceive greater control. This, in turn, would encourage the more frequent occurrence of challenge appraisals.

WHERE NEXT?

Before concluding this chapter, it is worth considering where gaps remain in the literature and the directions in which scholars are encouraged to take research next. These avenues include: the assessment of thriving, individual versus collective thriving, and thriving in other performers in sport.

Assessment of Thriving

Thriving is a subjective experience, meaning that it is personally attributed and determined. Take for example, Jonny, whose lacrosse team has just lost the cup final. Objectively, the defeat suggests that the team has not thrived. Moreover, the coach believes that the team has under-performed and, therefore, does not believe that any of her players have thrived. However, Jonny set himself some personal goals prior to the match and believed that he achieved these through his performance. In addition, he enjoyed the game, was energised by it, and felt that he acted with a positive mindset—Jonny believes that he thrived. Whose opinion do we consider as being correct? Given we are interested in Jonny's experience of thriving, it's his account which is most appropriate.

The subjective judgement of thriving raises challenging questions for measurement and pre-diction, as it means that only personal accounts (e.g., via self-report) can be used to determine its occurrence. Presently, various approaches have been used to assess thriving in sport. For example, Gucciardi et al. (2017) used an adapted version of the thriving at work scale, whereas McNeill et al. (2018) used multiple functioning indices to establish coaches who were fully functioning. No approach is without its critics, meaning that future work is needed to improve the accuracy and relevance of thriving assessments.

Individual Versus Collective Thriving

Existing literature on thriving in sport has been conducted at the individual level; that is, it has considered the occurrence of thriving within specific performers. Yet, as noted in the Introduc-tion, we often read media headlines or marketing slogans which suggest a collective aspect to some experiences of thriving. Sport performers often compete in pairs or teams with growing evidence now documenting the shared experiences of individuals and, significantly, the effect that one performer can have another performer (e.g., emotional contagion; Clarkson et al., 2020). While sport-based researchers have yet to examine whether a similar transference or contagion exists for thriving in sport, better understanding how one performer's experience of thriving impacts their teammates' experience of thriving is likely to represent an important avenue for future work.

In addition to understanding how thriving may be transferred between teammates, it will also be important to explore how to identify and promote thriving teams. For example, do all members of a team need to be personally thriving in order for their team to be labelled as *thriving*? On what dimensions do we determine team or collective thriving? Do we need to consider interpersonal processes as indicators of team functioning, along with performance and wellbeing metrics? The process of answering these questions will be complex, but it will also support coaches' and practi-tioners' understanding of how they can promote these desirable experiences across teams, as well as within themselves.

Thriving in Other Performers in Sport

Moving forwards, it is also important to remember that athletes are not the only 'performers' in sport, with coaches and support staff also exposed to personal and environmental demands which require them to cope effectively to perform at their best (e.g., Norris et al., 2017). While some early work has been conducted to guide our identification of coaches who thrive (e.g., McNeill et al., 2018) and to capture the experiences of applied sport psychologists who are thriving (e.g., Tod et al., 2011), much remains to be done to enhance our understanding of thriving in these 'non-playing' performers and of how environments should be devised to enable thriving for all those who operate within it.

CLOSING THOUGHTS

For many individuals involved in sport (e.g., athletes, coaches, support staff, performance directors), their continued employment and receipt of funding is contingent on success. Typically, success has been determined by the performances delivered in sporting arenas (e.g., football grounds, athletics stadia) and the subsequent victories, medals, and championships achieved. These criteria have driven a high-performance agenda which, in some cases, has fostered a win-at-all-costs mentality. As is becoming increasingly apparent through the media, a 'cost' or victim of this mentality has been athlete welfare and wellbeing (see Chapter 14).

The thriving agenda offers an alternative approach in that it does not prefer either performance or wellbeing above the other; instead, it calls for a joint agenda where athletes can function fully and experience *both* performance and wellbeing. Whilst it is recognised that this agenda is in its early stages and much work remains to be done, a greater hurdle persists. So long as the livelihoods of those involved in sport continue to depend on performance metrics, the more likely it is that performance will continue to be prioritised over athlete wellbeing. Thus, the challenge for thriving researchers will be to demonstrate that athletes who experience high levels of wellbeing can, simultaneously, deliver high-level performances. Or, better still, that those experiencing high wellbeing exhibit *greater* levels of performance than those who experience lower levels. More simply put: fulfilled performers are better performers.

REFERENCES

Benson, P. L. (1997). *All kids are our kids: What communities must do to raise caring and responsible children and adolescents.* Jossey-Bass.

Benson, P. L. (2002). Adolescent development in social and community context: A program of research. *New Directions for Youth Development, 2002*(95), 123–148. https://doi.org/10.1002/yd.19

Benson, P. L., & Scales, P. C. (2009). The definition and preliminary measurement of thriving in adolescence. *The Journal of Positive Psychology, 4*(1), 85–104. https://doi.org/10.1080/17439760802399240

Bowers, E. P., Geldhof, G. J., Johnson, S. K., Lerner, J. V., & Lerner, R. M. (2014). Special issue introduction: Thriving across the adolescent years: A view of the issues. *Journal of Youth and Adolescence, 43*(6), 859–868. https://doi.org/10.1007/s10964-014-0117-8

Brown, D. J., & Arnold, R. (2019). Sports performers' perspectives on facilitating thriving in professional rugby contexts. *Psychology of Sport and Exercise, 40*, 71–81. https://doi.org/10.1016/j.psychsport.2018.09.008

Brown, D. J., Arnold, R., Fletcher, D., & Standage, M. (2017). Human thriving: A conceptual debate and literature review. *European Psychologist, 22*, 167–179. https://doi.org/10.1027/1016-9040/a000294

Brown, D. J., Arnold, R., Reid, T., & Roberts, G. (2018). A qualitative inquiry of thriving in elite sport. *Journal of Applied Sport Psychology, 30*(2), 129–149. https://doi.org/10.1080/10413200.2017.1354339

Brown, D. J., Arnold, R., Standage, M., & Fletcher, D. (2017). Thriving on pressure: A factor mixture analysis of sport performers' responses to competitive sporting encounters. *Journal of Sport & Exercise Psychology, 39*(6), 423–437. https://doi.org/10.113/jsep.2016-0293

Brown, D. J., Arnold, R., Standage, M., Turner, J. E., & Fletcher, D. (2020). The prediction of thriving in elite sport: A prospective examination of the role of psychological need satisfaction, challenge appraisal, and salivary biomarkers. *Journal of Science and Medicine in Sport.* Advance online publication. https://doi.org/10.1016/j.jsams.2020.09.019

Brown, D. J., Passaportis, M., & Hays, K. (2021). Chapter 13: Thriving in sport. In R. Arnold & D. Fletcher (Eds.), *Stress, well-being, and performance in sport.* Taylor & Francis.

Brown, D. J., Sarkar, M., & Howells, K. (2020). Growth, resilience, and thriving: A jangle fallacy? In R. Wadey, M. Day, & K. Howells (Eds.), *Growth following adversity in sport: A mechanism to positive change in sport* (pp. 59–72). Routledge.

Bull, S. J., Shambrook, C. J., James, W., & Brooks, J. E. (2005). Towards an understanding of mental toughness in elite English cricketers. *Journal of Applied Sport Psychology, 17*(3), 209–227. https://doi.org/10.1080/10413200591010085

Carver, C. S. (1998). Resilience and thriving: Issues, models, and linkages. *Journal of Social Issues, 54*(2), 245–266. https://doi.org/10.1111/0022-4537.641998064

Clarkson, B. G., Wagstaff, C. R. D., Arthur, C. A., & Thelwell, R. C. (2020). Leadership and the contagion of affective phenomena: A systematic review and mini meta-analysis. *European Journal of Social Psychology, 50*(1), 61–80. https://doi.org/10.1002/ejsp.2615

Didymus, F. F., & Jones, M. V. (2021). Chapter 2: Cognitive appraisals. In R. Arnold & D. Fletcher (Eds.), *Stress, well-being, and performance in sport.* Taylor & Francis.

Feeney, B. C., & Collins, N. L. (2015). A new look at social support: A theoretical perspective on thriving through relationships. *Personality and Social Psychology Review, 19*(2), 113–147. https://doi.org/10.1177/1088868314544222

Gucciardi, D. F., Gordon, S., & Dimmock, J. A. (2009). Development and preliminary validation of a mental toughness inventory for Australian football. *Psychology of Sport and Exercise, 10*(1), 201–209. https://doi.org/10.1016/j.psychsport.2008.07.011

Gucciardi, D. F., Jackson, B., Hodge, K., Anthony, D. R., & Brooke, L. E. (2015). Implicit theories of mental toughness: Relations with cognitive, motivational, and behavioral correlates. *Sport, Exercise, and Performance Psychology, 4*(2), 100–112. https://doi.org/10.1037/spy0000024

Gucciardi, D. F., & Jones, M. I. (2012). Beyond optimal performance: Mental toughness profiles and developmental success in adolescent cricketers. *Journal of Sport & Exercise Psychology, 34*(1), 16–36. https://doi.org/10.1123/jsep.34.1.16

Gucciardi, D. F., Stamatis, A., & Ntoumanis, N. (2017). Controlling coaching and athlete thriving in elite adolescent netballers: The buffering effect of athletes' mental toughness. *Journal of Science and Medicine in Sport, 20*(8), 718–722. https://doi.org/10.1016/j.jsams.2017.02.007

Harris, M., Myhill, M., & Walker, J. (2012a). A promising career? The thriving transition cycle. *International Journal of Sports Science, 2*(3), 16–23. https://doi.org/10.5923/j.sports.20120203.01

Harris, M., Myhill, M., & Walker, J. (2012b). Thriving in the challenge of geographical dislocation: A case study of elite Australian footballers. *International Journal of Sports Science, 2*(5), 51–60. https://doi.org/10.5923/j.sports.20120205.02

Jones, G., Hanton, S., & Connaughton, D. (2002). What is this thing called mental toughness? An investigation of elite sport performers. *Journal of Applied Sport Psychology, 14*(3), 205–218. https://doi.org/10.1080/10413200290103509

Jones, M. I., & Lavellee, D. (2009). Exploring the life skills needs of British adolescent athletes. *Psychology of Sport and Exercise, 10*(1), 159–167. https://doi.org/10.1016/j.psychsport.2008.06.005

Kerr, G., Stirling, A., & Gurgis, J. (2017). An athlete-centred approach to enhance thriving within athletes and coaches. In S. Pill (Ed.), *Perspectives on athlete-centred coaching* (pp. 24–36). Routledge.

Kleine, A.-K., Rudolph, C. W., & Zacher, H. (2019). Thriving at work: A meta-analysis. *Journal of Organizational Behavior, 40*(9–10), 973–999. https://doi.org/10.1002/job.2375

Lazarus, R. S., & Folkman, S. (1984). *Stress, appraisal, and coping.* Springer.

Lerner, R. M., Dowling, E. M., & Anderson, P. M. (2003). Positive youth development: Thriving as a basis of personhood and civil society. *Applied Developmental Science, 7*(3), 172–180. https://doi.org/10.1207/S1532480XADS0703_8

Lerner, R. M., Lerner, J. V., & Institute for Applied Research in Youth Development. (2006). Toward a new vision and vocabulary about adolescence: Theoretical, empirical, and applied bases of a "positive youth development" perspective. In N. Eisenberg, R. Fabes, L. Balter, & C. Tamis-LeMonda (Eds.), *Child psychology: A handbook of contemporary issues* (2nd ed., pp. 445–469). Psychology Press.

Lerner, R. M., von Eye, A., Lerner, J. V., Lewin-Bizan, S., & Bowers, E. P. (2010). The meaning and measurement of thriving: A view of the issues. *Journal of Youth and Adolescence, 39*(7), 707–719. https://doi.org/10.1007/s10964-010-9531-8

Linley, P. A., Joseph, S., Harrington, S., & Wood, A. M. (2006). Positive psychology: Past, present, and (possible) future. *The Journal of Positive Psychology, 1*(1), 3–16. https://doi.org/10.1080/17439760500372796

Mahoney, J., Ntoumanis, N., Mallett, C., & Gucciardi, D. (2014). The motivational antecedents of the development of mental toughness: A self-determination theory perspective. *International Review of Sport and Exercise Psychology, 7*(1), 184–197. https://doi.org/10.1080/1750984X.2014.925951

McHenry, L. K., Cochran, J. L., Zakrajsek, R. A., Fisher, L. A., Couch, S. R., & Hill, B. S. (2020). Elite figure skaters' experiences of thriving in the coach-athlete relationship: A person-centered theory perspective. *Journal of Applied Sport Psychology*, Advance online publication. https://doi.org/10.1080/10413200.2020.1800862

McNeill, K., Durand-Bush, N., & Lemyre, P.-N. (2018). Thriving, depleted, and at-risk Canadian coaches: Profiles of psychological functioning linked to self-regulation and stress. *International Sport Coaching Journal, 5*(2), 145–155. https://doi.org/10.1123/iscj.2017-0042

Norris, L. A., Didymus, F. F., & Kaiseler, M. (2017). Stressors, coping, and well-being among sports coaches: A systematic review. *Psychology of Sport and Exercise, 33*(Supplement C), 93–112. https://doi.org/10.1016/j.psychsport.2017.08.005

O'Leary, V. E., & Ickovics, J. R. (1995). Resilience and thriving in response to challenge: An opportunity for a paradigm shift in women's health. *Womens Health, 1*(2), 121–142.

Park, C. L. (1998). Stress-related growth and thriving through coping: The roles of personality and cognitive processes. *Journal of Social Issues, 54*(2), 267–277. https://doi.org/10.1111/0022-4537.651998065

Porath, C., Spreitzer, G., Gibson, C., & Garnett, F. G. (2012). Thriving at work: Toward its measurement, construct validation, and theoretical refinement. *Journal of Organizational Behavior, 33*(2), 250–275. https://doi.org/10.1002/Job.756

Roberts, R., Woodman, T., Hardy, L., Davis, L., & Wallace, H. M. (2013). Psychological skills do not always help performance: The moderating role of narcissism. *Journal of Applied Sport Psychology, 25*(3), 316–325. https://doi.org/10.1080/10413200.2012.731472

Ryan, R. M., & Deci, E. L. (2017). *Self-determination theory: Basic psychological needs in motivation, development, and wellness.* Guilford Press.

Sarkar, M., & Fletcher, D. (2014). Ordinary magic, extraordinary performance: Psychological resilience and thriving in high achievers. *Sport, Exercise, and Performance Psychology, 3*, 46–60. https://doi.org/10.1037/spy0000003

Scott, L. (2020, August 20). Former Olympic cyclist appointed British athletics performance director. *BBC Sport.* www.bbc.co.uk/sport/athletics/53808069

Seligman, M. E. P. (1999). The president's address. *American Psychologist, 54*(8), 559–562. https://doi.org/10.1037/0003-066X.54.8.537

Seligman, M. E. P., & Csikszentmihalyi, M. (2000). Positive psychology: An introduction. *American Psychologist, 55*(1), 5–14. https://doi.org/10.1037/0003-066x.56.1.89

Spreitzer, G., Sutcliffe, K., Dutton, J., Sonenshein, S., & Grant, A. M. (2005). A socially embedded model of thriving at work. *Organization Science, 16*(5), 537–549. https://doi.org/10.1287/orsc.1050.0153

Su, R., Tay, L., & Diener, E. (2014). The development and validation of the Comprehensive Inventory of Thriving (CIT) and the Brief Inventory of Thriving (BIT). *Applied Psychology: Health and Well-Being, 6*(3), 251–279. https://doi.org/10.1111/aphw.12027

Tod, D., Andersen, M. B., & Marchant, D. B. (2011). Six years up: Applied sport psychologists surviving (and thriving) after graduation. *Journal of Applied Sport Psychology, 23*(1), 93–109. https://doi.org/10.1080/10413200.2010.534543

van Rens, F. E. C. A., & Filho, E. (2020). Realising, adapting, and thriving in career transitions from gymnastics to contemporary circus arts. *Journal of Clinical Sport Psychology, 14*(2), 127–148. https://doi.org/10.1123/jcsp.2018-0075

Wadey, R., & Hanton, S. (2014). Psychology of sport injury: Resilience and thriving. In F. G. Conner & R. Wilder (Eds.), *Running medicine* (pp. 932–951). Healthy Learning.

CHAPTER 14

Athlete Welfare for Optimal Athletic Development

Daniel J. A. Rhind

Recent media reports and anecdotal evidence from across a range of sports has led to questions about whether welfare and safety really are being given the priority they deserve in elite sport. At a time of success for British sport in terms of medals, championships, and profile, this raises challenging questions about whether the current balance between welfare and winning is right and what we are prepared to accept as a nation.

(Grey-Thompson, 2017, p. 4)

Recent high profile cases of abuse have served to shine an intense light on the darker side of sport (Kavanagh et al., 2020). For example, people have been found guilty of sexual abuse over prolonged periods of time in the contexts of US Gymnastics (Fisher & Anders, 2020) and football in the UK (BBC, 2019). Investigations into cycling, rowing, canoeing, and gymnastics in the UK have also identified organisational cultures which did not prioritise athlete welfare (Phelps et al., 2017). It is important to emphasise that there are threats to athlete wellbeing in all sports, irrespective of whether specific cases have come to light. This chapter will define athlete welfare as well as a range of related terms. The ways in which athlete welfare can be threatened by individual, relational, and organisational risks will be outlined. The need for organisations in sport to fulfil their duty of care will also be explained before the various ways in which athlete welfare can be promoted are discussed.

While promoting athlete welfare is important from moral, ethical, and legal perspectives, it is also important because of the range of associated outcomes. On the positive side, promoting athlete welfare can potentially enhance athlete wellbeing and performance (Seligman, 2008). Whereas, on the negative side, the impact of jeopardising an athlete's welfare can be severe and long-lasting. Negative implications include depression, anxiety, maladaptive eating behaviour, social withdrawal, self-harm, detriments to academic or work performance, and long-term post-traumatic stress symptomatology (Mountjoy et al., 2016). Furthermore, the impact can go beyond the athlete to have negative relational implications for their friends, families, and teammates (McMahon & McGannon, 2020).

WHAT IS 'ATHLETE WELFARE'?

Athlete welfare is a broad concept which encompasses a range of issues. It fundamentally concerns promoting the health and wellbeing of an athlete. It has both positive and negative aspects. On the one hand, steps can be taken to facilitate the health and wellbeing of an athlete. On the

TABLE 14.1 Defining key terms related to athlete welfare

Key Term	Definition
Athlete welfare	'The protection of the health and wellbeing of athletes. Welfare practices focus on either promoting aspects of well-being or on preventing aspects of ill-being' (Rhind, 2019, p. 12).
Safe sport	'An athletic environment that is respectful, equitable and free from all forms of non-accidental violence to athletes' (Mountjoy et al., 2015, p. 1).
Violence	'The intentional use of force or power, threatened or actual, against one-self, another person, or against a group or community, that either results in or has a high likelihood of resulting in injury, death, psychological harm, maldevelopment or deprivation' (World Health Organisation, 2002, p. 4).
Child maltreatment	'All forms of physical and/or emotional ill-treatment, sexual abuse, ne-glect or negligent treatment or commercial or other exploitation, resulting in actual or potential harm to the child's health, survival, development or dignity in the context of a relationship of responsibility, trust or power' (Butchart et al., 2006, p. 59).
Child abuse	'Acts of commission or omission which lead to children experiencing harm' (Rhind et al., 2016, p. 73).
Child protection	'A set of activities that are required for specific children who are at risk of/or are suffering from significant harm' (Rhind et al., 2016, p. 73).
Safeguarding	'The reasonable actions taken to ensure that everyone involved in sport are safe from harm' (Rhind et al., 2016, p. 73).

other hand, measures can be implemented which prevent potential negative impacts on an athlete's health or wellbeing.

There are a range of concepts which are often discussed when talking about issues of athlete welfare. These are summarised in Table 14.1.

You will note from the table that some of the terms specifically refer to children. This is because the vast majority of work to promote athlete welfare has been focused on children because organisations who have shown leadership in this area are child-focused. For example, in England, much of this work has been led by the Child Protection in Sport Unit which was established in 2001 through a collaboration between the National Society for the Prevention of Cruelty to Children (NSPCC) and Sport England (Brackenridge, 2001). However, it is important to emphasise that the promotion of wellbeing is relevant to all athletes and not just children. From an international perspective, significant progress has been made through collaborations involving organisations such as the United Nations Children's Fund (UNICEF). Such collaborations have proved important as they facilitate the sharing of knowledge, resources, and promising practices (Rhind & Owusu-Sekyere, 2018).

Early work in this field was primarily focused on identifying and protecting children who were deemed to be at increased risk. These strategies drew upon the broader concept of child protection as developed in the context of social work. Efforts were targeted at the reduction of potential harm in sport using terms such as violence, child maltreatment, and abuse. Since this time there has been a shift in strategy towards a more proactive approach called safeguarding. This aims to promote positive experiences in sport as well as prevent the more negative aspects as outlined previously (Mountjoy et al., 2015). There will be a more detailed discussion on safeguarding later in this chapter.

Also, there is a growing recognition that welfare issues are relevant to everyone in sport and that the need to safeguard individuals does not stop when someone turns 18 years old. Organisations continue to have a duty of care to protect the wellbeing of athletes of all ages. As a result, in the UK, national governing bodies and organisations such as the Ann Craft Trust now offer resources, training, and advice regarding how to safeguard adults within sport. This trend has been evident internationally—for example, the International Olympic Committee (IOC) emphasises that their mission is to protect the safety and wellbeing of athletes and state that everyone

> should take care that sport is practiced without danger to the health of the athletes and with respect for fair play and sports ethics . . . [and should take] measures necessary to protect the health of participants and to minimize the risks of physical injury and psychological harm.
>
> (Mountjoy et al., 2015, p. 883)

The IOC have also released a series of consensus statements related to athlete welfare (e.g., consensus statement on harassment and abuse; Mountjoy et al., 2016).

Why Is Athlete Welfare Important for Athletic Development?

When one considers the four key elements which characterise the conceptualisation of athletic development adopted in this book (see Chapter 1), the critical role played by athlete welfare seems clear. The first aspect concerns sustained coaching relationships over a period of time. As discussed in this chapter, there is scope for this critical relationship to be abusive in a range of ways which would jeopardise an athlete's welfare. The second aspect concerns outcomes of confidence and competence. Through ensuring that an athlete's welfare is prioritised, one can help to ensure that they develop confidence and athletic competence. Third, athletic development relates to sustainable sport participation and success at a range of levels. Whilst issues of athlete welfare are important throughout an athlete's career, research indicates that an athlete may be more likely to experience abuse as they progress through the levels (Alexander et al., 2011). Finally, athletic identity is another important consideration. Achieving an appropriate balance between an individual's identity as an athlete and other aspects of their life will be a key welfare concern during the different stages of their athletic career through to retirement.

When considering the behaviour of people, such as coaches, towards athletes, judgements of acceptability are not always black and white. Rather, there are many shades of grey that make this a complex issue. The scenario in the following case study was used in an experimental study conducted by Gervis et al. (2016). A series of scenarios similar to this were presented and participants were asked to rate the acceptability of the behaviour. The researchers manipulated key information within the scenarios to assess the impact on perceptions. Specifically, the competitive level (i.e., recreational, county, or national) and performance outcome (i.e., a successful outcome such as a medal or a negative outcome such as a poor performance) were changed. Where would you draw the line?

CASE STUDY 14.1

Where Do You Draw the Line?

Amy, age 14:

> I started swimming when I was four and absolutely loved it, I was a natural. Now, I train twice a day, six days a week and swimming is my only passion. My local swimming club is home to one of the best national coaches in the country, so I know how lucky I am to be part of her team. Regularly, she can be completely crazy and will order me to get out of 'her practice' for no reason at all. Her voice completely changes when she shouts, it's got such a scary tone. She is really unpredictable, so I never know what to expect. Sometimes, she will single me out and tell the other swimmers my faults. It's so embarrassing, and it makes me feel like I'm not as good as everyone else and that I don't deserve to be there. Her criticisms are really negative and sometimes pretty spiteful, and she very rarely explains what she has said. I can never talk to her about it after the session because she will think I am questioning her knowledge as a coach, and I don't want that. I just won the national junior championships with a personal best time and so I know that she is a great coach.

Having read the case study, answer the following questions:

- Is the coach's behaviour acceptable?
- Is it having an impact on performance and, if so, is this positive or negative?
- Is it having an impact on the athlete's wellbeing and, if so, is this positive or negative?
- Would your answers be different if we changed the age of the athlete? (e.g., 8, 18, or 28)
- Would your answers be different if we changed the competitive level? (e.g., recreational, regional, or the Olympic Games)

In the Gervis et al. (2016) study, the data revealed interesting findings in that the potentially psychologically abusive behaviour of the coach was viewed as being more acceptable in the scenarios which depicted the higher competitive levels and a successful performance outcome. This demonstrates that perceptions of where we draw the line of acceptability are complex and are influenced by a range of contextual factors. This finding is supported by subsequent empirical research which has demonstrated that athletes who have competed at the higher levels are more likely to report experiencing a range of abusive behaviours (Vertommen et al., 2016). These findings may also help us to explain the recent high profile cases of abuse which have been highlighted in the media, such as those mentioned in the introduction to this chapter. The variety of potential threats to an athlete's wellbeing go far beyond the behaviour of the coach and the next section discusses the wide range of possible threats to an athlete's welfare.

THREATS TO ATHLETE WELFARE

Athlete welfare can be conceptualised as occurring at the (a) individual, (b) relational, and (c) organisational levels and these are outlined in more detail here.

Individual Threats

Sport can represent a context within which athletes can have experiences which have negative consequences for their welfare. Firstly, there are risks to an athlete's physical welfare, such as the possibility of getting injured. This can have consequences for their short- and longer-term welfare. Secondly, sport may contribute to an athlete developing a range of psychological issues including depression, anxiety, and self-harm. Indeed, this may be associated with a range of problematic behaviours including disordered eating, alcoholism, drug-taking, or gambling addictions (Mountjoy et al., 2015).

Relational Threats

Athletes will have a large number of influential relationships throughout their development including relationships at home (such as those with their parents and siblings), in the context of sport (with teammates, training partners, opponents, and coaches), and a network of other relationships as an athlete progresses to the more elite level (such as with sports scientists, agents, sponsors, or senior executives). Whilst these relationships could be nurturing, all of these relationships have the potential to become abusive and threaten an athlete's welfare. Kavanagh et al. (2021) define the main forms of relational abuse as follows:

- Sexual abuse—Any sexual interaction or conduct of a sexual nature with person(s) of any age that is perpetrated against the victim's will, where consent is coerced/manipulated or is not or cannot be provided.
- Psychological abuse—Sustained and repeated pattern of deliberate non-contact behaviours by a person in a critical relationship role that has the potential to be harmful to an individual's affective, behavioural, cognitive, or physical wellbeing. While often referred to as emotional abuse, the adoption of the term psychological abuse recognises the broader impact of this abuse type beyond emotional affect. It also consists of cognitions, values, and beliefs about oneself, and the world. 'The behaviours that constitute psychological abuse target a person's inner life in all its profound scope' (Mountjoy et al., 2016, p. 1021).
- Physical abuse—Non-accidental trauma or physical injury caused by punching, beating, kicking, biting, burning, or otherwise harming an athlete which can be experienced as contact or non-contact abuse.

    (i) **Contact** abuse can relate to non-accidental trauma or physical injury inflicted by a person or caregiver (examples include punching, striking with an object, or shoving).

    (ii) **Non-contact** physical abuse can stem from punishments or actions that can cause physical discomfort but do not necessarily have to involve physical contact from the perpetrator (examples here include physically aggressive displays, the use of physical punishments, doping practices).

- Negligence—Acts of omission regarding the provision of safety for an athlete. For example, depriving an athlete of food/or drink, insufficient rest and recovery, failure to provide a safe physical training environment, or developmental age-inappropriate or physique-inappropriate training methods.

- Bullying—This could occur in peer-to-peer relationships or between coach and athlete and can include physical, verbal, or psychological attacks or intimidations that are intended to cause fear, distress, or harm which can include overt and covert hostility, such as repeated criticism or belittling, making threats, spreading rumours, verbal, and/or physical attacks.

Organisational Threats

There is a significant body of research within the context of youth sport which demonstrates how toxic environments can develop. For example, a review by Fraser-Thomas and Côté (2007) revealed that young athletes can feel an excessive pressure to win, that they are not included within a team, and can be exposed to poor sportsmanship. Additionally, Raakman et al. (2010) highlighted how children can be exposed to what the authors defined as indirect abuse. In other words, this involves incidents when young athletes may witness examples of physical or psychological abuse within the sports context. Examples were reported of young athletes witnessing two adults physically fighting in front of them or seeing an adult psychologically abuse another child.

Threats to athlete welfare can also be present due to the way in which sport is organised through the structures and procedures which are put in place. For instance, the ways in which athletes are developed may promote over-training. This can have negative consequences for an athlete's physical and psychological welfare. Organisations can actively promote initiations for new athletes (e.g., by funding team-building events which involve the consumption of unhealthy levels of alcohol). Organisations can also passively facilitate such behaviours through not taking action when they become aware of such threats to athlete welfare. The use of both legal and illegal drugs may also be promoted. The ways in which training programmes or competition calendars may be arranged could serve to neglect the physical, educational, psychological, or social development of an athlete. There are clearly many potential rewards associated with athletic success, but we must also consider the costs. Such costs are explored in Case Study 14.2.

CASE STUDY 14.2

What Is the True Cost of a Medal?

Diver Tom Daley gained a considerable amount of publicity when he competed at the 2008 Beijing Olympics at just 14 years old. He went on to have a very successful career which included winning bronze medals at both the London 2012 and Rio 2016 Olympics. However, there are very important welfare-related aspects to Tom's athletic development which need to be considered.

When Tom returned from the Beijing Olympics, he faced increasingly stressful bouts of bullying from his school peers: one peer allegedly said 'How much are those legs worth?

We're going to break your legs' (de Bruxelles & Eason, 2009). His father had to move Tom to another school as a result. Tom said:

> It's gone on a long time now but it reached a peak after the Olympics and has just stayed there. They've been taking the mick for ages, calling me 'Diver Boy', but now they spend most of their time throwing stuff at me. . . . It's sad and annoying that I can't have a normal life. But I put up with it because I'm doing something I love.
>
> (McRae, 2009, p. 13)

This leads one to question the true cost of an Olympic medal. In financial terms, UK Sport invested over £264m in the four-year cycle leading up to the London 2012 Olympic Games. Team GB won a total of 65 medals (29 gold, 17 silver, and 19 bronze). UK Sport then invested over £274m in the four-year cycle leading up to the Rio 2016 Olympic Games. Team GB increased their medal tally to 67 (27 gold, 23 silver, and 17 bronze). Overall, the investment of £538m contributed to a total of 132 medals. From a financial perspective, each medal therefore cost over £4m.

What other psychological and social costs do you think could be associated with an Olympic medal?

This chapter has highlighted the range of potential threats to athlete welfare. Organisations have a responsibility to take measures to protect athlete welfare and promote their wellbeing. This responsibility is referred to as a 'duty of care'.

DUTY OF CARE

The previous sections have illustrated the nature, scope, and importance of athlete welfare. As a result, there has been a growing recognition over recent years that organisations in sport have a duty of care to protect athletes (Wagstaff, 2018). In the UK this issue has gained particular attention since the publication of the *Duty of Care in Sport Review* (Grey-Thompson, 2017). This review was led by the highly successful Paralympian, Baroness Tanni Grey-Thompson. The review was established in response to high profile cases in which athlete welfare had been jeopardised.

The report emphasised the need to ensure that a duty of care for athletes is considered at all stages of an athlete's journey from initial participation and talent identification to athletic development and elite performance to transition out of the sport. The report identified seven key themes related to different elements of the duty of care in sport as follows (Grey-Thompson, 2017, p. 6).

1. Education—e.g., elite child athletes should be supported to access appropriate education
2. Transition—e.g., athletes should be supported through key transitions on their athletic journey such as from junior to senior sport or through retirement from sport

3. Representation of the athlete's voice—e.g., in all decisions which impact the athlete as well as ensuring representation at the organisational level on relevant committees

4. Equality, diversity, and inclusion—e.g., ensuring that all athletes are treated equally, that diversity is valued and all athletes feel included

5. Safeguarding—e.g., from the intrapersonal, interpersonal, and organisational threats to athlete welfare

6. Mental welfare—e.g., to ensure that measures to optimise the mental welfare of all athletes are implemented

7. Safety, injury, and medical issues—e.g., athletes are provided with access to appropriate medical care

Fundamentally, the report emphasised that 'Putting people—their safety, wellbeing, and welfare—at the centre of what sport does' is what is required to ensure that sports organisations fulfil their duty of care (Grey-Thompson, 2017, p. 5). It is therefore important to consider the specific steps which can be taken to promote athlete welfare.

PROMOTING ATHLETE WELFARE

Now that the importance of athlete welfare has been outlined, there is a need to ask the question: what are the practical measures that should be put in place to promote athlete welfare? This question was the focus of a large research programme which has been ongoing since 2013. It has involved the development, implementation, and evaluation of what are called the International Safeguards for Children in Sport (Rhind & Owusu-Sekyere, 2018). The International Safeguards explain the structures, procedures, and resources which should be implemented by any organisation providing sports activities to children and young people (Rhind & Owusu-Sekyere, 2018). The International Safeguards are grounded in the belief that all children have rights which should be protected and realised. These are outlined in the United Nations Convention on the Rights of the Child (United Nations, 1989). Whilst the International Safeguards were originally developed with a focus on children, the underlying principles are relevant to all athletes. The safeguards are based on the following principles (Rhind & Owusu-Sekyere, 2018, pp. 44–45) and are summarised in Table 14.2.

*   All children have the right to participate, enjoy, and develop through sport, in a safe and inclusive environment, free from all forms of abuse, violence, neglect, and exploitation.
*   Children have the right to have their voices heard and listened to. They need to know who they can turn to when they have a concern about their participation in sport.
*   Everyone, organisations and individuals, service providers and funders, has a responsibility to support the care and protection of young people.
*   Organisations providing sports activities to children and young people have a duty of care to them.
*   There are certain factors that leave some children more vulnerable to abuse, and steps need to be taken to address this (e.g., children with a disability or lack of social support).
*   Children have a right to be involved in shaping safeguarding policy and practice.
*   Organisations should always act in the best interests of the child.

- Everyone has the right to be treated with dignity and respect and not be discriminated against based on gender, race, age, ethnicity, ability, sexual orientation, and beliefs, religious, or political affiliation.
- The processes and activities for the creation, development, and implementation of safeguarding measures should be inclusive.

TABLE 14.2 The International Safeguards for Children in Sport

Safeguard	Description	Rationale
1. Developing Your Policy	Any organisation providing or with responsibility for sports activities for children and young people under the age of 18 should have a safeguarding policy. This is a statement of intent that demonstrates a commitment to safeguard children involved in sport from harm, and provides the framework within which procedures are developed.	A safeguarding policy makes clear to all what is required in relation to the protection of children and young people. It helps to create a safe and positive environment for children and to show that the organisation is taking its duty of care seriously. It also takes into account specific factors that may leave some children more vulnerable.
2. Procedures for Responding to Safeguarding Concerns	Procedures describe the operational processes required to implement organisational policy and provide clear step-by-step guidance on what to do in different circumstances. They clarify roles and responsibilities, and lines of communication. Effective systems are required which help to process any complaints or concerns and support any victims of violence. You should build on existing systems and understand your role with regards to relevant national systems and legislation.	For safeguarding to be effective, procedures have to be credible for children. Procedures help to ensure a prompt response to concerns about a child's safety or wellbeing. They also help you to comply with and implement legislation and guidance. Violence against children is distressing and can be difficult to deal with. Organisations have a duty to ensure that advice and support is in place to help people to play their part in safeguarding children.
3. Advice and Support	Arrangements made to provide essential information and support to those responsible for safeguarding children. Children and young people are advised on where to access help and support.	You have a duty to ensure advice and support is in place to help people to play their part in safeguarding children such that they know who they can turn to for help.
4. Minimising Risks to Children	Measures to assess and minimise the risks to children.	Some people, who work or seek to work in sport in a paid or voluntary capacity, pose a risk to children. Children are also at risk when placed in unsuitable places or asked to participate in unsuitable activities, including age-inappropriate activities, over-training and through unrealistic expectations being placed on them. It is possible to minimise these risks by putting safeguards in place.

TABLE 14.2 (Continued)

Safeguard	Description	Rationale
5. Guidelines for Behaviour	Codes of conduct to describe what an acceptable standard of behaviour is and promote current best practice.	Children's sport should be carried out in a safe, positive, and encouraging atmosphere. Standards of behaviour set a benchmark of what is acceptable for all.
6. Recruiting, Training, and Communicating	Recruiting appropriate members of staff, creating opportunities to develop and maintain the necessary skills, and communicating regarding safeguarding.	Everyone in contact with children has a role to play in their protection. They can only do so confidently and effectively if they are aware, have the necessary understanding of, and the opportunity to develop, practice, and implement key skills. Organisations providing sporting activities for children have a responsibility to provide training and development opportunities for staff and volunteers.
7. Working With Partners	Action taken by the organisation to influence and promote the adoption and implementation of measures to safeguard children by partner organisations.	A number of sports organisations have both a strategic and a delivery role in relation to children and young people. Where organisational partnership, membership, funding, or commissioning relationships exist or develop with other organisations, the organisation should use its influence to promote the implementation of safeguarding measures. The organisation should provide or signpost support and resources in relation to implementing adequate safeguarding measures. The organisation should actively promote the adoption of the International Safeguards for Children in Sport.
8. Monitoring and Evaluating	The ongoing monitoring of compliance and effectiveness, involving all relevant groups.	Organisations need to know whether safeguarding is effective and where improvements and adaptations are needed, or recognise patterns of risk.

Source: Adapted from Rhind & Owusu-Sekyere, 2018

These eight safeguards provide a set of strategies that organisations can use to promote athlete welfare. For example, with reference to Case Study 14.1 (Amy), the safeguards would help, through supporting the organisation, to develop clear guidelines for behaviour as well as establishing procedures for managing concerns. In relation to the case study about Tom (Box 14.2), the safeguards can help to ensure that advice and support are in place. They can also facilitate the development of relationships between key stakeholders, such as the national governing bodies and the school, to protect athlete welfare.

A global study was conducted to evaluate the impact of working towards the International Safeguards for Children in Sport (Rhind & Owusu-Sekyere, 2020). The experiences of people within 32 organisations from a diverse range of sports contexts were captured over two years. Half of this sample were organisations who worked directly with children. Self-audits demonstrated that these organisations had progressed from having 45% to 64% of the safeguards fully in place. The other half of the sample were organisations who governed other organisations which worked directly with children through providing funding, governance, or the co-ordination of member organisations. These participating organisations also improved based on the self-audits from 25% to 53%. Participants reported that there had been positive changes with respect to how people felt about safeguarding and their knowledge of what is required of them within their role as well as observable changes in safety-related behaviours. The number of safeguarding concerns which were being reported also increased across all of the organisations. This was an important indicator of how the International Safeguards were impacting the organisation because it suggests that people now knew how to report concerns and that they felt confident in making disclosures. These important impacts have contributed to a global engagement with the International Safeguards such that they are now endorsed by 125 organisations who work with a total of over 35 million children worldwide. More recent work has started to focus on expanding safeguarding to include adults and this has highlighted interesting issues, such as those related to coach-athlete sexual relationships, which are explored in the spotlight box.

Spotlight On: Coach-Athlete Sexual Relationships

The coach-athlete relationship is a close working relationship and central to an athlete's performance. This partnership can involve high levels of trust, liking, and respect. There are increasing examples within the media and in research of how coach-athlete sexual relationships can develop. There are interesting questions related to this topic with respect to morality, ethics, and professional practice. Also, there are debates around the concept of consent. These perspectives range from the argument that social forces render every sexual interaction between a coach and an athlete non-consensual due to the power imbalance, through to arguments based on civil liberties and people having the right to choose their sexual partner.

There is a particular grey area when the athlete in question is just over the age of consent for sexual activity in the given country. Some countries have the concept of a 'position of trust'. In such cases, the age of consent is increased, for example from 16 to 18, due to one person in the relationship being in a position of trust in relation to the other person (e.g., a teacher or care worker). In some countries, the position of sports coach is defined as a position of trust (e.g., Australia) but in other countries it is not (e.g., Canada).

Do you think that coaches should be included within the position of trust legislation?

CLOSING THOUGHTS

Debates related to athlete welfare in sport have often portrayed that a choice has to be made between protecting an athlete's welfare and achieving peak performance. People point to examples of athletes who have achieved elite performance having been trained in a way which did not prioritise their welfare. This is particularly salient with examples of psychological abuse. However, athlete welfare and performance are not mutually exclusive. An athlete who is experiencing high levels of wellbeing is likely to be able to achieve better performances. Likewise, a very good performance is likely to facilitate areas of the athlete's wellbeing. Clearly the athletes in the cited examples may have achieved their peak performances despite their treatment rather than because of it. Furthermore, it is logical that an athlete whose welfare has been protected and promoted will enjoy optimal athletic development.

Cases of historical abuse continue to come to light around the world. Research suggests that this increased level of disclosure can be attributed to a range of factors including increased awareness of the procedures through which concerns can be highlighted, increased confidence to make a disclosure, improved levels of support to help people through the process, as well as athletes being inspired to tell their story by seeing media coverage of other athletes who are survivors of abuse (Rhind & Owusu-Sekyere, 2020). There are clear challenges to navigate going forward in terms of future research in this area. There is a need to explore the effectiveness of other research methods which go beyond the use of surveys, such as qualitative methodologies (e.g. collaborative autoethnography; Owton & Sparkes, 2017). There is also a need to identify ways of effectively assessing the impact of efforts to promote athlete wellbeing through the application of rigorous research designs. Psychologists can play a key role in this domain and are well placed to deliver proactive measures to protect athletes as well as to provide support when safeguarding concerns are disclosed. It is useful to reflect on the topics discussed in this chapter and consider how they inter-link with the other chapters in this book. However you engage with sport in the future, you can play an important role in helping to be a champion for athlete wellbeing, perhaps as a coach, a psychologist, or any other role within a sports organisation.

REFERENCES

Alexander, K., Stafford, A., & Lewis, T. L. (2011). *The experiences of children participating in organized sport in the UK.* NSPCC Child Protection Research Centre.

BBC. (2019, August 6). *Football's child sex abuse scandal: A timeline.* www.bbc.co.uk/news/uk-49253181

Brackenridge, C. H. (2001). *Spoilsports: Understanding and preventing sexual exploitation in sport.* Routledge.

Butchart, A., Putney, H., Furniss, T., & Kahane, T. (2006). *Preventing child maltreatment: A guide to taking action and generating evidence.* World Health Organisation.

de Bruxelles, S., & Eason, K. (2009, April 24). Olympic start Tom Daley quits school after bully says 'I'll break your legs'. *Times Online.* www.thetimes.co.uk/article/olympic-star-tom-daley-quits-school-after-bully-says-ill-break-your-legs-mgn0c8v3ksq

Fisher, L. A., & Anders, A. D. (2020). Engaging with cultural sport psychology to explore systemic sexual exploitation in USA Gymnastics: A call to commitments. *Journal of Applied Sport Psychology, 32,* 129–145. https://doi.org/10.1080/10413200.2018.1564944

Fraser-Thomas, J., & Côté, J. (2007). Youth sports: Implementing findings and moving forward with research. *Athletic Insight.* www.athleticinsight.com/Vol8Iss3/YouthSports.htm

Gervis, M., Rhind, D. J. A., & Luzar, A. (2016). Factors influencing perceptions of emotional abuse in the coach-child athlete relationship. *International Journal of Sports Science and Coaching, 11,* 772–779.

Grey-Thompson, T. (2017). Duty of care in sport: Independent report to government. *HMSO.* www.gov.uk/government/publications/duty-of-care-in-sport-review

Kavanagh, E. J., Lock, D., Adams, A., Stewart, C., & Clelland, J. (2020). Managing abuse in sport: An introduction to the special issue. *Sport Management Review, 21,* 1–7. https://doi.org/10.1016/j.smr.2019.12.002

Kavanagh, E. J., Rhind, D. J. A., & Gordon-Thompson, G. (2021). Duties of care and welfare practices. In R. Arnold & D. Fletcher (Eds.). *Stress, well-being and performance in sport.* Routledge.

McMahon, J., & McGannon, K. R. (2020). Acting out what is inside of us: Self-management strategies of an abused ex-athlete. *Sport Management Review, 23,* 28–38. https://doi.org/10.1016/j.smr.2019.03.0 08.

McRae, D. (2009, April 18). It's sad I can't have a normal life. They throw stuff at me. *The Observer.*

Mountjoy, M., Brackenridge, C., Arrington, M., Blauwet, C., Carska-Sheppard, A., Fasting, K., & Budgett, R. (2016). The IOC consensus statement: Harassment and abuse (non-accidental violence) in sport. *British Journal of Sports Medicine, 50,* 1019–1029. http://doi.org/10.1136/bjsports-2016-096121.

Mountjoy, M., Rhind, D. J. A., Tiivas, A., & Leglise, M. (2015). Safeguarding the child athlete in sport: A review, a framework and recommendations for the IOC youth athlete development model. *British Journal of Sports Medicine, 49,* 883–886. http://doi.org/10.1136/bjsports-2015-094619

Owton, H., & Sparkes, A. (2017). Sexual abuse and the grooming process in sport: Learning from Bella's story. *Sport, Education and Society, 22,* 732–743.

Phelps, A., Kelly, J., Lancaster, S., Mehrzad, J., & Panter, A. (2017). *Report of the independent review panel into the climate and culture of the world class programme in British cycling.* UK Sport.

Raakman, E., Dorsch, K., & Rhind, D. J. A. (2010). The development of a typology of abusive coaching behaviours within youth sport. *International Journal of Sports Science and Coaching, 5,* 503–515.

Rhind, D. J. A. (2019). Athlete welfare. In D. Hackford, R. J. Schinke & B. Strauss (Eds.). *Dictionary of sport psychology.* Academic Press.

Rhind, D. J. A., Brackenridge, C. H., Kay, T., & Owusu-Sekyere, F. (2016). Child protection and SDP: The post-MDG agenda for policy, practice and research. In L. Hayhurst, T. Kay & M. Chawansky (Eds.), *Beyond sport for development and peace: Transitional perspectives on theory policy and practice* (pp. 72–86). Routledge.

Rhind, D. J. A., & Owusu-Sekyere, F. (2018). *International safeguards for children in sport: Developing and embedding a safeguarding culture.* Routledge.

Rhind, D. J. A., & Owusu-Sekyere, F. (2020). Evaluating the impacts of working towards the International Safeguards for Children in Sport. *Sport Management Review, 23,* 104–116.

Seligman, M. E. P. (2008). Positive health. *Applied Psychology: An International Review, 57,* 3–18.

United Nations General Assembly. (1989). *United Nations rights of the child.* www.unicef.org.uk/what-we-do/un-convention-child-rights//

Vertommen, T., Schipper-Van Veldhoven, N., Wouters, K., Kampen, J. K., Brackenridge, C., Rhind, D. J. A., Neels, K., & Van Den Eede, F. (2016). Interpersonal violence against children in sport in the Netherlands and Belgium. *Child Abuse and Neglect, 51,* 223–236.

Wagstaff, C. R. D. (2018). A commentary and reflections on the field of organizational sport psychology. *Journal of Applied Sport Psychology, 31,* 134–146. https://doi.org/10.1080/10413 200.2018.1539885

World Health Organisation. (2002). *World report on violence and health: Summary.* World Health Organisation.

SECTION IV

Conclusions

CHAPTER 15

Effective Athletic Development
Closing Thoughts

Ben Oakley, Caroline Heaney, and Nichola Kentzer

A final concluding chapter, such as this, is often read with a view that neat conclusions are arrived at and pithy solutions to issues and dilemmas are presented. Here though we offer a series of closing thoughts that recognise the complexity of athletic development. Since athletic development involves people, relationships, responses to maturation, and developmental challenges, the insights from this book need to be contextualised to the situation and individuals involved. Perhaps the best way practitioners can construct effective athletic development environments is to use psychologically informed design decisions that are based on some of the principles and themes discussed through the book. This chapter will discuss six broad ideas from the book regarding context, principles, and themes, and highlight some of the limitations of athletic development research.

1. ATHLETE NEEDS: CONTEXT IS KING

The needs of athletes differ markedly in early career contexts to when they are more experienced athletes, as we illustrate in the example that follows. Perhaps it is useful to revisit some of the elements discussed in Chapter 1 used to help clarify athletic development. As a reminder these were: sustained coaching relationships, outcomes of confidence and competence, sustainable sport participation and success at a range of levels, and an athletic identity. For us, a developing early career athlete is likely to show evidence of most of these elements when they fully commit to sport, often beyond their early years of training. If they start a sport in childhood, this commitment to a sport may be evident as young as 15 or 16 years of age in professional sports: we might term this as an 'early career' context (typically this is an educational, academy, or club environment). If we think about this and other distinct contexts which have arguably very different athletic development needs at least four varied contexts spring to mind:

- Early career contexts (as discussed previously).
- Training contexts.
- Competition contexts.
- Challenge or adversity contexts.

Therefore, we need to consider how the content of this book and other wider contributions are adapted to each of these different environments. For example, the coach-athlete relationship in 'early career' contexts is likely to be very different to that for an experienced athlete. Also, their capacity to negotiate episodes of challenge or adversity will also be very different based on life experiences and any psychological skills they have developed. Context is most definitely king.

2. INFLUENCING FACTORS: HELPING OR HINDERING DEVELOPMENT

This book has outlined research insights and factors that contribute to the ecology of athletic development environments. For instance, exploring the relationship between coach and athlete (see Chapter 6), their communication (see Chapter 7), and creating an optimal motivational climate (Chapter 8), along with consideration of family (see Chapter 9) and school environment influences (see Chapter 10). Social relationships and environmental influences such as these can often facilitate or impact an athlete's development. We also noted (see Chapter 2) that an individual athlete's personality traits, such as perfectionism, can have a dual effect; it can be helpful for development but in moderation (Hill et al., 2019).

Contributing to the athlete's experience on their sporting journey are the topics of mental health (see Chapter 11), resilience (see Chapter 12), thriving (see Chapter 13), and welfare (see Chapter 14). These also have a range of positive or negative aspects that can contribute to or harm an athlete's development.

3. ADAPTING TO ADVERSITY

One of the consistent themes illustrated through the book is that the capacity for athletes to adapt to change and to cope with adversity is fundamental for their progress. This underpins being able to respond to career transitions and other developmental challenges (see Chapters 3 and 4). Psychologists have referred to this capacity in different ways such as 'coping strategies', 'coping skills', 'resilience', 'personal assets', or 'psychological characteristics' and place emphasis on how these can be learnt and developed over time. We termed this a 'psychosocial attitudes, behaviours and skills perspective' in Chapter 2.

4. ATHLETES AS 'LEARNERS'

One theme that re-occurs through this book is how closely athletic development and learning are intertwined. Throughout their career an athlete needs to learn new physical skills, to adapt to new situations, and to respond to adversity. We contend that if more people in sport viewed athletes as 'learners', coaches as 'learning facilitators', and the places they inhabit as 'learning environments', then the culture and focus of sport would be more likely to be effective developmentally. We are not alone in this view; Barker-Ruchti et al. (2016) introduced a special issue on cultural learning in the *Physical Education and Sport Pedagogy* journal. A range of articles discussed cultural learning in a number of high-performance sports and settings including coaches for a professional sports team and a national sports institute. For Barker-Ruchti et al., (2016), a cultural learning theoretical framework "shifts the focus of much contemporary research from coaching effectiveness and performance enhancement to a focus on learning in a multidimensional sense" (p. 6). Imagine if there was also an emphasis for grassroots coaches to explore more about learning, learners, and designing pedagogically appropriate environments. We note how there is already considerable use of external coaches teaching primary physical education in many nations which partly resonates with this (see Chapter 10).

5. AVOID GENERALISING TOO FAR

Whilst most chapters make suggestions about designing effective athlete development environments we acknowledge, here and in several other chapters, that development is the product of dynamic interactions between an individual and their environment (e.g., Gagné, 2015) and that context is important. Generalising research to different athletes and environments is therefore often inappropriate. For example, some athletic development research is based on a single country and has small athlete samples, often in only one sport. When reading about research it is worth taking note of the cultural context and the extent of diversity in any athletes studied since this alerts us to avoid generalising too far. For example, the results of a study of a cricket academy in the UK might not apply that well to a basketball academy in the Philippines. Also, as Schorer et al. (2017) highlight "discussions about 'building optimal environments' tend to gravitate toward talent development" (p. 471). This is clearly also evident in the historical evolution of athletic development research perspectives (see Chapter 2).

A further observation about athletic development research was made in Chapter 5. The majority of studies within the field involve the collection of data at one point in time, such as in cross-sectional designs. However, as Cobley and Till (2017) suggest these "cannot detect development change, causal effects, interactions between variables or identify variables associated with onward learning or improvement" (p. 251). For this reason, they and others (e.g., Schorer et al., 2017) identify the desirability of more longitudinal designs with repeated observations of the same participants over two years or more. Funding of such projects is difficult to achieve and typically lead coaches move on to pursue new opportunities which make staff buy-in and continuity problematic. However, more longitudinal studies would enhance the field.

6. HOLISTIC STUDY CLAIMS

Finally, an observation about claims of a holistic approach to athlete careers. The term has a very broad reach: studies which are multidimensional and apply to athletes' whole careers, considering the whole person and their whole environment (see Section I Introduction). If you have read this book cover to cover, your holistic view may have been enhanced depending on your baseline knowledge. However, we would be wary of claiming the full multidimensional, multidisciplinary insight that the term can imply. For instance, we know that athlete development is complex yet we have only looked at psychological aspects, so the other parts of the multidimensional map include physiological adaptions and maturation aspects along with strength and conditioning considerations such as training load and fatigue, rest, and recovery.

In essence, there is so much more to the puzzle and each chapter represents only one way of investigating athletic development. Also, if you were to gather sport psychologists into a room and ask them to distinguish between sound psychological skills, mental toughness, resilience, thriving, mental health, and athlete welfare you would be unlikely to reach a clear consensus quickly: there is considerable overlap between these constructs. This book, then, represents part of the picture not the holistic whole.

FINALLY . . .

We introduced this book by highlighting the use of journey metaphors. Now at the end of your path and experience of using this book it is perhaps time to think about how sport at the end of the 2020s will be viewed in hindsight. There is no doubt that athlete welfare and mental health will have gained further prominence compared to the previous decade. This will perhaps help restore some balance in competitive sport between the urge for athletes and coaches to push forwards and pursue success compared to developing healthy well-rounded people. Surely, one of the legacies of sport should be for athletes to look back with a fondness for their activity and a deep connection to meaningful relationships in sport. Psychologically informed environments can, we believe, contribute towards this.

REFERENCES

Barker-Ruchti, N., Barker, D., Rynne, S. B., & Lee, J. (2016). Learning cultures and cultural learning in high-performance sport: Opportunities for sport pedagogues. *Physical Education and Sport Pedagogy, 21*(1), 1–9.

Cobley, S., & Till, K. (2017). Longitudinal studies of athlete development. In J. Baker, S. Cobley, J. Schorer & N. Wattie (Eds.), *Routledge handbook of talent identification and development in sport* (pp. 250–268). Routledge.

Gagné, F. (2015). From genes to talent: The DMGT/CMTD perspective. De los genes al talento: la perspectiva DMGT/CMTD. *Revista de Educación, 368*, 12–37.

Hill, A., MacNamara, Á., & Collins, D. (2019). Development and initial validation of the Psychological Characteristics of Developing Excellence Questionnaire version 2 (PCDEQ2). *European Journal of Sport Science, 19*(4), 517–528.

Schorer, J., Wattie, N., Cobley, S., & Baker, J. (2017). Concluding, but definitely not conclusive, remarks on talent identification and development. In J. Baker, S. Cobley, J. Schorer & N. Wattie (Eds.), *Routledge handbook of talent identification and development in sport* (pp. 466–476). Routledge.

Index

Note: Page numbers in *italics* indicate a figure and page numbers in **bold** indicate a table on the corresponding page.